NEUROLOGY - LABORATORY AND CLINICAL RESEARCH DEVELOPMENTS

PRIMARY CENTRAL NERVOUS SYSTEM LYMPHOMA (PCNSL): INCIDENCE, MANAGEMENT AND OUTCOMES

NEUROLOGY - LABORATORY AND CLINICAL RESEARCH DEVELOPMENTS

Additional books in this series can be found on Nova's website
under the Series tab.

Additional eBooks in this series can be found on Nova's website
under the eBook tab.

NEUROLOGY - LABORATORY AND CLINICAL RESEARCH DEVELOPMENTS

PRIMARY CENTRAL NERVOUS SYSTEM LYMPHOMA (PCNSL): INCIDENCE, MANAGEMENT AND OUTCOMES

RYUYA YAMANAKA
EDITOR

New York

Library of Congress Cataloging-in-Publication Data

ISBN: 978-1-63485-322-4
Library of Congress Control Number: 2016939456

Published by Nova Science Publishers, Inc. † New York

CONTENTS

PREFACE

Primary central nervous system lymphoma (PCNSL) is an extranodal form of non-Hodgkin's lymphoma occurring in the craniospinal axis that accounts for 1–3% of all central nervous system malignancies and for approximately 5% of non-Hodgkin's lymphomas. The majority of PCNSLs are high-grade B-cell non-Hodgkin's lymphomas, and differ from systemic B-cell non-Hodgkin's lymphomas in their less favorable prognosis. It is widely accepted that MTX-based chemotherapy achieves high response rates and improves survival; however, the optimal chemotherapy regimen and the role of whole brain irradiation (WBIR) are not well established. Molecular studies over the past decades have identified a variety of genetic aberrations that are specifically associated with PCNSL. In addition, certain molecular abnormalities have been linked to therapeutic responses, thereby establishing clinical biomarkers and molecular targets; the use of novel agents is being investigated.

At present, there is no comprehensive overview of the potential and challenges concerning the biology and clinical management of PCNSL patients. Since progress in this field has been astonishing over the last decade, we felt that a comprehensive textbook presenting the advances in PCNSL would be appropriate. In this book, we present an in depth discussion on the potential of these innovative methods, particularly in the broad field of PCNSL, in a manner that will be appealing to postgraduate students, clinicians, clinical scientists and basic scientists as well as to health professionals. The chapters review the basic and clinical background of the disease, and proceed from basic science at the bench to the patient's bedside in order to provide a realistic evaluation of PCNSL patients. Internationally distinguished experts in basic science and clinical neurooncology, mainly from Japan and South Korea, have contributed comprehensive chapters to this book covering the major topics of current research in the field.

The first part of the book focuses on recent progress in the etiology, biology and pathology of PCNSL. In the first chapter, K. Makino describes epidemiology, while Y. Sugita and Y. Komohara address the pathological aspect of the disease. The subsequent chapters by K. Yoshida provide an update on the genetics of PCNSL. The second part of the book focuses on the diagnostic approaches to PCNSL. Imaging, serum markers, gene expression signature, miRNA, and cross image analysis are the topics covered by K. Miyake, T. Sasayama, A. Kawaguchi, T. Kanayama, and M. Kinoshita, respectively. The third part of the book focuses on therapeutic approaches. Y. Shibamoto contributes a critical review on the role of radiation therapy; J.H. Jang addresses HD-MTX combined chemotherapy without radiotherapy, and Y. Iwadate discusses first-line treatment. Chapters by K. Makino, H. Kanno, and R. Yamanaka discuss second-line treatment. Finally, emerging molecularly targeted drugs that implicated as promising future treatments for PCNSL are discussed by K. Kawamoto. The fourth part of the book focuses on specific subtypes of PCNSL. Ocular lymphoma, intravascular lymphomatosis, and post-transplant lymphoproliferative disorder are the topics covered by T. Oyama, S. Koyano, and M. Honda, respectively. J. Fukai and R. Yamanaka specifically devote the final part of the book to the outcome and quality of life in patients with PCNSL.

Finally, I would like to thank all authors for their enormous contributions to this book.

Ryuya Yamanaka, MD, PhD.
Kyoto Prefectural University of Medicine
Kyoto, Japan

I. Epidemiology, Pathology and Biology

In: Primary Central Nervous System Lymphoma (PCNSL) ISBN: 978-1-63485-322-4
Editor: Ryuya Yamanaka

Chapter 1

EPIDEMIOLOGY OF PRIMARY CENTRAL NERVOUS SYSTEM LYMPHOMA

Keishi Makino* and Junichi Kuratsu
Department of Neurosurgery, Kumamoto University, Kumamoto, Japan

ABSTRACT

Primary central nervous system lymphoma (PCNSL) is an extranodal form of non-Hodgkin's lymphoma that accounts for approximately 3-4% of newly diagnosed central nervous system tumors. The incidence of PCNSL in immunocompetent populations appears to be increasing in some countries, whereas it is stable in others. The annual incidence ranges from 0.17 to 0.47/100,000, and the incidence is higher in males compared with females. Moreover, there is a trend for an increase in incidence in the elderly. Human immunodeficiency virus (HIV) infection is one of the prominent risk factors for the development of PCNSL. However, new AIDS therapies, primarily the highly active retroviral therapies, are associated with a decreased incidence of PCNSL in AIDS patients.

Keywords: primary central nervous system lymphoma, epidemiology, incidence

INTRODUCTION

Primary central nervous system lymphoma (PCNSL) accounts for less than 5% of all primary central nervous system (CNS) tumors and for 1-2% of all lymphomas [1]. It is an uncommon subtype of extranodal non-Hodgkin's lymphoma arising in the brain, spinal cord, leptomeninges, or eyes; at the time of diagnosis, patients are free of lymphoma outside the nervous system. The majority of PCNSLs are of the highly aggressive diffuse large cell subtypes, usually of B-cell origin. Although most cases of PCNSL occur sporadically, a

* Corresponding author: Keishi Makino, Department of Neurosurgery, Kumamoto University. Email: kmakino@fc.kuh.kumamoto-u.ac.jp.

prominent risk factor for the development of PCNSL is immunodeficiency, which includes congenital disorders, iatrogenic immunosuppression, and infection by human immunodeficiency virus (HIV). The incidence of PCNSL increases with age, and PCNSL is becoming more common in regions with an aging population [2]. On the other hand, this disease occurs at a younger age in immunocompromised patients. In this chapter, we review studies regarding the epidemiology of PCNSL.

EPIDEMIOLOGY OF PCNSL

Overall PCNSL Incidence

The incidence of PCNSL has been increasing steadily since the 1970s. Data from the Surveillance, Epidemiology and End Results (SEER) database of the National Cancer Institute in the US show that PCNSL significantly increased more than 10-fold from 0.025/10,000 in 1973 to 0.3/100,000 in 1991 [3]; after the incidence peaked in 1995, a non-significant reduction was observed. Between 1995 and 1999, the incidence rate of PCNSL significantly decreased [4]. According to data acquired between 2000 and 2008, the overall incidence of PCNSL was 0.47/10,000 [4]. Moreover, recent data from the Central Brain Tumor Registry of the United States showed an annual age-adjusted PCNSL incidence of 0.44/100,000 [5]. In other countries, the overall age-adjusted incidence in an immunocompetent population was 0.47/100,000 in Kumamoto, Japan [6], 0.17/100,000 in Korea [7], and 1.49/million in Norway [8].

PCNSL Incidence Is Higher in Males Than in Females

Studies have consistently shown a higher incidence in males compared with females. For instance, in the US, the incidence in males was significantly higher than that in females in the late 1990s (males, 0.55/100,000; females, 0.39/100,000) [4] and in data from 2007-2011 (males, 0.51/100,000; females, 0.39/100,000) [5]. The incidence in males is also higher in Kumamoto, Japan (males, 0.55/100,000, females, 0.41/100,000) [6] and Korea (males, 0.22/100,000; females, 0.14/100,000) [7].

PNSCL Incidence Increases with Advancing Age

There are also several reports that PCNSL incidence increases with advancing age [2, 4, 9]. For instance, the incidence of PCNSL was highest in those over the age of 75 years (1.90/100,000) [4], among those age over 65 years (1.41/100,000) [2].

Other systemic lymphomas have also increased in incidence in the elderly. Data from SEER demonstrated that the rate of diffuse large B-cell lymphoma (DLBCL) in the elderly increased 1.4% per year from 1992 to 2001 [10]. The increased incidence of DLBCL in the elderly has been attributed to a possible reduction in immunological surveillance or an increased number of somatic mutations that accrue over a lifetime. It is possible that the increasing incidence of PCNSL in the elderly could be attributed to similar mechanisms [11, 12]. Because of the relatively recent implementation of more aggressive diagnostic practices among the elderly, Legler et al. pointed to ascertainment bias: between 1986 and 1994, there was a demonstrable increase in the number of aged patients subjected to brain magnetic resonance imaging, computed tomography, and stereotactic biopsy studies [13].

Country-Specific Increases in PCNSL Incidence

The incidence of PCNSL reportedly increased in some countries, but remained stable in others. For instance, the incidence in Kumamoto, Japan increased from 0.29/100,000 during the period of 1989-1994 to 0.72/100,000 during the period of 2005-2008 [6]. Moreover, the incidence in Norway increased from 0.89/million during the period of 1989 to 1993, to 1.74/ million during the period of 1994-1998, to 1.82/million during the period of 1999-2003 [8]. In addition, the incidence in Korea increased from 0.11/100,000 in 1999 to 0.25/100,000 in 2009, an annual percent increase of 8.8% [7]. In contrast, PCNSL incidence has remained stable in Canada, Denmark, Scotland, and Hong Kong [14-17]. Hao et al. reported that annual age-standardized PCNSL incidence from 1975 to 1996 in Alberta, Canada ranged from 0.178 to 1.631 per million, with no change in incidence over time [14]. Similarly, using a Danish lymphoma registry, Krogh-Jensen et al. showed that the average annual incidence of non-AIDS-related PCNSL during the period 1971-1990 was 1.56/million, also with no change in incidence over time [15].

Immunodeficiency Is a Risk Factor for PCNSL

A prominent risk factor for the development of PCNSL is immunodeficiency, which includes congenital disorders, iatrogenic immunosuppression, and most notably, HIV. PCNSL is one of the four AIDS-defining malignancies, and HIV infection carries a 3600-fold increased risk of developing PCNSL compared with the general population [18]. The median age of AIDS patients at diagnosis is 37-39 years, and an AIDS diagnosis is more preponderant in men [19, 20]. There has been a significant increase in the incidence of PCNSL from the 1960s, which peaked in the mid-1990s [2, 8, 21]. This increase is generally attributed to the concurrent increased incidence of HIV/AIDS, and the decrease since 1999 has been attributed to the subsequent development of effective ant-retroviral therapies. Besson et al. showed that the incidence of AIDS-related lymphomas before and after the use of highly active retroviral therapies in HIV-infected patients in the French HIV Hospital Database decreased between 1993-1994 and 1997-1998 from 86.0/10,000 to 42.9/10,000 person-years [22].

Conclusion

PCNSL is an increasingly diagnosed malignancy, not only in Western countries, but also in Asian countries. Since there is an increased incidence with advancing age, increased awareness of this tumor should help to improve treatment strategies for the elderly.

References

[1] Miller DC, Hochberg FH, Harris NL, Gruber ML, Louis DN, Cohen H: Pathology with clinical correlations of primary central nervous system non-Hodgkin's lymphoma. The Massachusetts General Hospital experience 1958-1989. *Cancer* 74: 1383-1397, 1994.

[2] Olson JE, Janney CA, Rao RD, Cerhan JR, Kurtin PJ, Schiff D, Kaplan RS, O'Neill BP: The continuing increase in the incidence of primary central nervous system non-Hodgkin lymphoma: a surveillance, epidemiology, and end results analysis. *Cancer* 95: 1504-1510, 2002.

[3] Corn BW, Marcus SM, Topham A, Hauck W, Curran WJ, Jr.: Will primary central nervous system lymphoma be the most frequent brain tumor diagnosed in the year 2000? *Cancer* 79: 2409-2413, 1997.

[4] Villano JL, Koshy M, Shaikh H, Dolecek TA, McCarthy BJ: Age, gender, and racial differences in incidence and survival in primary CNS lymphoma. *Br J Cancer* 105: 1414-1418, 2011.

[5] Ostrom QT, Gittleman H, Liao P, Rouse C, Chen Y, Dowling J, Wolinsky Y, Kruchko C, Barnholtz-Sloan J: CBTRUS statistical report: primary brain and central nervous system tumors diagnosed in the United States in 2007-2011. *Neuro Oncol* 16 Suppl. 4: iv1-63, 2014.

[6] Nakamura H, Makino K, Yano S, Kuratsu J: Epidemiological study of primary intracranial tumors: a regional survey in Kumamoto prefecture in southern Japan-20-year study. *Int J Clin Oncol* 16: 314-321, 2011.

[7] Shin SH, Jung KW, Ha J, Lee SH, Won YJ, Yoo H: Population-based Incidence and Survival for Primary Central Nervous System Lymphoma in Korea, 1999-2009. *Cancer research and treatment: official journal of Korean Cancer Association* 47: 569-574, 2015.

[8] Haldorsen IS, Krossnes BK, Aarseth JH, Scheie D, Johannesen TB, Mella O, Espeland A: Increasing incidence and continued dismal outcome of primary central nervous system lymphoma in Norway 1989-2003: time trends in a 15-year national survey. *Cancer* 110: 1803-1814, 2007.

[9] Norden AD, Drappatz J, Wen PY, Claus EB: Survival among patients with primary central nervous system lymphoma, 1973-2004. *J Neurooncol* 101: 487-493, 2011.

[10] Morton LM, Wang SS, Devesa SS, Hartge P, Weisenburger DD, Linet MS: Lymphoma incidence patterns by WHO subtype in the United States, 1992-2001. *Blood* 107: 265-276, 2006.

[11] Westin EH, Longo DL: Lymphoma and myeloma in older patients. *Semin Oncol* 31: 198-205, 2004.

[12] Muller AM, Ihorst G, Mertelsmann R, Engelhardt M: Epidemiology of non-Hodgkin's lymphoma (NHL): trends, geographic distribution, and etiology. *Ann Hematol* 84: 1-12, 2005.

[13] Legler JM, Ries LA, Smith MA, Warren JL, Heineman EF, Kaplan RS, Linet MS: Cancer surveillance series [corrected]: brain and other central nervous system cancers: recent trends in incidence and mortality. *J Natl Cancer Inst* 91: 1382-1390, 1999.

[14] Hao D, DiFrancesco LM, Brasher PM, deMetz C, Fulton DS, DeAngelis LM, Forsyth PA: Is primary CNS lymphoma really becoming more common? A population-based study of incidence, clinicopathological features and outcomes in Alberta from 1975 to 1996. *Ann Oncol* 10: 65-70, 1999.

[15] Krogh-Jensen M, D'Amore F, Jensen MK, Christensen BE, Thorling K, Pedersen M, Johansen P, Boesen AM, Andersen E: Clinicopathological features, survival and prognostic factors of primary central nervous system lymphomas: trends in incidence of primary central nervous system lymphomas and primary malignant brain tumors in a well-defined geographical area. Population-based data from the Danish Lymphoma Registry, LYFO, and the Danish Cancer Registry. *Leuk Lymphoma* 19: 223-233, 1995.

[16] Yau YH, O'Sullivan MG, Signorini D, Ironside JW, Whittle IR: Primary lymphoma of central nervous system in immunocompetent patients in south-east Scotland. *Lancet* 348: 890, 1996.

[17] Au WY, Chan AC, Srivastava G, Leung SY, Liang R: Incidence and pathology of primary brain lymphoma in Hong Kong Chinese patients. *Leuk Lymphoma* 37: 175-179, 2000.

[18] Cote TR, Manns A, Hardy CR, Yellin FJ, Hartge P: Epidemiology of brain lymphoma among people with or without acquired immunodeficiency syndrome. AIDS/Cancer Study Group. *J Natl Cancer Inst* 88: 675-679, 1996.

[19] Ling SM, Roach M, 3rd, Larson DA, Wara WM: Radiotherapy of primary central nervous system lymphoma in patients with and without human immunodeficiency virus. Ten years of treatment experience at the University of California San Francisco. *Cancer* 73: 2570-2582, 1994.

[20] Raez LE, Patel P, Feun L, Restrepo A, Raub WA, Jr., Cassileth PA: Natural history and prognostic factors for survival in patients with acquired immune deficiency syndrome (AIDS)-related primary central nervous system lymphoma (PCNSL). *Crit Rev Oncog* 9: 199-208, 1998.

[21] Schabet M: Epidemiology of primary CNS lymphoma. *J Neurooncol* 43: 199-201, 1999.

[22] Besson C, Goubar A, Gabarre J, Rozenbaum W, Pialoux G, Chatelet FP, Katlama C, Charlotte F, Dupont B, Brousse N, Huerre M, Mikol J, Camparo P, Mokhtari K, Tulliez M, Salmon-Ceron D, Boue F, Costagliola D, Raphael M: Changes in AIDS-related lymphoma since the era of highly active antiretroviral therapy. *Blood* 98: 2339-2344, 2001.

In: Primary Central Nervous System Lymphoma (PCNSL) ISBN: 978-1-63485-322-4
Editor: Ryuya Yamanaka

Chapter 2

PATHOLOGY OF PRIMARY CENTRAL NERVOUS SYSTEM LYMPHOMAS

Yasuo Sugita*
Department of Pathology, Kurume University School of Medicine, Kurume, Japan

ABSTRACT

Primary central nervous system (CNS) lymphomas are malignant lymphomas that arise primarily within the parenchyma of the CNS. Although primary diffuse large B-cell lymphomas (DLBCL) of the central nervous system are designated as primary CNS lymphomas according to the WHO Classification of Tumours of Haematopoietic and Lymphoid Tissue in 2008, a variety of other primary CNS lymphomas (Burkitt lymphomas, EBV-positive diffuse large B-cell lymphoma of the elderly, marginal zone B-cell lymphomas of mucosa-associated tissue type, lymphomatosis cerebri, peripheral T-cell lymphomas-NOS) have been described in recent years. Therefore, clinicopathological characteristics and key points for differentiation of these lymphomas are summarized in this chapter.

DLBCL of the CNS typically show patchy, poorly demarcated, angiocentric proliferation that differs from other systemic lymphomas. From these perivascular cuffs, tumor cells invade neural parenchyma or subarachnoid spaces, resembling encephalitis. The histopathology of primary CNS Burkitt lymphomas mimics that of primary DLBCL of the CNS after steroid administration. Therefore, for correct diagnosis of the involved lymphoma, comprehensive FISH analysis for *c-MYC* and *BCL2* is recommended in doubtful cases.

The pathological characteristics of primary CNS EBV-positive diffuse large B-cell lymphoma of the elderly have similarities with those of the latency phenotypes III, which are EBV lymphoproliferative disorders that arise in the setting of immunodeficiency.

In marginal zone B-cell lymphomas of the mucosa-associated tissue type, tumor cells are composed of small mildly atypical lymphocytes with clear cytoplasm and variable plasmacytic differentiation. These tumors predominantly occur in middle-aged women

* Corresponding author: Yasuo Sugita, MD, Department of Pathology, Kurume University School of Medicine, 67 Asahimachi, Kurume, Fukuoka 830-0011, Japan. Email: sugita_yasuo@med.kurume-u.ac.jp.

and usually present as dural-localized mass lesions that have often been clinically misdiagnosed as meningioma.

Lymphomatosis cerebri is designated as a diffuse infiltrating form of primary CNS lymphoma without evidence of mass lesions that resembles the form of gliomatosis cerebri.

Most primary T-cell lymphomas are classified as peripheral T-cell lymphoma, not otherwise specified (PTCL-NOS). The prognosis of primary CNS PTCL-NOS is worse compared with other primary CNS lymphomas. However, a small number of cases with low grade may show a more indolent clinical course.

On the other hand, intravascular large B-cell lymphoma involvement of the CNS are important lymphomas that should be differentiated from other primary CNS lymphomas.

Finally, this chapter focuses on the concomitant use of intraoperative cytology and frozen sections that are helpful in rapid intraoperative diagnosis.

Keywords: primary CNS lymphomas, Burkitt lymphomas, EBV-positive diffuse large B-cell lymphoma of the elderly, marginal zone B-cell lymphomas, lymphomatosis cerebri intravascular B-cell lymphomas

INTRODUCTION

According to the WHO Classification of Tumours of the Nervous System, primary CNS lymphomas involve the leptomeninges, the eye, or the spinal cord without evidence of systemic disease, and they do not include systemic lymphomas that have spread to the CNS [1]. Recent advances in investigation of primary CNS lymphomas have provided clinicians and pathologists with new information about these diseases [1, 2]. Although primary diffuse large B-cell lymphomas are designated as primary CNS lymphomas according to the WHO Classification of Tumours of Haematopoietic and Lymphoid Tissue [2], a variety of other CNS lymphomas, such as primary CNS Burkitt lymphoma, [3, 4] primary CNS B-cell lymphomas that have features intermediate between diffuse large B-cell lymphomas and Burkitt lymphoma [5], and primary CNS EBV-positive diffuse large B-cell lymphoma of the elderly [6-10], have been reported in recent years. Pathological diagnosis of primary CNS lymphoma is often difficult because pathologists are generally required to make neurosurgical diagnoses by using very small tissue sections [11, 12]. In addition, primary CNS lymphoma, glioblastomas and demyelinating disease should be differentiated, because, histopathologically, these diseases show atypical cells and/or contain polymorphic astrocytes [12]. Therefore, this chapter is focused on the pathological characteristics and diagnostic key-points of primary CNS lymphomas and discusses differential diagnosis regarding varied primary CNS lymphomas.

DIFFUSE LARGE B-CELL LYMPHOMAS

The majority of primary CNS lymphoma are classified as diffuse large B-cell lymphoma of the CNS [2]. Histopathologically, diffuse large B-cell lymphomas of the CNS are composed of large blastic cells, pleomorphic nuclei and distinct nucleoli. Diffuse large B-cell lymphomas of the CNS typically show patchy, poorly demarcated, angiocentric proliferation that differs from other systemic lymphomas. From these perivascular cuffs, tumor cells invade neural parenchyma or subarachnoid spaces, resembling encephalitis (Figure 1a, 1b) [13, 14]. Immunohistochemically, the tumor cells express B cell markers (CD19, CD20, CD79a), BCL6, MUM-1 and SHP-1 (Figure 1c, 1d), and show very low expression of CD10 [15, 16].

Based on these immunophenotypes, tumor cells of diffuse large B-cell lymphoma of the CNS are considered to originate from a late germinal center to an early postgerminal center [15, 16]. In addition, tumor cells usually express BCL2, which is not indicative of the t (14; 18) (q32;q21) translocation [17]. Several studies have recently shown the genomic basis of tumorigenesis in diffuse large B-cell lymphoma of the CNS. These studies have reported that diffuse large B-cell lymphoma of the CNS exhibit remarkably high prevalence of oncogenic *MYD88* and/or *CD79B* mutations that trigger NF-κB signaling in these lymphomas [18, 19].

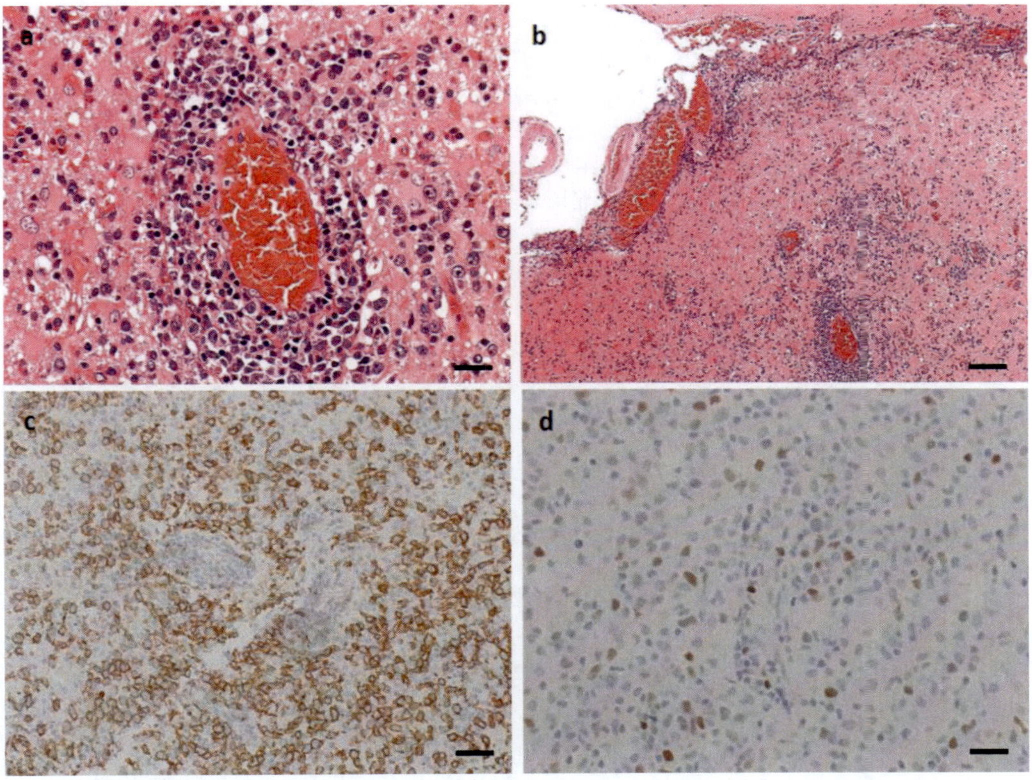

Figure 1. Histopathological findings of diffuse large B-cell lymphomas of the CNS. a) Diffuse large B-cell lymphomas of the CNS showing typical patchy, poorly demarcated, angiocentric proliferation (hematoxylin and eosin staining; bar, 20 μm). b) Lymphoma cells invading neural parenchyma or subarachnoid spaces resembling encephalitis (hematoxylin and eosin staining; bar, 100 μm). c) Lymphoma cells showing positive immunohistochemical staining for CD20 (bar, 50 μm). d) Lymphoma cells showing positive immunohistochemical staining for MUM-1 (bar, 20 μm).

BURKITT LYMPHOMAS

There have been a few reports of primary Burkitt lymphoma or a lymphoma that is intermediate between diffuse large B-cell and Burkitt lymphoma in the CNS [3-5]. In general, Burkitt lymphomas are defined as B-cell lymphomas that often present in extranodal sites or as an acute leukemia [20]. The tumor has an extremely high proliferation fraction as well as a high fraction of apoptosis. These tumors usually show a "starry sky" appearance, which is imparted by numerous macrophages that have ingested apoptotic tumor cells [3-5, 20]. The tumors are composed of monomorphic basophilic medium-sized transformed cells, and the nuclei are round with finely clumped and dispersed chromatin (Figure 2). An important thing to remember is that tumor cells of diffuse large B-cell lymphoma of the CNS fragment and die easily, leaving behind cellular debris that is comprised of apoptotic cells [15, 16]. In particular, many diagnostic lymphoma cells undergo apoptosis early in the course of steroid administration [15]. Therefore, pathologists should be careful to differentiate this histopathological feature of diffuse large B-cell lymphoma of the CNS from the true "starry sky" appearance of Burkitt lymphomas. In addition, pathologists should perform immunohistochemical and cytogenetic studies of doubtful cases according to the WHO Classification of Tumours of Heamtopoietic and Lymphoid Tissue [20]. Thus, to make the correct diagnosis of primary Burkitt lymphoma or an intermediate between diffuse large B-cell and Burkitt lymphoma of the CNS, comprehensive FISH analysis for *c-MYC* and *BCL2* should be performed in all primary CNS lymphoma cases that show aggressive clinical course, multifocal involvment of the CNS, and a high proliferation index.

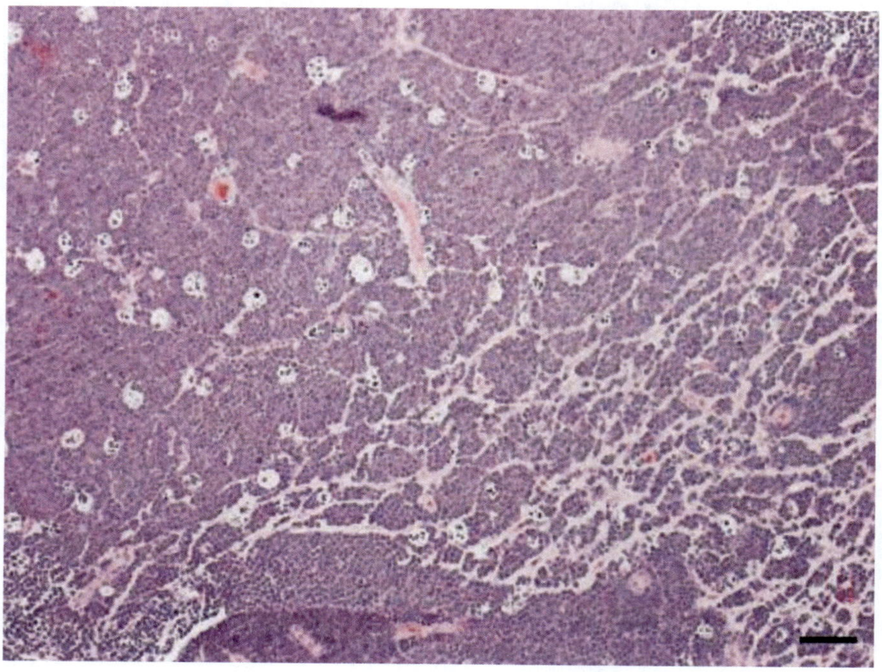

Figure 2. Histopathological findings of Burkitt lymphoma of the CNS. The tumor is composed of monomorphic basophilic medium-sized transformed cells, and the nuclei are round with finely clumped and dispersed chromatin. Burkitt lymphoma cells show a "starry sky" appearance (hematoxylin and eosin staining; bar, 100 μm).

EBV-Positive Diffuse Large B-Cell Lymphomas of the Elderly

Oyama et al. documented 22 cases in 2003 termed senile Epstein-Barr virus (EBV) associated B-cell lymphoproliferative disorders that arose in elderly patients aged ≥60 years without predisposing immunodeficiencies, suggesting that this disease has a relationship with an immunological deterioration derived from the aging process [21]. However, taking into consideration the existence of rare young patients with this disease, they subsequently renamed this new entity as age-related EBV-associated B-cell lymphoproliferative disorders (AELDs) [22]. AELDs have a distinctive histopathology of polymorphic tumor cells with extensive necrosis and reactive inflammatory cells. AELDs have been classified into two subtypes: a polymorphic lymphoproliferative disorder with favorable clinical outcome, and a large cell lymphoma subtype with a tendency towards an aggressive and fatal clinical course. In addition, the current WHO classification of Tumours of Haematopoietic and Lymphoid Tissue defines EBV-positive diffuse large B-cell lymphoma of the elderly as EBV+ clonal B-cell lymphoid proliferation occurring in patients >50 years [23]. Furthermore in the original and additional descriptions of EBV-positive diffuse large B-cell lymphoma of the elderly, nodal and extranodal sites such as skin, stomach, and lung were affected, but not the CNS [21, 22]. However, in a review of the reported cases, EBV-positive diffuse large B-cell lymphoma of the elderly did occur in the CNS of immunocompetent patients, arising in elderly patients aged >50 years without predisposing immunodeficiencies, suggesting that this disease in the CNS also has a relationship with an immunological deterioration derived from the aging process. Therefore, taking into consideration additional common clinicopathological features, several investigators have recently considered that EBV presence in primary CNS B-cell lymphomas in immunocompetent elderly patients should be categorized with primary CNS EBV-positive diffuse large B-cell lymphoma of the elderly [6-10]. Jamal et al. investigated the prevalence and clinicopathological features of primary CNS EBV-positive diffuse large B-cell lymphoma of the elderly in a large cohort study, and reported that five of the 134 (4%) lymphomas that occurred in immunocompetent patients expressed EBV sequences by *in situ* hybridization [10]. In addition, Jamal et al. concluded that primary CNS-EBV positive diffuse large B-cell lymphoma of the elderly is uncommon in primary CNS B-cell lymphoma in the Eastern United States. Kitai et al. observed EBER-1 expression in three of 22 (13.6%) primary CNS B-cell lymphomas, and speculated that the incidence of EBV-associated primary CNS B-cell lymphomas in the Fukui area of Japan is higher than that previously reported from Western countries [7]. Saglam et al. also reported that six of 26 (12.5%) primary CNS B-cell lymphomas that occurred in immunocompetent patients expressed EBV sequences by *in situ* hybridization [9]. They also reported that the incidence of EBV in primary CNS B-cell lymphomas from Turkey appears to be higher than that observed in Western countries. On the other hand, Mahadevan et al. recently studied EBV sequences in 24 primary CNS B-cell lymphomas from Southern Indian patients, and found that all cases were negative for EBV using both *in situ* hybridization and LMP1 immunohistochemistry [24]. Therefore, geographical differences in the incidence of primary CNS-EBV positive diffuse large B-cell lymphoma of the elderly should be investigated using a large cohort study in the future. It is unknown if EBV presence in primary CNS B-cell lymphomas is associated with patient prognosis [6-8]. Kitai et al. described shorter overall survival for patients with EBV positivity in their series [7]. In addition, Utsuki et al. classified the tumor cells from patients into three groups based on EBV expression by *in situ* hybridization; strongly positive, slightly positive, or negative for EBV, and compared the prognosis of these 3 groups [8]. The outcome was poorest for patients whose tumor cells were strongly positive for EBV whereas patients whose tumor cells were EBV-negative had the best outcome.

Regarding EBV-host interactions, four different forms of virus latency have been recognized based on the rate of expression of EBV-encoded proteins and RNA [25]. Type 1, which is observed in Burkitt lymphoma, shows exclusive expression of EBV-encoded nuclear antigen 1 (small non-polyadenylated RNA (EBER) molecules and EBV-encoded nuclear antigen 1 (EBNA-1); type II, which is observed in Hodgkin's lymphoma, shows additional expression of latent membrane proteins (LMP); type III, which is observed in lymphoproliferative disorders in immunocompromised patients, shows expression of all six EBNAs, all three LMPs, and the two EBERs; type IV latency is less strictly defined and pertains to infectious mononucleosis and post-transplantation LPD. The pathological characteristics of primary CNS EBV-positive diffuse large B-cell lymphoma of the elderly have similarities with those of the latency phenotypes III, which are EBV lymphoproliferative disorders that arise in the setting of immunodeficiency. Thus, pathologically, primary CNS EBV-positive diffuse large B-cell lymphoma of the elderly shows a broad range of B-cell maturation, from immunoblasts to plasma cells, with inflammatory and necrotic background, and are positive for EBV using *in situ* hybridization (Figure 3).

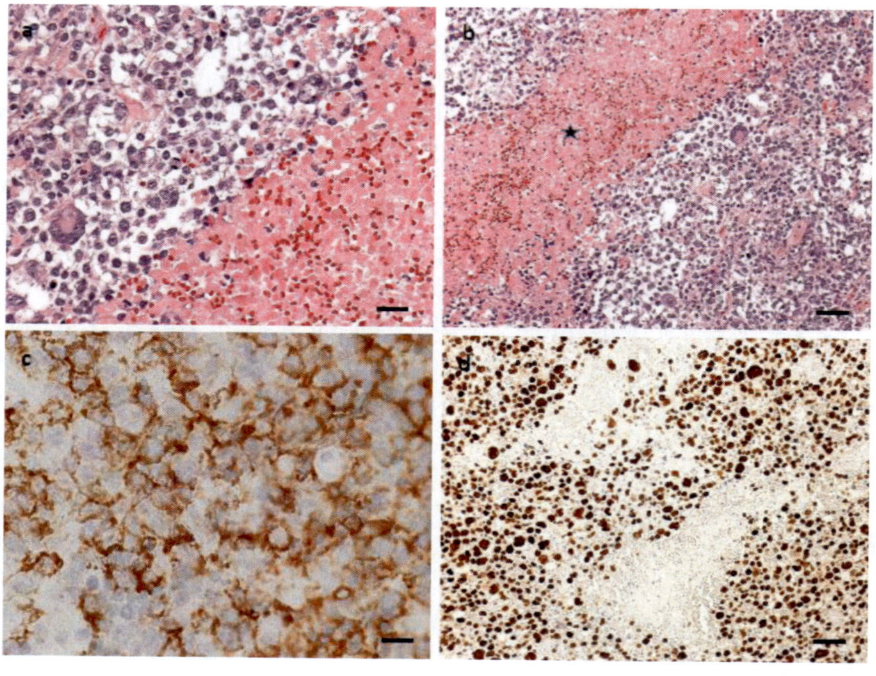

Figure 3. Histopathological findings of primary CNS EBV-positive diffuse large B-cell lymphoma of the elderly. a) Diffuse mixed small-cleaved and large cell lymphoma showing polymorphous features (hematoxylin and eosin staining; bar, 20 μm). b) Section showing angiocentric pattern with extensive necrosis (hematoxylin and eosin stain; bar, 50 μm; asterisks, necrosis). c) Lymphoma cells showing positive immunohistochemical staining for CD20 (bar: 20 μm). d) Lymphoma cells showing positive signals for EBV-encoded small RNAs (EBERs) by *in situ* hybridization (bar, 50 μm).

Marginal Zone B-Cell Lymphomas of Mucosa-Associated Tissue Type

Marginal zone B-cell lymphoma (MZBCL) is a subtype of B-cell lymphomas that originate primarily in the marginal zone. Extranodal MZBCL of the mucosa-associated lymphoid tissue (MALT) type usually present localized mass lesions with no lesions of the bone marrow or lymph node [26-28]. This lymphoma was first described in the MALT of the gastrointestinal tract but its presence in lung, thyroid, salivary gland, breast and the CNS is also currently recognized. In the CNS, MZBCL of the MALT type predominantly occurs in middle-aged women and is usually present as dural-localized mass lesions [26-28]. Therefore, extranodal MZBCL of the MALT type has often been clinically misdiagnosed as meningioma. However, the location of this type of lymphoma has been also reported as cortical, cavernous sinus, cerebellopontine angle, and right hemisphere mass [26-28].

The pathogenesis of MZBCL of the MALT type is considered to be the result of chronic inflammation by microorganisms. An alternative viewpoint is that dura-associated lymphoid tissue may arise from chronic stimuli, analogous to the MALT of other organs. Other studies have speculated that meningothelial cells or arachnoid cap cells play the role of epithelial cells in the development of MZBCL of the MALT type at non-mucosal sites [26-28]. Microscopically, the tumor cells are composed of small mildly atypical lymphocytes with clear cytoplasm and variable plasmacytic differentiation (Figure 4a). Lymphoid follicles may be seen in the tumor. Immunohistochemically, the tumor cells express B cell markers (CD19, CD20, CD79a), (Figure 4b) but do not express CD3, CD10 or CD23. Regarding the prognosis of low grade lymphomas including MZBCL of the MALT type, some studies have reported a favorable prognosis by combining surgery and radiochemotherapy [26-28].

Lymphomatosis Cerebri

Lymphomatosis cerebri is designated as a diffuse infiltrating form of primary CNS lymphoma without evidence of mass lesions that resembles the form of gliomatosis cerebri [29-31].

In general, primary CNS lymphomas usually present focal or multifocal mass lesions. On the other hand, a characteristic of the neuroimaging of lymphomatosis cerebri is diffuse infiltrating leukoencephalopathy in both hemispheres [29-31]. Therefore, diagnosis of lymphomatosis cerebri by clinicians and pathologists is often confused with the diagnosis of Binswanger's disease, infectious leukoencephalitis, toxic and metabolic abnormalities, or gliomatosis cerebri. Microscopically, the lesion reveals increased cellularity in the white matter without causing tissue destruction. The atypical lymphoid cells are not cohesive; they spread along the white matter tracts without a mass lesion and occasionally cluster around blood vessels (Figure 4c). Immunohistochemically, the tumor cells express B cell markers (CD20, CD79a) (Figure 4d) and MUM-1, but do not express CD3 [30, 31].

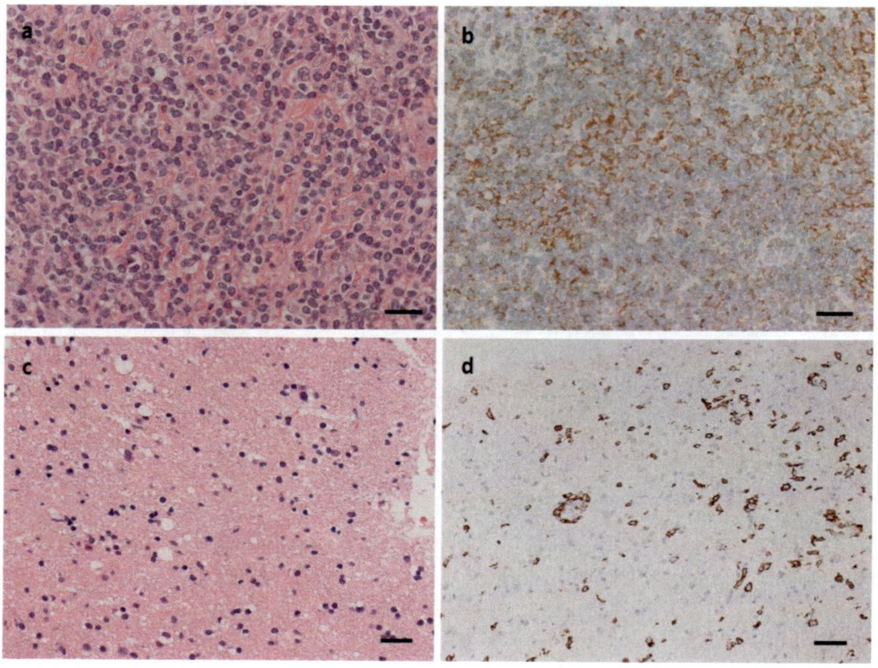

Figure 4. Histopathological findings of marginal zone B-cell lymphoma of the mucosa-associated lymphoid tissue type (a,b). a) Tumor cells consist of small mildly atypical lymphocytes with clear cytoplasm and variable plasmacytic differentiation. Lymphoid follicles may be seen in the tumor (hematoxylin and eosin staining; bar, 20 μm). b) Atypical lymphoid cells showing positive immunohistochemical staining for CD20 (bar, 20 μm). Histopathological findings of lymphomatosis cerebri (c,d). c) The atypical lymphoid cells are not cohesive, are spread along the white matter tracts without mass lesion and are occasionally clustered around blood vessels (bar, 20 μm). d) The tumor cells express the B cell marker, CD20 (bar, 50 μm).

From the clinical point of view, in the background of a rapidly progressive subcortical dementia and extensive white matter disease, neoplastic disorders of the brain, especially lymphomatosis cerebri, should be considered. On the other hand, Sugie et al. showed that most of the previously reported cases of lymphomatosis cerebri were diagnosed only by performing a brain biopsy, and detailed neuropathological studies were not performed [32]. They therefore considered that lymphomatosis cerebri without any enhanced lesions at early stages of the condition might be accompanied by typical mass lesions of primary CNS lymphomas in their later clinical courses more frequently than has been previously considered.

PERIPHERAL T-CELL LYMPHOMAS-NOS

Primary T-cell lymphoma is quite rare, and the incidence of this tumor accounts for only 2-9% of all CNS lymphomas [17, 33]. Most primary T-cell lymphomas are classified as peripheral T-cell lymphoma, not otherwise specified (PTCL-NOS) [17, 33]. Microscopically, tumor cells of PTCL-NOS are composed of small or intermediate-sized mild atypical lymphocytes with irregular nuclei, often indistinct nucleoli, and scanty cytoplasm (Figure 5a). [17, 33] Prominent perivascular infiltration and perivascular cuffing are seen.

Immunohistochemically, the tumor cells usually are positive for CD3 (Figure 5b) and they may be positive for CD4 or/and CD8. The tumor cells show aberrant T cell phenotype with frequent downregulation of CD5 and CD7 and they may express T-cell receptor α/β or γ/δ chains. The expression of TIA-1 and granzyme B indicates a cytotoxic T-lymphocyte phenotype. Clonal TCR rearrangements suggest a lymphoproliferative disorder or a neoplastic disorder [17, 33].

The prognosis of primary CNS PTCL-NOS is worse compared with other primary CNS lymphomas. However, a small number of cases with a low grade may show a more indolent clinical course [17, 33].

CNS Involvment of Intravascular Large B-Cell Lymphomas

Intravascular large B-cell lymphomas (IVLBCL) are designated as a rare type of extranodal large B-cell lymphoma and are characterized by the selective growth of lymphoma cells within the lumina of vessels, particularly capillaries, with the exception of the lumina of larger arteries and veins (Figure 5c). Immunohistochemically, the tumor cells express the B cell marker, CD20 (Figure 5d) [17, 34-36]. Several cases of intravascular T-cell or natural-killer cell lymphoma have been reported and some of these cases have been associated with EBV infection. However, these cases are considered as different diseases from IVLBCL [17].

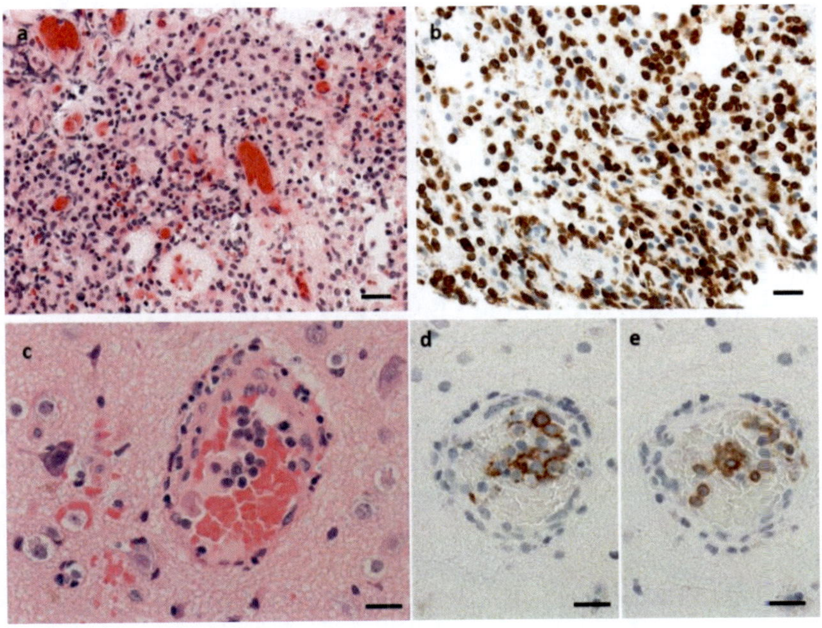

Figure 5. Histopathological findings of peripheral T-cell lymphoma, not otherwise specified (a,b). a) Tumor cells showing perivascular infiltration and perivascular cuffing. The tumors consist of small or intermediate-sized mildly atypical lymphocytes with irregular nuclei, often indistinct nucleoli, and scanty cytoplasm (bar, 20 μm). b) Tumor cells are positive for CD3 (bar, 20 μm). Histopathological findings of intravascular large B-cell lymphomas (c,d). d) Lymphoma cells showing selective growth within the lumina of vessels, particularly of capillaries (bar, 20 μm). e) Tumor cells express the B cell marker, CD20(d) and CD79a(b) (bar, 20 μm).

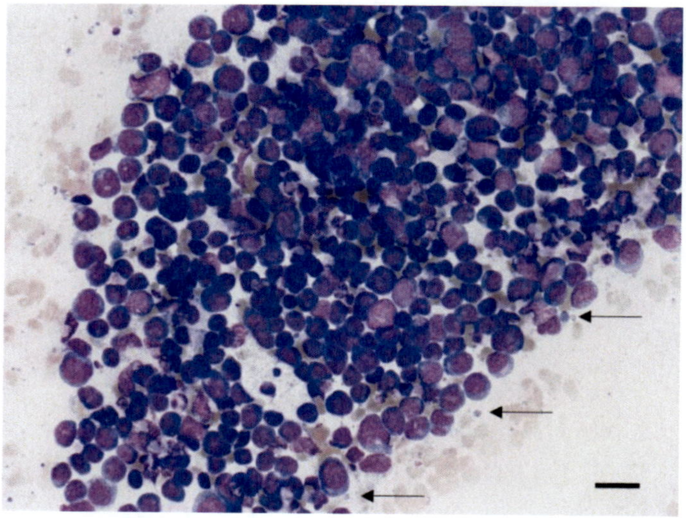

Figure 6. A cytological preparation showing the characteristic LGB (arrows) and the morphology of the lymphoma cells (Giemsa stain; bar, 20 μm).

Tumor cells of IVLBCL can be involved in extranodal sites including any organ. In addition, IVLBCL shows a tendency to present more frequently with CNS and skin symptoms in Western countries or with hemophagocytic syndrome in Asian countries. Therefore, strictly speaking, IVLBCL does not satisfy the definition of primary CNS lymphomas. However, it is well known that IVLBCL commonly affect the CNS as describe above. In addition, CNS involvement, particularly recurrence including progression during treatment usually represents serious and/or fatal complications. Furthermore, a recently published autopsy report showed the coexistence of IVLBCL and lymphomatosis cerebri, which suggests a possible link between IVLBCL and lymphomatosis cerebri [36]. Therefore, clinicians and pathologists should recognize the clinicopathological characteristics of CNS involvement of IVLBCL.

Intraoperative Cytopathology of Primary CNS Lymphomas

The imaging modalities employed for the diagnostic work-up of primary CNS lymphomas include contrast-enhanced cranial computed tomography and MRI. MRI in particular can detect the typical features of these tumors, including intra-axial homogeneous single- or multiple-contrast enhancing lesions with marked surrounding edema and restricted diffusion, usually in contact with a surface exposed to cerebrospinal fluid [37, 38]. Neuroimaging thus provides crucial information to intraoperative pathologists. An intraoperative smear also provides key information about primary CNS lymphomas. Thus, when examining intraoperative preparations, pathologists should note the key feature that cells from primary CNS lymphomas do not adhere to each other in smears. In addition, primary CNS lymphomas cells fragment and die easily, leaving behind cellular debris that is comprised of apoptotic cells and lymphoglandular bodies (LGB) [12, 39, 40]. These LGB are small, membrane-delimited fragments of cytoplasm that often contain a slightly more basophilic core. These bodies are highly characteristic of high-grade lymphoma [12, 39, 40]. Characteristic LGB are readily apparent, and the morphology of neoplastic cells in primary CNS lymphomas are readily seen in cytopathological preparations (Figure 6)

Primary CNS lymphomas are sometimes histologically indistinguishable from malignant gliomas or demyelinating diseases, particularly in the frozen sections used for intraoperative rapid diagnosis. However, several studies have reported the diagnostic utility of cytopathology in intraoperative rapid diagnosis of primary CNS lymphomas [11, 12, 39,40]. Therefore, the concomitant use of both intraoperative cytopathology and frozen sections is recommended in intraoperative rapid diagnosis when primary CNS lymphomas are considered.

CONCLUSION

The diagnosis of primary CNS lymphomas in the CNS is challenging, especially considering that various subtype of lymphomas (Burkitt lymphomas, EBV-positive diffuse large B-cell lymphoma of the elderly, marginal zone B-cell lymphomas, Intravascular B-cell lymphomas, lymphomatosis cerebri) can occur in the CNS. Therefore, both pathologists and clinicians need to know the clinicopathological characteristics of each lymphoma. In addition, a combination of morphologic assessment, immunohistochemical study and genetic investigation helps in establishing the diagnosis of primary CNS lymphomas.

REFERENCES

[1] Deckert M, Paulus W (2007) Malignant lymphomas. In: Louis DN, Ohgaki H, Wiestler OD, Cavenee WK (eds.) *WHO Classification of Tumours of the Central Nervous suystem.* Lyon: International Agency for Research on Cancer Press, Lyon, pp. 188-192.

[2] Kluin PM, Deckert M, Ferry JA (2008) Primary diffuse large B-cell lymphoma of the CNS. In:Swerdlow SH, Campo E, Harris NL, Jaffe ES, Pileri SA, Stein H, Thiele J, Vardiman JW (eds.) *WHO Classification of Tumours of the Haematopoietic and Lymphoid Tissues.* International Agency for Research on Cancer, Lyon, pp. 240-241.

[3] Jiang M, Zhu J, Guan YS, Zou LQ. Primary central nervous system Burkitt lymphoma with non-immunogloublin heavy chain translocation in right ventricle. *Pediatr Hematol Oncol* 2011; 28: 454-458.

[4] Gu Y, Hou Y, Zhang XB, Hu F. Primary central nervous system Burkitt lymphoma as conomitant lesions in the third and the left ventricles: a case study and literature review. *J Neurooncol* 2010; 99: 277-281.

[5] Jiang L, Li Z, Finn LE, Personnet DA, Edenfield B, Foran JM, Jaeckle KA, Reimer R, Menke DM, Ketterling RP, Tun HW. Primary central nervous system B cell lymphoma with features intermediate between diffuse large B cell lymphoma and Burkitt lymphoma. *Int J Clin Exp Pathol* 2012; 5: 72-76.

[6] Sugita Y, Terasaki M, Niino D, Ohshima K, Fumiko A, Shigemori M, Sato Y, Asano N. Epstein-Barr virus-associated primary central nervous system lymphomas in

immunocompetent elderly patients: analysis for latent membrane protein-1 oncogene deletion and EBNA-2 strain typing. *J Neuro-oncol* 2010; 100: 271-279.

[7] Kitai R, Matsuda K, Adachi E, Saito Y, Nakajima T, Takeuchi H, Sato K, Imamura Y, Kubota T. Epstein-Barr virus-associated primary central nervous system lymphoma in the Japanese population. *Neurol Med Chir* 2010; 50: 114-118.

[8] Utsuki S, Oka H, Miyajima Y, Kijima C, Yasui Y, Fujii K. Epstein-Barr virus-associated primary central nervous system lymphoma: is incidence of EBV expression associated with median survival time? *Brain Tumor Pathol* 2011; 28: 145-149.

[9] Saglam A, Akyurek N, Soylemezoglu F, Uner A. Epstein-Barr virus frequency in primary central nervous system lymphomas in Turkey. *APMIS* 2013; 121: 232-238.

[10] Jamal SE, Li S, Bajaj R, Wang Z, Kenyon L, Glass J, Pang CS, Bhagavathi S, Peiper, SC, Gong JZ. Primary central nervous system Epstein-Barr virus-positive large B-cell lymphoma of the elderly: a clinicopathologic study of five cases. *Brain Tumor Pathol* 2014; 31: 265-273.

[11] Powell SZ. Intraoperative consultation, cytologic preparation, and frozen section in the central nervous system. *Arch Pathol Lab Med* 2005; 129: 1635-1652.

[12] Sugita Y, Terasaki M, Nakashima S, Ohshima K, Morioka M, Abe H. Intraoperative rapid diagnosis of primary central nervous system lymphomas: Advantages and pitfalls. *Neuropathol* 2014; 34: 438-445.

[13] Sugita Y, Takase Y, Mori D, Tokunaga O, Nakashima A, Shigemori M. Endoglin (CD 105) is expressed on endothelial cells in the primary central nervous system lymphoma and correlates with survival. *J Neurooncol* 2007; 82: 249-256.

[14] Rubenstein JL, Fridlyand J, Shen A, Aldape K, Ginzinger D, Batchelor T, Treseler P, Berger M, McDermott M, Prados M, Karch J, Okada C, Hyun W, Parikh S, Haqq C, Shuman M. Gene expression and angiotropism in primary CNS lymphoma. *Blood* 2006; 107: 3716-3723.

[15] Sugita Y, Tokunaga O, Nakashima A, Shigemori M. SHP-1 expression in primary central nervous system B-cell lymphomas in immunocompetent patients reflects maturation stage of normal B cell counterparts. *Pathol Int* 2004; 54: 659-666.

[16] Camillëri-Broet, Crinière E, Broët P, Delwail V, Mokhtari K, Moreau A, Kujas M, Raphaël M, Iraqi W, Sautès-Fridman C, Colombat P, Hoang-Xuan K, Martin A. A uniform activated B-cell-like immunophenotype might explain the poor prognosis of primary central nervous system lymphomas: analysis of 83 cases. *Blood* 2006; 107: 190-196.

[17] Giannini C, Dogan A, Salomão DR. CNS lymphoma: A practical diagnostic approach. *J Neuropathol Exp Neurol* 2014;78:478-494.

[18] Yamada S, Ishida Y, Matsuno A, Yamazaki K. Primary diffuse large B-cell lymphomas of central nervous system exhibit remarkably high prevalence of oncogenic MYD88 and CD79B mutations. *Leuk Lymphoma* 2014;56:2141-2145.

[19] Nakamura T, Tateishi K, Niwa T, Matsushita Y, Tamura K, Kinoshita M, Tanaka K, Fukushima S, Takami H, Arita H, Kubo A, Shuto T, Ohno M, Miyakita Y, Kocialkowski S, Sasayama T, Hashimoto N, Maehara T, Shibui S, Ushijima T, Kawahara N, Narita Y, Ichimura K. Recurrent mutations of CD79B and MYD88 are the hallmark of primary central nervous system lymphomas. *Neuropathol Appl Neurobiol* 2015; [Epub. ahead of print].

[20] Leoncini L, Raphaël M, Stain H, Harris NL, Jaffe ES, Kluin PM (2007) Burkitt lymphoma. In:Swerdlow SH, Campo E, Harris NL, Jaffe ES, Pileri SA, Stein H, Thiele J, Vardiman JW (eds.) *WHO Classification of Tumours of the Haematopoietic and Lymphoid Tissues*. International Agency for Research on Cancer, Lyon pp. 262-264.

[21] Oyama T, Ichimura K, Suzuki R, Suzumiya J, Ohshima K, Yatabe Y, Yokoi T, Kojima M, Kamiya Y, Taji H, Kagami Y, Ogura M, Saito H, Morishima Y, Nakamura S. Senile EBV+B-cell lymphoproliferative disorders: A clinicopathological study of 22 patients. *Am J Surg Pathol* 2003; 27: 16-26.

[22] Oyama T, Yamamoto K, Asano N, Oshiro A, Suzuki R, Kagami Y, Morishima Y, Takeuchi K, Izumo T, Mori S, Ohshima K, Suzumiya J, Nakamura N, Abe M, Ichimura K, Sato Y, Yoshino T, Naoe T, Shimoyama Y, Kamiya Y, Kinoshita T, Nakamura S. Age-related EBV-associated B-cell lymphoproliferative disorders constitute a distinct clinicopathologic group: A study of 96 patients. *Clin Cancer Res* 2007; 13: 5124-5132.

[23] Nakamura S, Jaffe ES, Swerdlow SH (2007) EB positive diffuse large B-cell lymphoma of the elderly. In:Swerdlow SH, Campo E, Harris NL, Jaffe ES, Pileri SA, Stein H, Thiele J, Vardiman JW (eds.) *WHO Classification of Tumours of the Haematopoietic and Lymphoid Tissues*. International Agency for Research on Cancer Lyon, pp. 243-244.

[24] Mahadevan A, Rao CR, Shanmugham M, Shankar SK. Primary central nervous system diffuse large B-cell lymphoma in the immunocompetent immunophenotypic subtypes and Epstein Barr-virus association. *J Neurosci Rural Pract* 2015; 6: 8-14.

[25] Nomura Y, Lavu EK, Muta K, Niino D, Takeshita M, Hirose S, Nakamura, S Yoshino T, Kikuchi M, Ohshima K Histological characteristics of 21 Papua New Guinean children with high-grade B-cell lymphoma, which is frequently associated with EBV infection. *Pathol Int* 2008; 58: 695-700.

[26] Bayraktar S, Stefanovic A, Montague N, Davis J, Murray T, Lossos IS. Central nervous system manifestations of marginal zone B-cell lymphoma. *Ann Hematol* 2010;89:1003-1009.

[27] Ueba T, Okawa M, Abe H, Inoue T, Takano K, Hayashi H, Nabeshima K, Ohshima K. Central nervous system marginal zone B-cell lymphoma of mucosa-associated lymphoid tissue type involving the brain and spinal cord parenchyma. *Neuropathology* 2013;33:306-311.

[28] Choi JY, Chung JH, Park YJ, Yoon TW, Kim YJ, Lim TK, Kim B, Nam S-H. Extranodal marginal zone B-cell lymphoma of mucosa-associated tissue type involving the Dura. *Cancer Res Treat* 2015; [Epub. ahead of print].

[29] Raz E, Tinelli E, Antonelli M, Canevelli M, Fiorelli M, Bozzao L, Di Piero V, Caramia F. MRI findings in lymphomatosis cerebri: description of a case and revision of the literature. *Neuroimaging* 2011; 21:e183-e186.

[30] Pandit L, Chickabasaviah Y, Raghothaman A, Mustafa S, Vasudevan A. Lymhomatosis cerebri-a rare cause of leukoencephalopathy. *J Neurol Sci* 2010;293:122-124.

[31] Kitai R, Hashimoto N, Yamate K, Ikawa M, Yoneda M, Nakajima T, Arishima H, Takeuchi H, Sato K, Kikura K. Lymphomatosis cerebri: clinical characteristics, neuroimaging, and pathological findings. *Brain Tumor Pathol* 2012;29:47-53.

[32] Sugie M, Ishihara K, Kato H, Nakano I, Kawamura M. Primary central nervous system lymphoma initially mimicking lymphomatosis cerebri: an autopsy case report. *Neuropathology* 2009;29:704-707.

[33] Menon MP, Nicolae A, Meeker H, Raffeld M, Xi L, Jegalian AG, Miller DC, Pittaluga S, Jaffe ES. Primary CNS T-cell Lymphomas: A Clinical, Morphologic, Immunophenotypic, and Molecular Analysis. *Am J Surg Pathol* 2015;39:1719-1729.

[34] Shimada K, Kinoshita T, Naoe T, Nakamura S. Presentation and management of intravascular large B-cell lymphoma. *Lancet Oncol* 2009;10:895-902.

[35] Ponzoni M, Ferreri AJ, Campo E, Facchetti F, Mazzucchelli L, Yoshino T, Murase T, Pileri SA, Doglioni C, Zucca E, Cavalli F, Nakamura S. Definition, diagnosis, and management of intravascular large B-cell lymphoma: proposals and perspectives from an international consensus meeting. *J Clin Oncol* 2007;25:3168-3173.

[36] Hishikawa N, Niwa H, Hara T, Hara K, Ito M, Shimada S, Yoshida M, Hashizume Y, Murakami N. An autopsy case of lymphomatosis cerebri showing pathological changes of intravascular large B-cell lymphomas in visceral organs. *Neuropathology* 2011;31: 612-619.

[37] Küker W, Nägele T, Korfel A, Heckl S, Thiel E, Bamberg M, Weller M, Herrlinger U. Primary central nervous system lymphomas (PCNSL): MRI features at presentation in 100 patients. *J Neurooncol* 2005; 72: 169-177.

[38] Yap KK, Sutherland T, Liew E, Tartaglia CJ, Pang M, Trost N. Magnetic resonance imaging in the immunocompetent patient: a pictorial essay. *J Med Imaging Radiat Oncol* 2012; 56: 179-186.

[39] Joseph JT. Hematological tumors. In: Joseph JT ed. *Diagnostic Neuropathology Smears*. Philadelphia: Lippincott Williams and Wilkins, 2007: 145-164.

[40] Sharma S, Deb P. Intraoperative neurocytology of primary central nervous system neoplasia: a simplified and practical diagnostic approach. *J Cytol* 2011; 28: 147-158.

In: Primary Central Nervous System Lymphoma (PCNSL) ISBN: 978-1-63485-322-4
Editor: Ryuya Yamanaka

Chapter 3

The Role of Tumor-Associated Microglia/Macrophages in Primary Central Nervous System Lymphoma: A New Target for Anti-Lymphoma Therapy?

Yoshihiro Komohara*

Department of Cell Pathology, Graduate School of Medical Sciences,
Kumamoto University, Kumamoto, Japan

Abstract

In hematological malignancies including primary central nervous system lymphoma (PCNSL), tumor-associated macrophages (TAMs) infiltrated in lymphoma/leukemia tissues are suggested to be involved in the progression, and phenotypical changes of TAMs have been studied by many researchers. Cell-cell interactions between protumoral TAMs and lymphoma/leukemia cells are suggested to play an important role in lymphoma/leukemia microenvironment. Although detail molecular mechanisms of cell-cell interaction have never been clarified, targeting TAMs might be a new strategy for treating malignant hematological diseases.

Keywords: macrophage, microglia, TAM, CD163, M2

Introduction

It is well known that many leukocytes including macrophages and lymphocytes infiltrate in lymphoma/leukemia tissues [1-3]. To our knowledge, the observation that macrophages are detected in tumor tissues was first reported around 50 years ago. Following the technique of

* Corresponding author: Yoshihiro Komohara, M.D., Ph.D. Honjo 1-1-1, Chuoku, Kumamoto, 860-8556, Japan. Tel: +81-96-373-5095 FAX: +91-96-373-5096. E-mail: ycomo@kumamoto-u.ac.jp.

immunohistochemistry had been established in 1990s, many articles has been published and demonstrated that many macrophages are detected in several malignant tumors including lymphoma/leukemia in recent decade [3]. Infiltrated macrophages were previously considered to have tumorcidal activity, however, recent advances demonstrate macrophages have protumor functions by secreting the several factors [1, 2]. Macrophages infiltrating into tumor tissues are generally named as tumor-associated macrophages (TAMs). Intratumoral infiltration of monocytes or macrophages is induced by various chemokines including chemokine (C-C motif) ligand (CCL)2, CCL5, CCL7, chemokine (C-X3-C motif) ligand (CX3CL)1 as well as cytokines such as macrophage colony-stimulating factor (M-CSF) and granulocyte-macrophage colony-stimulating factor, and these molecules are mainly secreted by tumor cells [4].

Macrophage Heterogeneity

Macrophage activation is well known to be involved in the pathogenesis of several diseases. The heterogeneity of macrophage differentiation was suggested from late 1990s based on the difference of surface markers or nitric oxide (NO)/Ornithine production or surface markers such as CD206 [5, 6]. Macrophage activation has been considered to be broadly divided into classically activated macrophages and alternatively activated macrophages. Classically activated (M1) macrophages preferentially express pro-inflammatory molecules such as NO, IL-12, CXCL9, CXCL10, CXCL11, and reactive oxygen species (ROS), and contribute to inflammatory responses and Th1-type immune reaction. On the other hands, alternatively activated (M2) macrophages express anti-inflammatory molecules such as Ornithine, IL-10, CCL17, CCL18, CCL22, and scavenger receptors, and are considered to be related to Th2-type immune reactions and tumor promotion by inducing angiogenesis, immunosuppression and tumor cell activation. CD163 (hemoglobin scavenger receptor), CD204 (Class A macrophage scavenger receptor), CD206 (mannose receptor, C type 1) are known to be highly expressed on M2 macrophages, and widely used as markers for M2 macrophages. M-CSF, IL-4, IL-10, IL-13, and corticosteroids are known to be involved in the differentiation of alternatively activated macrophages [1-3].

TAMs in PCNSL

Since there was no research study investigating the role or M1/M2 balance of TAMs in PCNSL, we tried to uncover the significance of M2 TAMs using human materials [7]. We first performed immunostaining for CD68, CD163, CD204, and pStat3 with paraffin-embedded PCNSL specimens obtained from 43 patients. Stat3 is one of the main molecules involved in lymphoma cell survival and is also known to be related to poor clinical prognosis of patients with lymphoma. Activation of Stat3 in tumor cells is caused by several receptor-type tyrosine kinases including vascular endothelial growth factor, platelet-derived growth factor, epidermal growth factor receptor, and Src, and Stat3 induces anti-apoptotic proteins such as Bcl-2, Bcl-XL, and surviving [8]. CD163 and CD204 served as markers of the M2 phenotype (Figure 1). All samples showed infiltration of many CD68$^+$ cells, and 29 and 25 cases evidenced high numbers of CD163+ and CD204+ M2 TAMs, respectively. Stat3 activation in lymphoma cells increased in patients with high infiltration of CD163+ TAMs, but not in those of CD204+ M2 TAMs [7]. Our *in vitro* co-culture experiment to investigate cell-cell interactions between macrophages and lymphoma cells found that Stat3 in lymphoma cells was strongly activated by co-culture with macrophages [7, 9]. BrdU incorporation in lymphoma cells was also increased by co-culture with macrophages, and notably strong activation of lymphoma cells was induced by M2 macrophages. Stat3 activation was also observed in macrophages co-cultured with lymphoma cells, and direct contact with lymphoma cells was seemed to be related to macrophage activation [9]. The fact that blocking Stat3 in macrophages abrogated the co-culture-induced lymphoma cell activation indicated that Stat3 activation in macrophages is key step for the cell-cell interaction between macrophages and lymphoma cells. We also found that macrophage derived soluble factors including IL-6, TNF-alpha, GRO-alpha, I-309, and C5a were closely involved in the activation of lymphoma cells [10]. However, our observation of human tissue samples showed that the numbers of CD68+, CD163+, and CD204+ TAMs and Stat3 activation in lymphoma cells were not correlated with prognosis [7]. Further studies are necessary to uncover the significance of cell-cell interaction between TAMs and lymphoma cells in the pathogenesis of PCNSL (Figure 2).

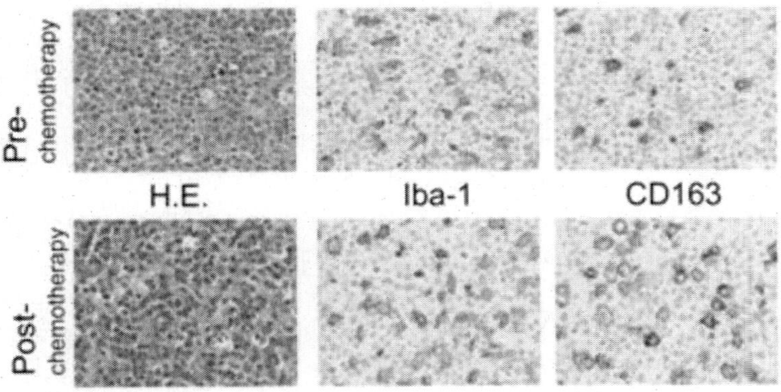

a

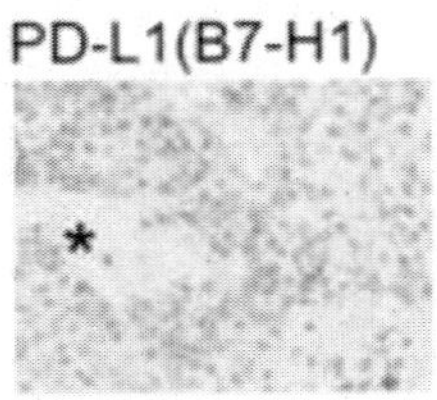

b

Figure 1. Immunostaining of macrophages in lymphoma tissues. Immunostaining of Iba-1 (pan-macrophage marker), CD163 (M2 marker), and PD-L1 (B7-H1) were performed on serial sections of chemo-resistant PCNSL. Iba-1 is a more useful marker for pan-macrophage than CD68. In a presented case of PCNSL, TAM infiltration was significantly increased after chemotherapy and TAMs expressed CD163 (A) and PD-L1 (B). PD-L1 is known to be related to immunosuppression by binding to PD-1 (one of immune checkpoint molecule). PD-L1-positive TAMs are preferentially detected around vessels (*).

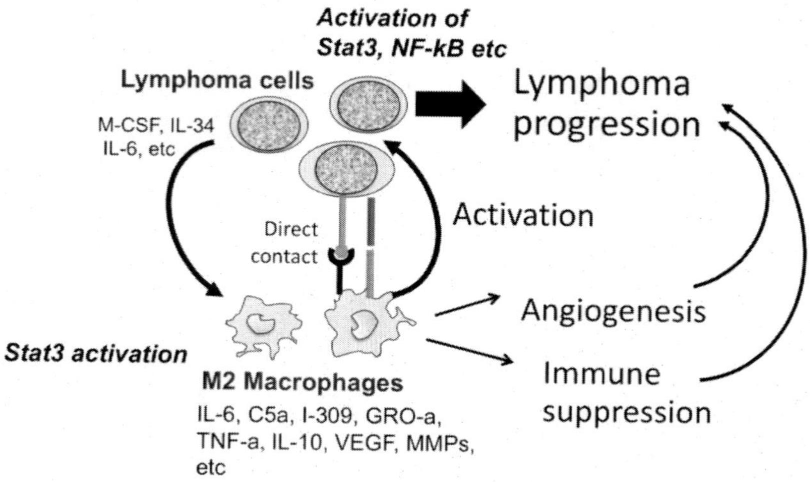

Figure 2. Schema of the functions and molecules related to cell-cell interaction between TAMs and lymphoma cells are summarized.

TARGETING TAMS

Several macrophage-targeting agents that inhibit macrophage recruitment into tumor tissues and/or inhibit macrophage differentiation into the M2 phenotype are currently under investigation [11]. It is well known that CSF-1 is required for macrophage differentiation, and some CSF-1R inhibitors have been developed by pharmaceutical companies. These inhibitors significantly suppressed tumor progression by inhibiting macrophage differentiation into the M2 phenotype and macrophage-related angiogenesis and immune suppression. We originally screened for compounds that would inhibit macrophage differentiation into the M2 phenotype using a new compound screening system. We found that triterpenoid compounds significantly inhibited macrophage differentiation into the M2 phenotype. Corosolic acid, a triterpenoid compound that is contained in apple pomace and banaba leaves, significantly suppressed subcutaneous tumor development and lung metastasis in a murine sarcoma model [12]. We are now studying other compounds which potentially useful for the therapy for patients with malignant tumor including lymphoma.

CONCLUSION

TAMs, especially M2 TAMs are considered to be involved in lymphoma progression by accelerating angiogenesis, lymphoma cell activation, and immunosuppression. Macrophage-targeting agents have just recently been developed by some companies, macrophage differentiation into the protumor M2 phenotype is also considered to be a promising target for treating patients with malignant tumors. Further investigation regarding the detailed mechanisms of macrophage activation is necessary for the advancement of anti-lymphoma therapy.

Disclosure Statement: All authors have no conflict of interest regarding this manuscript.

References

[1] Komohara, Y., Jinushi, M., Takeya, M., (2014). Clinical significance of macrophage heterogeneity in human malignant tumors. *Cancer. Sci.* 105, 1-8.

[2] Jinushi, M., Komohara, Y., (2015). Tumor-associated macrophages as an emerging target against tumors: Creating a new path from bench to bedside. *Biochim. Biophys. Acta.*, 1855, 123-30.

[3] Komohara, Y., Niino, D., Ohnishi, K., Ohshima, K., Takeya, M., (2015). Role of tumor-associated macrophages in hematological malignancies. *Pathol. Int.* 65, 170-6.

[4] Kitamura, T., Qian, B.Z., Pollard, J.W., (2015). Immune cell promotion of metastasis. *Nat. Rev. Immunol.* 15, 73-86.

[5] Gordon, S., (2003). Alternative activation of macrophages. *Nat. Rev. Immunol.* 3, 23-35.

[6] Mills, C.D., (2015). Anatomy of a discovery: m1 and m2 macrophages. *Front. Immunol.* 6, 212.

[7] Komohara, Y., Horlad, H., Ohnishi, K., Ohta, K., Makino, K., Hondo, H., Yamanaka, R., Kajiwara, K., Saito, T., Kuratsu, J., Takeya, M., (2011). M2 macrophage/microglial cells induce activation of Stat3 in primary central nervous system lymphoma. *J. Clin. Exp. Hematop.* 51, 93-9.

[8] Yu, H., Pardoll, D., Jove, R., (2009). STATs in cancer inflammation and immunity: a leading role for STAT3. *Nat. Rev. Cancer.* 9, 798-809.

[9] Bai, B., Horlad, H., Saito, Y., Ohnishi, K., Fujiwara, Y., Takeya, M., Komohara, Y., (2013). Role of Stat3 activation in cell-cell interaction between B-cell lymphoma and macrophages: the in vitro study. *J. Clin. Exp. Hematop.* 53, 127-33.

[10] Komohara, Y., Niino, D., Saito, Y., Ohnishi, K., Horlad, H., Ohshima, K., Takeya, M., (2013) Clinical significance of CD163$^+$ tumor-associated macrophages in patients with adult T-cell leukemia/lymphoma. *Cancer. Sci.* 104, 945-51.

[11] Komohara, Y., Fujiwara, Y., Ohnishi, K., Takeya, M., (2016) Tumor-associated macrophages: Potential therapeutic targets for anti-cancer therapy. *Adv Drug Deliv Rev.* 99,180-5.

[12] Fujiwara, Y., Takeya, M., Komohara, Y., (2014) A novel strategy for inducing the antitumor effects of triterpenoid compounds: blocking the protumoral functions of tumor-associated macrophages via STAT3 inhibition. *Biomed Res Int.* 2014, 348539.

In: Primary Central Nervous System Lymphoma (PCNSL) ISBN: 978-1-63485-322-4
Editor: Ryuya Yamanaka

Chapter 4

GENETICS OF PRIMARY CENTRAL NERVOUS SYSTEM LYMPHOMA

Kenichi Yoshida*
Department of Pathology and Tumor Biology, Graduate School of Medicine,
Kyoto University, Kyoto, Japan

ABSTRACT

Most primary central nervous system lymphomas (PCNSLs) are pathologically classified as diffuse large B-cell lymphomas (DLBCLs). Recently, the genetic background of systemic DLBCL has been unraveled; thus, similar genetic abnormalities, particularly those involved in B-cell receptor and nuclear factor-κB signaling, have been frequently detected in PCNSL. The development of targeted treatment against these genetic lesions is anticipated. On the other hand, some genetic lesions leading to immune escape or somatic hypermutations in non-immunoglobulin genes have been frequently identified in PCNSL, highlighting that systemic DLBCL and PCNSL are distinct disease entities. In this chapter, I will summarize the recent insight into genetic abnormalities in PCNSL.

Keywords: mutation, BCR, NF-κB, HLA, SHM

INTRODUCTION

Approximately 95% of PCNSL cases show a typical histology of diffuse large B-cell lymphoma (DLBCL) [1], and the remaining cases are classified as peripheral T-cell or Burkitt's lymphomas [2]. On the other hand, PCNSL shows very different biological and clinical characteristics from systemic DLBCL. PCNSL presents a more aggressive clinical course and is rarely curable with conventional chemoradiotherapy. The mechanism of its

* Corresponding author: Kenichi Yoshida, Department of Pathology and Tumor Biology, Graduate School of Medicine, Kyoto University. Email: yoshiken-thk@umin.ac.jp.

confinement to the CNS, a putative immune-privileged site, has long been discussed but still poorly understood. In addition, whether PCNSL cells emerge from within the CNS-derived lymphoid compartment or are derived from the lymphoma cells in the systemic lymphoid organs remains controversial [3]. An increased incidence of PCNSL has been reported in individuals with congenital or acquired immunodeficiency and appears to be frequently associated with Epstein–Barr virus (EBV) infection, which is rare in patients with no apparent immunodeficiency [3].

The germinal center (GC) is thought to be the place where antigen- or T-cell-derived stimulation activate mature B-cells and a source of many subtypes of lymphomas. Similar to systemic DLBCL, PCNSL is also likely to originate from GC-derived B-cells as suggested by ongoing somatic hypermutations (SHMs) in immunoglobulin (Ig) genes. Moreover, frequent (50%-80%) usage of the V4-34 gene segment suggests that specific antigens trigger the development of PCNSL [4, 5]. On the other hand, systemic DLBCLs are divided into the following two groups based on their cell-of-origin: 1) activated B cell-like (ABC) DLBCL and 2) germinal center B cell-like (GCB) DLBCL [6]. Most PCNSLs are assigned to the ABC (non-GCB) DLBCL based on immunostaining. Expression of CD10, BCL6, and MUM1 (IRF4) were positive in approximately 10%—20%, 60%—80%, and 90% of PCNSL cases, respectively [7]. Recent advances in genetic research have unveiled the pathogenesis of systemic DLBCL and PCNSL. Comparative genomic hybridization (CGH) or single-nucleotide polymorphism (SNP) array karyotyping and whole-exome sequencing (WES) of PCNSL identified a number of genes/pathways frequently affected in PCSNL (Table 1).

CONSTITUTIVE NF-κB/B-CELL RECEPTOR ACTIVITY

Frequent mutations affecting the immunoreceptor tyrosine-based activation motifs (ITAMs) of CD79A and CD79B, signaling subunits of BCR, have been reported in ABC-DLBCL [8]. In PCNSL, *CD79B* mutations were also frequently identified (30%–83%) [9-12]. These mutations are likely to augment chronic active BCR signaling and activate multiple downstream pathways, including the mitogen-activated protein kinase pathway, the phosphoinositide 3-kinase (PI3K), mammalian target of rapamycin (mTOR), and nuclear factor of activated T cells pathways. Frequent chronic active B-cell-receptor signaling is an anticipated therapeutic target in ABC-DLBCL, which acts by inhibiting downstream signaling, the SRC-family kinases BTK, SYK and PKC or PI3K-mTOR pathway [13].

In addition, the nuclear factor-κB (NF-κB) pathway, which is one of the downstream targets of BCR signaling, is also activated in ABC-DLBCL and PCNSL. Myeloid differentiation primary response 88 (MYD88), an adaptor molecule that links Toll/IL-1 receptor to NF-κB activation, is mutated in 30-86% of ABC-DLBCLs [14], whereas *MYD88* is mutated in as many as 76% of PCNSL cases [9, 11, 12, 15-17].

Moreover, activating mutations in CARD11 [11, 17, 18], which transmit BCR signaling to NF-κB signaling together with BCL10 and MALT1 (CBM complex), and inactivating mutations of TNFAIP3 (A20), negative regulator of NF-κB signaling, have been reported in PCNSL [17].

Table 1. Recurrent genetic lesions in PCNSL

Pathway/gene	Type	Frequency	References
Constitutive NF-κB/BCR activity			
MYD88	Mutation	38-86%	[9, 11, 12, 16, 17]
Pathway/gene	Type	Frequency	References
CD79B	Mutation	30-83%	[9, 11, 12, 17]
CARD11	Mutation	29-30%	[11, 17]
TNFAIP3/A20	Mutation/deletion	20%	[17]
Immune escape			
HLA region	Deletion	22-79%	[17, 21]
B2M	Mutation/deletion	<20%*	[17]
CD58	Mutation/deletion	<20%*	[17]
Dysregulation of differentiation of B-cells			
BCL6	Translocation	23-47%	]23, 24]
PRDM1/BLMP1	Mutation/deletion	11-20%	[9, 17]
PRKCD	Deletion	20%	[17]
TOX	Deletion	28%	[17]
ETV6	Mutation/deletion	16-21%	[11, 12]
IRF4	Mutation	14-29%	[11, 12]
Cell cycle			
CDKN2A/2B	Deletion	50-83%	[17, 21, 33]
TP53	Mutation/deletion	7%	[11]
Histone/chromatin modification			
CREBBP	Mutation	20%	[9]
Others			
TBL1XR1	Mutation/deletion	19-36%	[11, 12]
TMEM30A	Mutation/deletion	<20%*	[17]
GNA13	Mutation/deletion	20%	[17]
SHMs			
PIM1	Mutation	22-71%	[11, 12, 17]
BTG1	Mutation	43%	[11]
OSBPL10	Mutation	33%	[10]

* indicates the frequency of homozygous deletions of each gene.

IMMUNE ESCAPE

B-cells express major histocompatibility complex class II (MHC II) molecules on their surface to present antigens to T cells. Frequent loss of MHC II expression due to the deletion of chromosome 6p has been identified in lymphomas that have occurred in immune-privileged sites, including PNCSL [19]. Copy number losses in 6p21.3 (*HLA* region) are more frequently observed in PCNSL compared with systemic DLBCL [19, 20], suggesting that immune escape caused by decreased or absent MHC I and II expressions play a role in the pathogenesis of PCNSL. Recent CGH analysis has reported loss of 6p21.3 in 22-79% of PCNSL cases [17, 21]. β2-microglobulin (B2M) comprises a part of the MHC class I molecule that is thought to be necessary for the recognition of tumor cells by cytotoxic T lymphocytes (CTLs). Mutations and deletions of *B2M* have been identified in 30% of systemic DLBCL [22] and PCNSL cases [17]. Moreover, mutations and deletions in a member of the immunoglobulin superfamily gene *CD58*, which function as C2 receptor ligand and interact and activate CTL or natural killer (NK) cells, were also reported in PCNSL [17] and systemic DLBCL [22].

Dysregulation of Differentiation of B-Cells

BCL6 is a transcriptional repressor, which regulates premature B-cell activation and exit from germinal center, is frequently targeted by rearrangement in systemic DLBCL, particularly ABC-DLBCL. In PCNSL, as many as 17%-23% of cases harbor *BCL6* translocations [23, 24], which places BCL6 under the control of the powerful immunoglobulin enhancers, leading to repressed BCL6 downregulation.

The PR domain zinc finger protein 1 (PRDM1 or BLIMP1) is a master regulator of terminal differentiation from B-cells to plasma cells, and is mutated and deleted in systemic DLBCL (25%) [25]. *PRDM1* is also mutated in 19% of PCNSL cases [26].

Moreover, recent WES studies identified a number of novel recurrently mutated genes associated with B cell differentiation, including *PRKCD*, *TOX*, *ETV6* as well as *IRF4* [12, 17].

Altered Histone/Chromatin Modification

Recent genetics studies using high-throughput sequencing technologies identified a number of novel driver genes in systemic DLBCL, including histone acetyltransferase *CREBBP* [27, 28], which was also mutated in PCNSL [9]. Regarding the mechanism through which *CREBBP* mutations contribute to the pathogenesis of DLBCL, it is suggested that mutations in *CREBBP* alter BCL6 and TP53 (both of which are substrates of CREBBP) acetylation, activate BCL6, and decrease TP53 activity [27].

Other Pathways

WES identified several recurrently mutated genes in other pathways in PCNSL. *TBL1XR1*, a transcription factor comprising the NCoR/SMRT transcription repressor complex, was mutated in 19-36% of the PCNSL cases [9, 11, 12]. *GNA13*, the gene encoding the G protein Gα13, and the flippase complex gene *TMEM30A* were also recurrently mutated and deleted in PCNSL [17] and systemic DLBCL [28, 29]. *TP53*, which is inactivated in the majority of human cancers, is rarely mutated in PNCSL [11].

ONGOING SHMS

SHM in the immunoglobulin variable region is a fundamental mechanism of generating an extreme diversity of immunoglobulin (Ig) molecules and has been mediated by activation-induced cytidine deaminase. Furthermore, SHM targets a number of non-immunoglobulin genes in both normal and neoplastic B-cells [30, 31] and is thought to be involved in the lymphomas pathogenesis. SHMs were identified in at least one gene among *PIM1*, *c-MYC*, *RhoH/TTF*, *PAX5* and *CD95*, which were previously reported targets of SHMs in systemic DLBCL [30], for almost all PCNSL cases (9/10), and ongoing SHMs was also confirmed along with SHMs in systemic DLBCL [32]. SHMs were 2–5 times more frequently observed in PCNSL when compared with those in systemic DLBCL. WES also identified novel targeted genes of SHMs in PCNSL, including *BTG1* [11], H1 linker histone genes, *KLHL14*,and *OSBPL10* [10].

CHROMOSOMAL ABNORMALITIES IN PCNSL

In addition to the above mentioned *BCL6* translocations and deletion in the *HLA* region, copy number analyses using CGH and SNP array karyotyping identified a number of recurrent copy number abnormalities in PCNSL. Deletions in 9p21 including CDKN2A/p16 were frequently observed in as many as 83% of PNCSL cases [17, 21, 33]. Moreover, deletions at 6q and gains at 12q, 22q and 18q21 (including *BCL2* and *MALT1*) were reported [34].

CLONAL ORIGIN OF PCNSL

As for the origin of PCNSL, several sets of evidence have suggested that premalignant clones entered into the central nervous system. It has been reported that genetic lesions in PCNSL cells are often detected in peripheral blood and/or bone marrow samples, suggesting that premalignant clone entered the central nervous system [35, 36]. Moreover, a substantial fraction of patients with ABC-DLBCL (11/39, 28.2%) and PCNSL (4/15, 26.7%) showed monoclonal B lymphocytosis (MBL) or bone marrow monoclonal small B-cell infiltration (MSBC) [37]. Malecka et al. have demonstrated that lymphoma cells originated from an MBL/MSBC clone in three of six DLBCL cases, on the basis of IgH rearrangement [38].

CONCLUSION

Recent advances in genetic analyses have revealed the genetic abnormalities in PCNSL, in which several functional pathways frequently undergo dysregulation. Most of these genetic lesions, including those involved in BCR/NF-κB signaling, were also commonly affected in ABC-DLBCL, showing concordant results with previous immunophenotypic analysis. On the other hand, several genetic legions, such as deletions in the *HLA* region and SHMs were more specific to PCNSL, highlighting the unique feature of PCNSL when compared with systemic

DLBCL. Further analysis of a larger cohort of PCNSL cases would demonstrate the full spectrum of genetic lesions and the PCNSL pathogenesis.

REFERENCES

[1] Swerdlow SH. WHO classification of tumours of haematopoietic and lymphoid tissues. Lyon: International Agency for Research on Cancer; 2008.

[2] Korfel A, Schlegel U. Diagnosis and treatment of primary CNS lymphoma. *Nat Rev Neurol.* 2013;9(6):317-27.

[3] Deckert M, Engert A, Brück W, Ferreri AJ, Finke J, Illerhaus G et al. Modern concepts in the biology, diagnosis, differential diagnosis and treatment of primary central nervous system lymphoma. *Leukemia.* 2011;25(12):1797-807.

[4] Montesinos-Rongen M, Küppers R, Schlüter D, Spieker T, Van Roost D, Schaller C et al. Primary central nervous system lymphomas are derived from germinal-center B cells and show a preferential usage of the V4-34 gene segment. *Am J Pathol.* 1999;155(6): 2077-86.

[5] Thompsett AR, Ellison DW, Stevenson FK, Zhu D. V(H) gene sequences from primary central nervous system lymphomas indicate derivation from highly mutated germinal center B cells with ongoing mutational activity. *Blood.* 1999;94(5):1738-46.

[6] Alizadeh AA, Eisen MB, Davis RE, Ma C, Lossos IS, Rosenwald A et al. Distinct types of diffuse large B-cell lymphoma identified by gene expression profiling. *Nature.* 2000; 403(6769):503-11.

[7] Camilleri-Broët S, Crinière E, Broët P, Delwail V, Mokhtari K, Moreau A et al. A uniform activated B-cell-like immunophenotype might explain the poor prognosis of primary central nervous system lymphomas: analysis of 83 cases. *Blood.* 2006;107(1): 190-6.

[8] Davis RE, Ngo VN, Lenz G, Tolar P, Young RM, Romesser PB et al. Chronic active B-cell-receptor signalling in diffuse large B-cell lymphoma. *Nature.* 2010;463(7277):88-92.

[9] Nakamura T, Tateishi K, Niwa T, Matsushita Y, Tamura K, Kinoshita M et al. Recurrent mutations of CD79B and MYD88 are the hallmark of primary central nervous system lymphomas. *Neuropathol Appl Neurobiol.* 2015.

[10] Vater I, Montesinos-Rongen M, Schlesner M, Haake A, Purschke F, Sprute R et al. The mutational pattern of primary lymphoma of the central nervous system determined by whole-exome sequencing. *Leukemia.* 2015;29(3):677-85.

[11] Chapuy B, Roemer MG, Stewart C, Tan Y, Abo RP, Zhang L et al. Targetable genetic features of primary testicular and primary central nervous system lymphomas. *Blood.* 2015.

[12] Bruno A, Boisselier B, Labreche K, Marie Y, Polivka M, Jouvet A et al. Mutational analysis of primary central nervous system lymphoma. *Oncotarget.* 2014;5(13):5065-75.

[13] Wilson WH, Young RM, Schmitz R, Yang Y, Pittaluga S, Wright G et al. Targeting B cell receptor signaling with ibrutinib in diffuse large B cell lymphoma. *Nat Med.* 2015.

[14] Ngo VN, Young RM, Schmitz R, Jhavar S, Xiao W, Lim KH et al. Oncogenically active MYD88 mutations in human lymphoma. *Nature*. 2011;470(7332):115-9.

[15] Montesinos-Rongen M, Godlewska E, Brunn A, Wiestler OD, Siebert R, Deckert M. Activating L265P mutations of the MYD88 gene are common in primary central nervous system lymphoma. *Acta Neuropathol.* 2011;122(6):791-2.

[16] Kraan W, Horlings HM, van Keimpema M, Schilder-Tol EJ, Oud ME Scheepstra C et al. High prevalence of oncogenic MYD88 and CD79B mutations in diffuse large B-cell lymphomas presenting at immune-privileged sites. *Blood Cancer J.* 2013;3:e139.

[17] Braggio E, Van Wier S, Ojha J, McPhail ER, Assmann Y, Egan JB et al. Genome-wide analysis uncovers novel recurrent alterations in primary central nervous system lymphomas. *Clin Cancer Res.* 2015.

[18] Montesinos-Rongen M, Schmitz R, Brunn A, Gesk S, Richter J, Hong K et al. Mutations of CARD11 but not TNFAIP3 may activate the NF-kappaB pathway in primary CNS lymphoma. *Acta Neuropathol.* 2010;120(4):529-35.

[19] Riemersma SA, Jordanova ES, Schop RF, Philippo K, Looijenga LH, Schuuring E et al. Extensive genetic alterations of the HLA region, including homozygous deletions of HLA class II genes in B-cell lymphomas arising in immune-privileged sites. *Blood.* 2000;96(10):3569-77.

[20] Booman M, Douwes J, Glas AM, Riemersma SA, Jordanova ES, Kok K et al. Mechanisms and effects of loss of human leukocyte antigen class II expression in immune-privileged site-associated B-cell lymphoma. *Clin Cancer Res.* 2006;12(9): 2698-705.

[21] Gonzalez-Aguilar A, Idbaih A, Boisselier B, Habbita N, Rossetto M, Laurenge A et al. Recurrent mutations of MYD88 and TBL1XR1 in primary central nervous system lymphomas. *Clin Cancer Res.* 2012;18(19):5203-11.

[22] Challa-Malladi M, Lieu YK, Califano O, Holmes AB, Bhagat G, Murty VV et al. Combined genetic inactivation of β2-Microglobulin and CD58 reveals frequent escape from immune recognition in diffuse large B cell lymphoma. *Cancer Cell.* 2011;20(6): 728-40.

[23] Montesinos-Rongen M, Zühlke-Jenisch R, Gesk S, Martín-Subero JI, Schaller C, Van Roost D et al. Interphase cytogenetic analysis of lymphoma-associated chromosomal breakpoints in primary diffuse large B-cell lymphomas of the central nervous system. *J Neuropathol Exp Neurol.* 2002;61(10):926-33.

[24] Cady FM, O'Neill BP, Law ME, Decker PA, Kurtz DM, Giannini C et al. Del(6)(q22) and BCL6 rearrangements in primary CNS lymphoma are indicators of an aggressive clinical course. *J Clin Oncol.* 2008;26(29):4814-9.

[25] Mandelbaum J, Bhagat G, Tang H, Mo T, Brahmachary M, Shen Q et al. BLIMP1 is a tumor suppressor gene frequently disrupted in activated B cell-like diffuse large B cell lymphoma. *Cancer Cell.* 2010;18(6):568-79.

[26] Courts C, Montesinos-Rongen M, Brunn A, Bug S, Siemer D, Hans V et al. Recurrent inactivation of the PRDM1 gene in primary central nervous system lymphoma. *J Neuropathol Exp Neurol.* 2008;67(7):720-7.

[27] Pasqualucci L, Dominguez-Sola D, Chiarenza A, Fabbri G, Grunn A, Trifonov V et al. Inactivating mutations of acetyltransferase genes in B-cell lymphoma. *Nature.* 2011; 471(7337):189-95.

[28] Morin RD, Mendez-Lago M, Mungall AJ, Goya R, Mungall KL, Corbett RD et al. Frequent mutation of histone-modifying genes in non-Hodgkin lymphoma. *Nature*. 2011;476(7360):298-303.

[29] Morin RD, Mungall K, Pleasance E, Mungall AJ, Goya R, Huff RD et al. Mutational and structural analysis of diffuse large B-cell lymphoma using whole-genome sequencing. *Blood*. 2013;122(7):1256-65.

[30] Pasqualucci L, Neumeister P, Goossens T, Nanjangud G, Chaganti RS, Küppers R et al. Hypermutation of multiple proto-oncogenes in B-cell diffuse large-cell lymphomas. *Nature*. 2001;412(6844):341-6.

[31] Liu M, Duke JL, Richter DJ, Vinuesa CG, Goodnow CC, Kleinstein SH et al. Two levels of protection for the B cell genome during somatic hypermutation. *Nature*. 2008; 451(7180):841-5.

[32] Montesinos-Rongen M, Van Roost D, Schaller C, Wiestler OD, Deckert M. Primary diffuse large B-cell lymphomas of the central nervous system are targeted by aberrant somatic hypermutation. *Blood*. 2004;103(5):1869-75.

[33] Cobbers JM, Wolter M, Reifenberger J, Ring GU, Jessen F, An HX et al. Frequent inactivation of CDKN2A and rare mutation of TP53 in PCNSL. *Brain Pathol*. 1998;8 (2):263-76.

[34] Weber T, Weber RG, Kaulich K, Actor B, Meyer-Puttlitz B, Lampel S et al. Characteristic chromosomal imbalances in primary central nervous system lymphomas of the diffuse large B-cell type. *Brain Pathol*. 2000;10(1):73-84.

[35] McCann KJ, Ashton-Key M, Smith K, Stevenson FK, Ottensmeier CH. Primary central nervous system lymphoma: tumor-related clones exist in the blood and bone marrow with evidence for separate development. *Blood*. 2009;113(19):4677-80.

[36] Jahnke K, Hummel M, Korfel A, Burmeister T, Kiewe P, Klasen HA et al. Detection of subclinical systemic disease in primary CNS lymphoma by polymerase chain reaction of the rearranged immunoglobulin heavy-chain genes. *J Clin Oncol*. 2006;24(29):4754-7.

[37] Tierens AM, Holte H, Warsame A, Ikonomou IM, Wang J, Chan WC et al. Low levels of monoclonal small B cells in the bone marrow of patients with diffuse large B-cell lymphoma of activated B-cell type but not of germinal center B-cell type. *Haematologica*. 2010;95(8):1334-41.

[38] Malecka A, Tierens A, Østlie I, Schmitz R, Trøen G, Spetalen S et al. Primary diffuse large B cell lymphoma associated with Clonally-related monoclonal B lymphocytosis indicates a common precursor cell. *Haematologica*. 2015.

II. DIAGNOSIS

In: Primary Central Nervous System Lymphoma (PCNSL)
Editor: Ryuya Yamanaka
ISBN: 978-1-63485-322-4

Chapter 5

DIAGNOSTIC IMAGING OF PRIMARY CENTRAL NERVOUS SYSTEM MALIGNANT LYMPHOMA

Keisuke Miyake** and Takashi Tamiya
Department of Neurological Surgery, Kagawa University Faculty of Medicine, Kagawa, Japan

ABSTRACT

This section summarizes diagnostic imaging of primary central nervous system malignant lymphoma (PCNSL). In a typical PCNSL case, diagnostic imaging is not difficult; e.g., common findings include high density on non-contrast computed tomography (CT); periventricular location, homogeneous contrast enhancement, and iso- to hypointensity when compared to gray matter on T2 weighted magnetic resonance (MR) imaging; and high intensity on diffusion weighted MR imaging. Hemorrhage is rare unlike a case of glioblastoma. ^{18}F-fluorodeoxyglucose ([^{18}F]FDG) positron emission tomography (PET) is useful for diagnosis of PCNSL. [^{18}F]FDG uptake in typical PCNSL is approximately 2.5 times higher than that in the normal gray matter, and the tumor can usually be identified visually. [^{18}F]FDG uptake pattern and value can be used to differentiate PCNSL from other enhancing malignant brain tumors, especially glioblastoma. In patients with acquired immunodeficiency syndrome (AIDS), irregular ring enhancement is noted on enhanced CT and MRI, and [^{18}F]FDG can be used to distinguish AIDS related brain disease such as cerebral toxoplasmosis from PCNSL. However, in atypical PCNSL cases such as disseminated or non-enhancing lesions, [^{18}F] FDG PET often fails to show the presence of tumor in the brain because [^{18}F]FDG uptake is faint. Most difficult to distinguish is a tumefactive multiple sclerosis. Most of the reported tumefactive multiple sclerosis cases are diagnosed by brain biopsy when the brain tumor, especially malignant lymphoma is suspected. In conclusion, [^{18}F]FDG PET is very useful for the diagnosis of typical PCNSL and can differentiate PCNSL from other malignant brain tumors. However, in case of atypical PCNSL, diagnosis by using [^{18}F]FDG PET is limited. Moreover, atypical MR findings such as disseminated lesions

* Corresponding author: Department of Neurological Surgery, Kagawa University Faculty of Medicine, 1750-1 Ikenobe, Miki-cho, Kita-gun, Kagawa, 761-0793, Japan. Tel: +81-87-891-2207, fax: +81-87-891-2208, email: keisuke@kms.ac.jp.

or no lesions are more prevalent in a recent study than formally reported in immunocompetent patients with PCNSL.

Keywords: primary central nervous system malignant lymphoma, diagnostic imaging, ^{18}F-fluorodeoxyglucose ([^{18}F]FDG)

INTRODUCTION

Although primary central nervous system lymphoma (PCNSL) is a rare tumor accounting for only 3-5% of all primary brain tumors, the incidence of PCNSL in developed countries is approximately 5 patients per 1 million people annually [32, 36]. Epidemiological data have shown a continuous increase over the past three decades in the population whereas the incidence seems to decline in patients with acquired immunodeficiency syndrome (AIDS) since the development of highly active antiretroviral therapies [14]. PCNSL affects all age group with the peak incidence in the fifth to seventh decades in non-AIDS patients. Therefore, the rising incidence of PCNSL may only represent the increased aging population. Recent studies have shown an encouraging improvement in the overall survival time when radiotherapy is combined with high-dose methotrexate-(MTX-) based chemotherapy [29, 40]. Young age and Karnofsky performance score (KPS) at the time of diagnosis are reported to be associated with longer survival time [2]. Therefore, early diagnosis of PCNSL is essential for starting early treatment before the decline of patient's performance status. Clinical diagnosis of PCNSL is sometimes difficult and delayed because common initial symptoms such as focal signs, raised intracranial pressure, and behavioral and personality changes especially in elderly patients are nonspecific [4]. Computed tomography (CT) and magnetic resonance (MR) images in PCNSL patients show single or multiple uniformly well-enhancing lesions that are usually located in the periventricular lesions and the basal ganglia and often involve the corpus callosum [8]. These radiological findings are not pathognomonic for PCNSL and cannot accurately differentiate PCNSL from other tumorous and nontumorous brain lesions.

Although CT and MRI imaging are still the most important modalities in the diagnosis of PCNSL, modern metabolic imaging modalities are increasingly used to improve accuracy of the diagnosis. Positron emission tomography (PET) with glucose analogue ^{18}F-fluorodeoxyglucose ([^{18}F]FDG) is one of the most attractive and widely used modalities for evaluating tumor metabolism noninvasively. PCNSL usually shows high uptake of [^{18}F]FDG, although normal high levels of [^{18}F]FDG in the cerebral cortex, basal ganglia and thalamus sometimes mask the presence of underlying PCNSL. Even in a rapid emerging clinical application, the role of [^{18}F]FDG PET in PCNSL is not fully defined and reviewed systemically. This section reviews the usefulness and limitation of neuroimaging for the diagnosis of PCNSL.

CT AND MRI IN THE DIAGNOSIS OF PCNSL

Characteristic images of PCNSL illustrate high cell density, high ratio of nucleo-cytoplasma, areas of the blood-brain barrier breakdown and a common site (the periventricular lesions, basal ganglia and the corpus callosum) [9]. Plain CT image (Figure 1) shows high density lesion in the typical PCNSL [6]. T2 weighted image (WI) and fluid attenuated IR (FLAIR) show slightly high intensity lesion with edema, and gadolinium-enhanced T1WI shows homogeneous enhanced lesion (Figure 2). In addition, calcification, bleeding and necrosis are rare. PCNSL may be associated with edema, but not as frequent as usual malignant glioma and meningioma. A delineation of PCNSL margin is clear, and multiple PCNSL is considered to be frequent occurrence in 20-40%. As approximately one third of non-enhancing gliomas are malignant, the clinical application of conventional imaging in brain tumor diagnosis is limited and nonspecific. Similarly, PCNSL with atypical MRI, such as disseminated or non-enhanced lesions, exhibit obscure images wherein a tumor cannot be clearly identified in the lesions [16]. ^{1}H-MR spectroscopy (MRS) provides information on metabolic changes *in vivo*. The most specific finding for typical PCNSL on MRS is an increase in lipid/lactate peak [10, 41]. PCNSL also demonstrated a raised choline peak relative to creatine and N-acetyl aspartate (NAA), which are nonspecific and also shown in astrocytic tumors [18]. Advanced MRI techniques, such as perfusion weighted imaging (PWI) or diffusion weighted imaging (DWI) allow more accurate analysis of PCNSL [7, 24]. DWI is a method that evaluates water diffusion in the extracellular space. The results of this examination are DWI images and apparent diffusion coefficient (ADC) maps It is a relatively short (1-5 minutes) sequence which does not require contrast administration. Generally, homogenous diffusion restriction (high signal on DWI images and low signal on ADC maps) is characteristic of highly cellular tumors such as PCNSLs. On the contrary, high-grade gliomas or metastases show only small areas of diffusion restriction corresponding with the most cellular and the most malignant parts of the tumor core [7]. PWI is an advanced MRI technique that enables measurements of cerebral hemodynamics at the capillary level. The dynamic susceptibility contrast (DSC) MRI technique is most widely used. It is based on MRI signal calculations evaluated from T2-weighted sequences after the first contrast passage through the microcirculation [37]. On the basis of these calculations, parametric maps of Cerebral Blood Volume (CBV) and perfusion curves are created. In tumors, the CBV parameter is measured within the lesion and normalized to the CBV parameter from the normal appearing white mater of the contralateral hemisphere (rCBV) [25, 45]. According to the literature, rCBV values correlate with the density of tumor vascularization and are elevated in lesions with increased pathological neoangiogenesis and increased malignancy such as high-grade gliomas and metastases [3]. The perfusion curves after contrast passage are created from the outlined regions of interest (ROIs), and in malignant tumors such as HGGs or metastases, the ROIs do not reach the baseline. PCNSLs present a typical perfusion pattern such as hypoperfusion and the characteristic shape of the signal intensity curves returning above the baseline level [24]. DSC perfusion and DWI sequences can help to better define malignant tumor biology. Reduced ADC metrics correlates with increased tumor cellularity [27]. PCNSL biology is reflected by physiologic MR imaging metrics. Physiologic MR imaging biomarkers can improve diagnostic capabilities in cases of PCNSL.

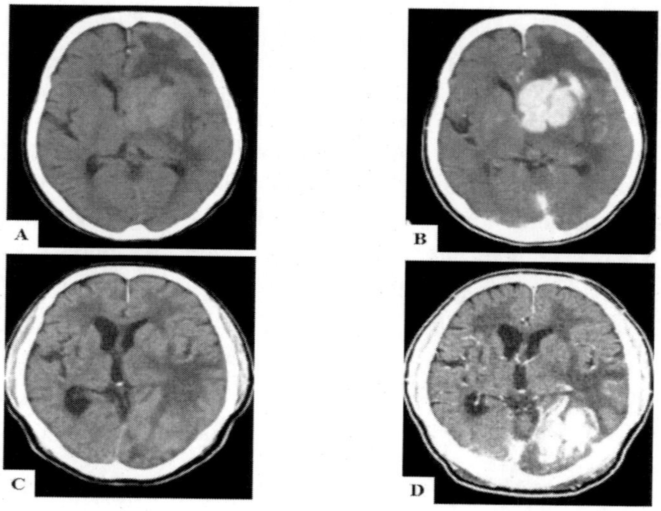

Figure 1. Plain CT (A, C) and contrast-enhanced CT (B, D) images in PCNSL. Plain CT shows a slightly high density in the lesions and contrast-enhanced CT shows a homogenous enhanced lesion in the left basal ganglia (B) and the left occipital white matter (D).

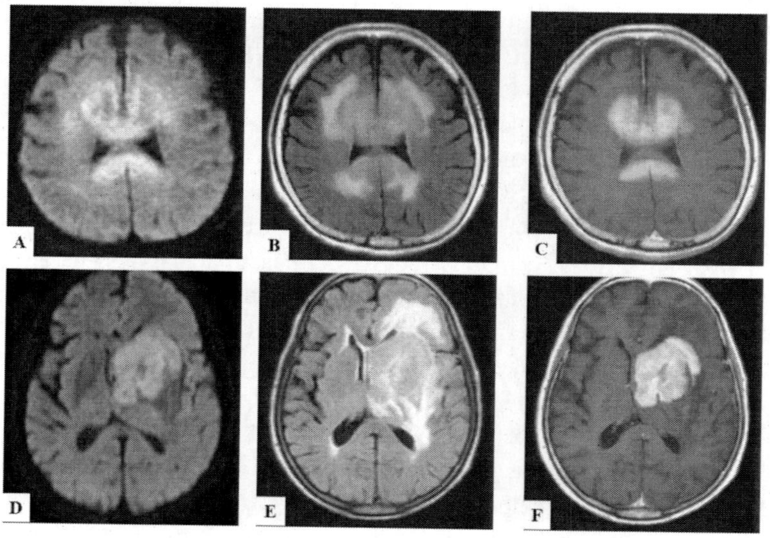

Figure 2. DWI in PCNSL shows a high intensity lesion in the corpus callosum (A) and the left basal ganglia (D). FLAIR images show a high intensity lesion (B, E) and contrast-enhanced T1-weighted MR images show a homogenous enhanced lesion (C, F).

FDG PET IN THE DIAGNOSIS OF PCNSL

Primary Diagnosis and Differentiation from Nontumorous Lesions

PCNSL is characterized by very high cellular density and increased glucose metabolism, usually associated with high uptake of [^{18}F]FDG in the tumor [17, 19, 20, 23, 33, 38]. The semiquantitative [^{18}F]FDG uptake values measured by maximum SUV (SUVmax) are reported to be 14-22 in PCNSL (Figure 3), and this value is approximately 2.5 times higher than the average SUV in the normal gray matter [17, 19, 20, 23]. A modified three-compartment model was used for the measurement of FDG kinetics in the brain [34]. The FDG kinetic parameters were calculated from the dynamic activities obtained from tissue ROIs. Five parameters (K_1, k_2, k_3, k_4, and blood volume) were estimated by use of nonlinear least-square fitting technique. The FDG influx rate constant (K_i) was calculated using the following formula: $K_i = ([K_1 \times k_3]/[k_2 + k_3])$. In this model, the movement of FDG from the plasma to the tissue compartment represents primarily the transporter-related transport of FDG and thus reflects the activity of the glucose transporter (GLUT-1). However, the K_1 value may also include extravasation of the tracer into the extracellular space through the disrupted blood brain barrier in the tumor. Once FDG is transported into the metabolic compartment, FDG phosphorylated by hexokinase and trapped inside the tissue as FDG-6-phosphate. The k_3 reflects the activity of FDG phosphorylation by hexokinase and is reporter to be elevated in PCNSL (Figure 4) [15, 28]. In patients with acquired immunodeficiency syndrome (AIDS), [^{18}F]FDG uptake in the lesions can be used to distinguish human-immunodeficiency-virus-(HIV)-related brain disease such as cerebral toxoplasmosis from PCNSL [11, 30, 44]. The use of [^{18}F]FDG PET in the diagnosis of PCNSL is not a new concept. In 1992, Rosenfeld et al. reported a high [^{18}F]FDG uptake in a group of 10 PCNSL patients [38]. They also reported a patient who showed dramatic disappearance of [^{18}F]FDG uptake in the tumor with steroid therapy [38]. Hustinx et al. examined SUVs in primary brain tumors on [^{18}F]FDG PET and concluded that SUV measurements were influenced by a variety of factors, such as plasma glucose level, steroid treatment, tumor size and heterogeneity, time after injection, and previous radiation therapy [12]. Steroids have a cytotoxic effect in lymphoma cells and reduce [^{18}F]FDG uptake in the tumor, significantly causing false negative results during the diagnosis of PCNSL [20]. Moreover, nonspecific uptake of [^{18}F]FDG has been reported in patients with nontumorous brain lesions such as intracerebral hematoma [5], brain abscess [43], and multiple sclerosis [39]. Animal studies have shown that inflammatory cells significantly contribute to [^{18}F]FDG uptake in tumors. Kubota et al. reported that approximately 30% of [^{18}F]FDG uptake was related to the non-tumorous tissue in a mouse malignant tumor model [21]. The extent of [^{18}F]FDG uptake in the non-tumorous lesions depends on the increased density of inflammatory cells as well as disruption of the BBB in the lesion.

Differentiation from Other Malignant Brain Tumors

Recent studies have revealed that [^{18}F]FDG PET can differentiate PCNSL from other malignant brain tumors such as glioblastoma and metastatic brain tumor [20, 23]. The [^{18}F]FDG uptake in PCNSL is usually homogenous in contrast to inhomogeneous uptake in other malignant brain tumors. Kosaka et al. showed that metastatic brain tumors and glioblastomas except for 1 case can be distinguished from PCNSL with [^{18}F]FDG PET when cutoff value was set at 15 SUVmax [20]. A recent study demonstrated the usefulness of [^{18}F] FDG PET for differentiating PCNSL and glioblastoma, showing similar MR findings. [^{18}F] FDG uptake in PCNSL (SUVmax of 16.8 ± 7.2) was significantly higher than that in glioblastoma (SUVmax of 8.2 ± 3.1; $P < 0.01$) [23]. The accuracy of [^{18}F]FDG PET for lesion differentiation was 0.86 when cutoff value was set at 12 SUVmax with a sensitivity of 100% and a specificity of 71.4% [23]. The overlying cortical gray matter sometimes shows glucose hypometabolism in PCNSL located in the deep white matter and the basal ganglia/thalamus. This finding is not specific for PCNSL, only reported in patients with gliomatosis cerebri due to disconnection of the cortical gray matter by tumor infiltration [35].

Diagnosis of Atypical PCNSL

PCNSL with typical radiological findings shows high [^{18}F]FDG uptake in almost all cases, and [^{18}F]FDG PET provides valuable information in the primary diagnosis of PCNSL. However, PCNSL sometimes demonstrates atypical radiological findings such as disseminated or non-enhancing lesions in contrast-enhanced MR or CT images [8, 22]. Such atypical findings in non-AIDS patients with PCNSL were more prevalent in a recent study, showing that 13% of the patients had no lesions and 7% of the patients had disseminated lesions [8]. Ring-like enhancement occurs in more than 50% of the lesions in AIDS-related PCNSL, but also in 6-13% of the lesions in non-AIDS PCNSL [8, 22]. [^{18}F]FDG uptake in PCNSL with atypical radiological findings is not increased sufficiently to visually detect the tumor because of normal high background uptake of [^{18}F]FDG in the brain. Kawai et al. revealed that 3 out of 4 [^{18}F]FDG PET tests failed to show the presence of PCNSL with atypical radiological findings. Quantitative FDG uptake values (K_i) in the tumors are significantly lower in atypical PCNSL compared with those in typical PCNSL (Figure 5) [17]. Therefore, [^{18}F]FDG PET is not a perfect tool, and caution is necessary, especially in the diagnosis of atypical PCNSL. To date, no imaging modality can definitively diagnose PCNSL, and early tumor biopsy is still recommended when PCNSL is suspected, especially with atypical radiological findings [42].

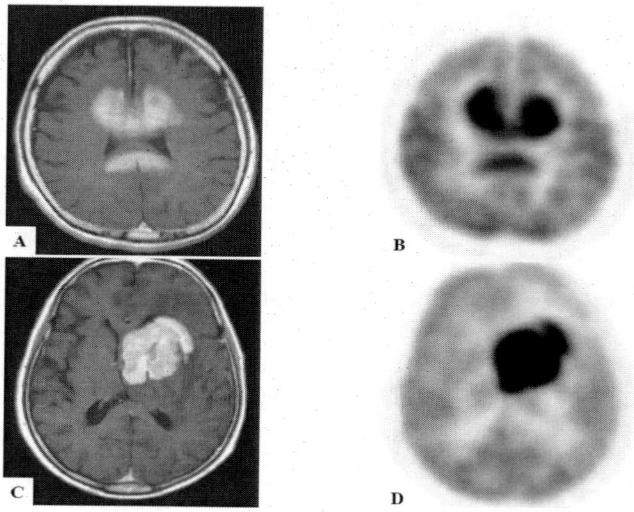

Figure 3. Contrast-enhanced T1-weighted MR (left) and ^{18}F-FDG PET (right) images in PCNSL patients with typical MR findings. MR images show a homogenous enhanced lesion in the corpus callosum (A) and the left basal ganglia (C). ^{18}F-FDG PET images show a strong ^{18}F-FDG uptake in the lesions (B, D).

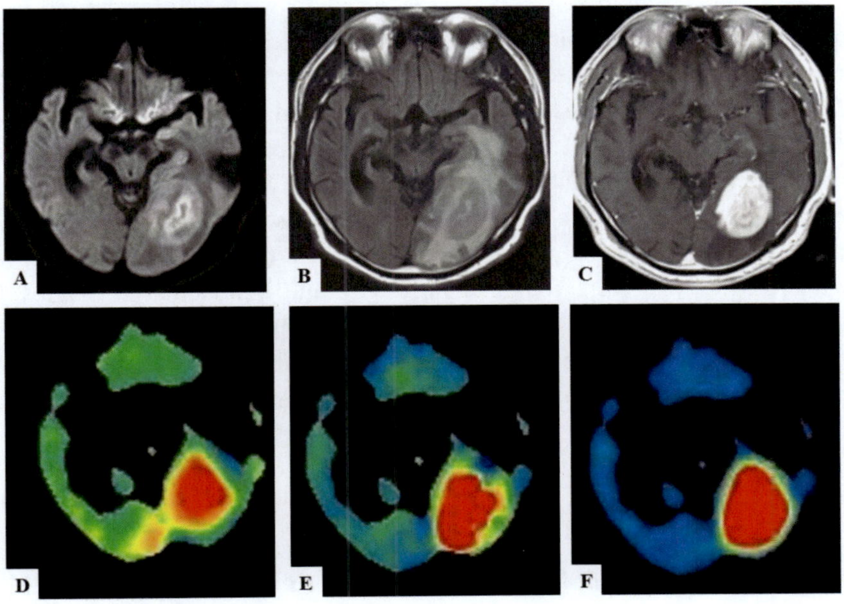

Figure 4. Representative MR image (upper) and ^{18}F-FDG-PET kinetic analysis (lower) in typical PCNSL. DWI shows a high intensity in the left occipital lesion (A). FLAIR shows a high intensity lesion with edema (B). Contrast-enhanced T1-WI shows a well-defined enhancing tumor in the left occipital lesion in the left occipital lesion (C). The tumor exhibits substantially higher ^{18}F-FDG uptake relative to the surrounding brain on ^{18}F-FDG *Ki* images (F). Corresponding lesion shows a markedly increased hexokinase activity (k_3) with a strong increased FDG transport ($K1$) in the kinetic analysis.

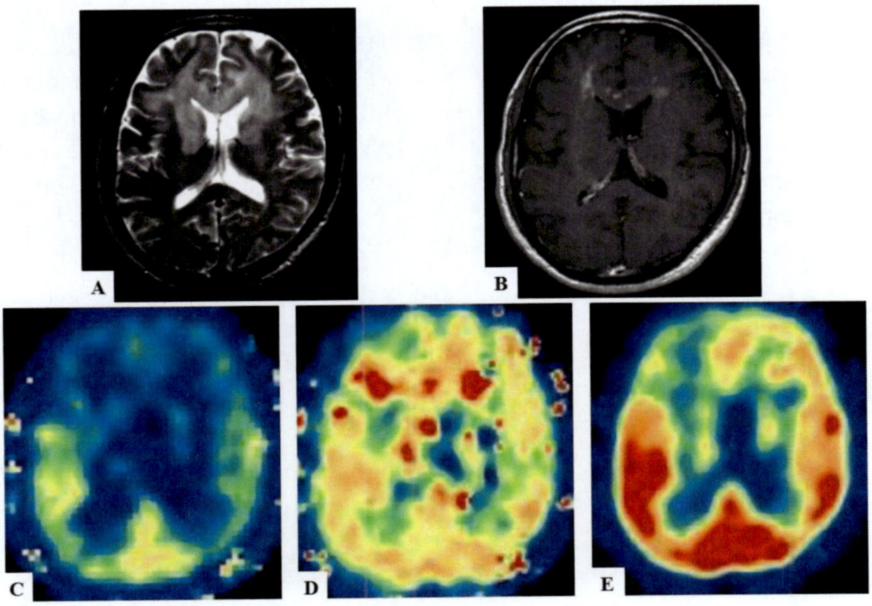

Figure 5. Representative MR image (upper) and ^{18}F-FDG-PET kinetic analysis (lower) in atypical PCNSL. T2-WI shows a high intensity lesion with edema in the corpus callosum (A). Contrast-enhanced T1-WI shows multiple small enhanced lesions (B). ^{18}F-FDG *Ki* images display an insignificant decrease in ^{18}F-FDG uptake in the lesions compared to the surrounding brain (E). Kinetic analysis of this scan shows decreased FDG transport (K_1) (C) and increased hexokinase activity (k_3) in the lesions (D).

PCNSL is a non-Hodgkin's lymphoma restricted to the CNS by definition. Standard staging for PCNSL needs to examine contrast enhanced CT of the chest, abdomen and pelvis, and sometimes bone marrow biopsy to exclude systemic lymphoma [1]. Conventional body staging in patients initially diagnosed with PCNSL showed an occult systemic lymphoma in about 4% of the patients [31]. The clinical significance of identifying systemic disease is uncertain, but at least 5% of PCNSL relapse outside the CNS [13]. [^{18}F]FDG PET may be more sensitive than conventional body staging and may disclose higher rates of concomitant systemic disease at initial PCNSL diagnosis. Mohile et al. demonstrated that 7% of patients initially diagnosed PCNSL were found to have systemic lymphoma by staging [^{18}F]FDG whole body PET scan even when body CT scans and bone marrow biopsies were negative [26]. Detection of systemic lymphoma at the time of initial PCNSL diagnosis may play important roles regarding the origin of the disease and treatment strategies.

CONCLUSION

CT and MRI in patients with PCNSL show single or multiple uniformly well-enhancing lesions that are usually located in the periventricular lesions. However, these radiological findings cannot accurately differentiate PCNSL from other tumorous and nontumorous brain lesions. The application of [^{18}F]FDG PET is currently increasing in clinical neurooncology. [^{18}F]FDG PET is very useful for the diagnosis of typical PCNSL, usually showing high uptake of [^{18}F]FDG in the tumor. The uptake value is approximately 2.5 times higher than that in the normal gray matter, and the tumors can visually be identified in the brain. The [^{18}F] FDG uptake pattern and value provide useful information to differentiate PCNSL from other enhancing malignant brain tumors, especially glioblastoma. However, the usefulness of [^{18}F] FDG PET is limited in the diagnosis of PCNSL with atypical radiological findings. In the modern metabolic imaging era, [^{18}F]FDG is useful when differential diagnoses of brain tumors are difficult. As [^{18}F]FDG PET is not a perfect tool, differential diagnoses are required for PCNSL; therefore, early tumor biopsy is still necessary, especially with atypical radiological findings.

Conflicts of interest disclosure: The authors have no personal, financial, or institutional interest. All authors are members of the Japan Neurosurgical Society (JNS), and have registered online Self-reported COI Disclosure Statements forms through website for JNS members.

REFERENCES

[1] Abrey, L. E., Batchelor, T. T., Ferreri, A. J., Gospodarowicz, M., Pulczynski, E. J., Zucca, E., Korfel, A., Soussain, C., DeAngelis, L. M., Neuwelt, E. A., O'Neill, B. P., Thiel, E., Shenkier, T., Graus, F., van den Bent, M., Seymour, J. F., Poortmans, P., Armitage, J. O., Cavalli, F. International Primary, C. N. S. L. C. G. (2005). Report of

an international workshop to standardize baseline evaluation and response criteria for primary CNS lymphoma. J Clin Oncol, 23, 5034-5043.

[2] Abrey, L. E., Ben-Porat, L., Panageas, K. S., Yahalom, J., Berkey, B., Curran, W., Schultz, C., Leibel, S., Nelson, D., Mehta, M., DeAngelis, L. M. (2006). Primary central nervous system lymphoma: the Memorial Sloan-Kettering Cancer Center prognostic model. J Clin Oncol, 24, 5711-5715.

[3] Aronen, H. J., Gazit, I. E., Louis, D. N., Buchbinder, B. R., Pardo, F. S., Weisskoff, R. M., Harsh, G. R., Cosgrove, G. R., Halpern, E. F., Hochberg, F. H. (1994). Cerebral blood volume maps of gliomas: comparison with tumor grade and histologic findings. Radiology, 191, 41-51.

[4] Bataille, B., Delwail, V., Menet, E., Vandermarcq, P., Ingrand, P., Wager, M., Guy, G., Lapierre, F. (2000). Primary intracerebral malignant lymphoma: report of 248 cases. J Neurosurg, 92, 261-266.

[5] Dethy, S., Goldman, S., Blecic, S., Luxen, A., Levivier, M., Hildebrand, J. (1994). Carbon-11-methionine and fluorine-18-FDG PET study in brain hematoma. J Nucl Med, 35, 1162-1166.

[6] Erdag, N., Bhorade, R. M., Alberico, R. A., Yousuf, N., Patel, M. R. (2001). Primary lymphoma of the central nervous system: typical and atypical CT and MR imaging appearances. AJR Am J Roentgenol, 176, 1319-1326.

[7] Guo, A. C., Cummings, T. J., Dash, R. C., Provenzale, J. M. (2002). Lymphomas and high-grade astrocytomas: comparison of water diffusibility and histologic characteristics. Radiology, 224, 177-183.

[8] Haldorsen, I. S., Krakenes, J., Krossnes, B. K., Mella, O., Espeland, A. (2009). CT and MR imaging features of primary central nervous system lymphoma in Norway, 1989-2003. AJNR Am J Neuroradiol, 30, 744-751.

[9] Haldorsen, I. S., Espeland, A., Larsson, E. M. (2011). Central nervous system lymphoma: characteristic findings on traditional and advanced imaging. AJNR Am J Neuroradiol, 32, 984-992.

[10] Harting, I., Hartmann, M., Jost, G., Sommer, C., Ahmadi, R., Heiland, S., Sartor, K. (2003). Differentiating primary central nervous system lymphoma from glioma in humans using localised proton magnetic resonance spectroscopy. Neurosci Lett, 342, 163-166.

[11] Hoffman, J. M., Waskin, H. A., Schifter, T., Hanson, M. W., Gray, L., Rosenfeld, S., Coleman, R. E. (1993). FDG-PET in differentiating lymphoma from nonmalignant central nervous system lesions in patients with AIDS. J Nucl Med, 34, 567-575.

[12] Hustinx, R., Smith, R. J., Benard, F., Bhatnagar, A., Alavi, A. (1999). Can the standardized uptake value characterize primary brain tumors on FDG-PET? Eur J Nucl Med, 26, 1501-1509.

[13] Jahnke, K., Thiel, E., Martus, P., Herrlinger, U., Weller, M., Fischer, L., Korfel, A., German Primary Central Nervous System Lymphoma Study, G. (2006). Relapse of primary central nervous system lymphoma: clinical features, outcome and prognostic factors. J Neurooncol, 80, 159-165.

[14] Kadan-Lottick, N. S., Skluzacek, M. C., Gurney, J. G. (2002). Decreasing incidence rates of primary central nervous system lymphoma. Cancer, 95, 193-202.

[15] Kawai, N., Nishiyama, Y., Miyake, K., Tamiya, T., Nagao, S. (2005). Evaluation of tumor FDG transport and metabolism in primary central nervous system lymphoma

using [18F] fluorodeoxyglucose (FDG) positron emission tomography (PET) kinetic analysis. Ann Nucl Med, 19, 685-690.

[16] Kawai, N., Okubo, S., Miyake, K., Maeda, Y., Yamamoto, Y., Nishiyama, Y., Tamiya, T. (2010). Use of PET in the diagnosis of primary CNS lymphoma in patients with atypical MR findings. Annals of Nuclear Medicine, 24, 335-343.

[17] Kawai, N., Zhen, H. N., Miyake, K., Yamamaoto, Y., Nishiyama, Y., Tamiya, T. (2010). Prognostic value of pretreatment 18F-FDG PET in patients with primary central nervous system lymphoma: SUV-based assessment. J Neurooncol, 100, 225-232.

[18] Kawai, N., Okada, M., Haba, R., Yamamoto, Y., Tamiya, T. (2012). Insufficiency of Positron Emission Tomography and Magnetic Resonance Spectroscopy in the Diagnosis of Intravascular Lymphoma of the Central Nervous System. Case Reports in Oncology, 5, 339-346.

[19] Kawase, Y., Yamamoto, Y., Kameyama, R., Kawai, N., Kudomi, N., Nishiyama, Y. (2011). Comparison of 11C-methionine PET and 18F-FDG PET in patients with primary central nervous system lymphoma. Mol Imaging Biol, 13, 1284-1289.

[20] Kosaka, N., Tsuchida, T., Uematsu, H., Kimura, H., Okazawa, H., Itoh, H. (2008). 18F-FDG PET of common enhancing malignant brain tumors. AJR Am J Roentgenol, 190, W365-369.

[21] Kubota, R., Yamada, S., Kubota, K., Ishiwata, K., Tamahashi, N., Ido, T. (1992). Intratumoral distribution of fluorine-18-fluorodeoxyglucose in vivo: high accumulation in macrophages and granulation tissues studied by microautoradiography. J Nucl Med, 33, 1972-1980.

[22] Kuker, W., Nagele, T., Korfel, A., Heckl, S., Thiel, E., Bamberg, M., Weller, M., Herrlinger, U. (2005). Primary central nervous system lymphomas (PCNSL): MRI features at presentation in 100 patients. J Neurooncol, 72, 169-177.

[23] Makino, K., Hirai, T., Nakamura, H., Murakami, R., Kitajima, M., Shigematsu, Y., Nakashima, R., Shiraishi, S., Uetani, H., Iwashita, K., Akter, M., Yamashita, Y., Kuratsu, J. (2011). Does adding FDG-PET to MRI improve the differentiation between primary cerebral lymphoma and glioblastoma? Observer performance study. Ann Nucl Med, 25, 432-438.

[24] Mangla, R., Kolar, B., Zhu, T., Zhong, J., Almast, J., Ekholm, S. (2011). Percentage signal recovery derived from MR dynamic susceptibility contrast imaging is useful to differentiate common enhancing malignant lesions of the brain. AJNR Am J Neuroradiol, 32, 1004-1010.

[25] Meshkini, A., Shahzadi, S., Zali, A., Tajeddini, A., Mirzayan, J., Hamdi, A. (2012). Systemic juvenile xanthogranuloma with multiple central nervous system lesions. J Cancer Res Ther, 8, 311-313.

[26] Mohile, N. A., Deangelis, L. M., Abrey, L. E. (2008). The utility of body FDG PET in staging primary central nervous system lymphoma. Neuro Oncol, 10, 223-228.

[27] Neska-Matuszewska, M., Zimny, A., Kalwak, K., Sasiadek, M. J. (2015). Central nervous system lymphoma in a 3-year-old male suffering from a severe juvenile xanthogranuloma - the usefulness of perfusion weighted imaging and diffusion weighted imaging in the diagnostics of pediatric brain tumors. Pol J Radiol, 80, 31-35.

[28] Nishiyama, Y., Yamamoto, Y., Monden, T., Sasakawa, Y., Kawai, N., Satoh, K., Ohkawa, M. (2007). Diagnostic value of kinetic analysis using dynamic FDG PET in

immunocompetent patients with primary CNS lymphoma. Eur J Nucl Med Mol Imaging, 34, 78-86.

[29] O'Brien, P. C., Roos, D. E., Pratt, G., Liew, K. H., Barton, M. B., Poulsen, M. G., Olver, I. N., Trotter, G. E., Trans-Tasman Radiation Oncology, G. (2006). Combined-modality therapy for primary central nervous system lymphoma: long-term data from a Phase II multicenter study (Trans-Tasman Radiation Oncology Group). Int J Radiat Oncol Biol Phys, 64, 408-413.

[30] O'Doherty, M. J., Barrington, S. F., Campbell, M., Lowe, J., Bradbeer, C. S. (1997). PET scanning and the human immunodeficiency virus-positive patient. J Nucl Med, 38, 1575-1583.

[31] O'Neill, B. P., Dinapoli, R. P., Kurtin, P. J., Habermann, T. M. (1995). Occult systemic non-Hodgkin's lymphoma (NHL) in patients initially diagnosed as primary central nervous system lymphoma (PCNSL): how much staging is enough? J Neurooncol, 25, 67-71.

[32] Olson, J. E., Janney, C. A., Rao, R. D., Cerhan, J. R., Kurtin, P. J., Schiff, D., Kaplan, R. S., O'Neill, B. P. (2002). The continuing increase in the incidence of primary central nervous system non-Hodgkin lymphoma: a surveillance, epidemiology, and end results analysis. Cancer, 95, 1504-1510.

[33] Palmedo, H., Urbach, H., Bender, H., Schlegel, U., Schmidt-Wolf, I. G., Matthies, A., Linnebank, M., Joe, A., Bucerius, J., Biersack, H. J., Pels, H. (2006). FDG-PET in immunocompetent patients with primary central nervous system lymphoma: correlation with MRI and clinical follow-up. Eur J Nucl Med Mol Imaging, 33, 164-168.

[34] Phelps, M. E., Huang, S. C., Hoffman, E. J., Selin, C., Sokoloff, L., Kuhl, D. E. (1979). Tomographic measurement of local cerebral glucose metabolic rate in humans with (F-18)2-fluoro-2-deoxy-D-glucose: validation of method. Ann Neurol, 6, 371-388.

[35] Plowman, P. N., Saunders, C. A., Maisey, M. N. (1998). Gliomatosis cerebri: disconnection of the cortical grey matter, demonstrated on PET scan. Br J Neurosurg, 12, 240-244.

[36] Ricard, D., Idbaih, A., Ducray, F., Lahutte, M., Hoang-Xuan, K., Delattre, J. Y. (2012). Primary brain tumours in adults. Lancet, 379, 1984-1996.

[37] Rosen, B. R., Belliveau, J. W., Vevea, J. M., Brady, T. J. (1990). Perfusion imaging with NMR contrast agents. Magn Reson Med, 14, 249-265.

[38] Rosenfeld, S. S., Hoffman, J. M., Coleman, R. E., Glantz, M. J., Hanson, M. W., Schold, S. C. (1992). Studies of primary central nervous system lymphoma with fluorine-18-fluorodeoxyglucose positron emission tomography. J Nucl Med, 33, 532-536.

[39] Schiepers, C., Van Hecke, P., Vandenberghe, R., Van Oostende, S., Dupont, P., Demaerel, P., Bormans, G., Carton, H. (1997). Positron emission tomography, magnetic resonance imaging and proton NMR spectroscopy of white matter in multiple sclerosis. Mult Scler, 3, 8-17.

[40] Sierra del Rio, M., Rousseau, A., Soussain, C., Ricard, D., Hoang-Xuan, K. (2009). Primary CNS lymphoma in immunocompetent patients. Oncologist, 14 526-539.

[41] Taillibert, S., Guillevin, R., Menuel, C., Sanson, M., Hoang-Xuan, K., Chiras, J., Duffau, H. (2008). Brain lymphoma: usefulness of the magnetic resonance spectroscopy. J Neurooncol, 86, 225-229.

[42] Tang, Y. Z., Booth, T. C., Bhogal, P., Malhotra, A., Wilhelm, T. (2011). Imaging of primary central nervous system lymphoma. Clin Radiol, 66, 768-777.

[43] Tsuyuguchi, N., Sunada, I., Ohata, K., Takami, T., Nishio, A., Hara, M., Kawabe, J., Okamura, T., Ochi, H. (2003). Evaluation of treatment effects in brain abscess with positron emission tomography: comparison of fluorine-18-fluorodeoxyglucose and carbon-11-methionine. Ann Nucl Med, 17, 47-51.

[44] Villringer, K., Jager, H., Dichgans, M., Ziegler, S., Poppinger, J., Herz, M., Kruschke, C., Minoshima, S., Pfister, H. W., Schwaiger, M. (1995). Differential diagnosis of CNS lesions in AIDS patients by FDG-PET. J Comput Assist Tomogr, 19, 532-536.

[45] Zimny, A., Sasiadek, M. (2011). Contribution of perfusion-weighted magnetic resonance imaging in the differentiation of meningiomas and other extra-axial tumors: case reports and literature review. J Neurooncol, 103, 777-783.

In: Primary Central Nervous System Lymphoma (PCNSL)
Editor: Ryuya Yamanaka
ISBN: 978-1-63485-322-4

Chapter 6

Cerebrospinal Fluid Interleukin-10 (IL-10) as a Diagnostic Marker in Primary Central Nervous System Lymphoma

Takashi Sasayama[1,*], Kazuhiro Tanaka[1], Katsu Mizukawa[1], Masamitsu Nishihara[2] and Eiji Kohmura[1]

[1]Department of Neurosurgery, Kobe University Graduate School of Medicine, Kobe, Japan

[2]Department of Neurosurgery, Nishikobe Medical Center, Kobe, Japan

Abstract

The diagnosis of primary central nervous system lymphoma (PCNSL) is commonly obtained via a stereotactic biopsy. However, PCNSL lesions are frequently located deep within the brain, and performing a stereotactic biopsy is not always feasible. The use of radiographic images (CT, MRI, and PET) frequently fails to distinguish PCNSLs from other brain tumors and inflammatory diseases. Although flow-cytometry based and cytological analyses of cerebrospinal fluid (CSF) are useful for the evaluation of leptomeningeal PCNSLs, these tests are usually insensitive to focal PCNSLs. A biomarker for the early diagnosis of PCNSL could permit early treatment and could attenuate disease progression and neurological deterioration. However, there is currently no useful diagnostic biomarker for PCNSL.

In this study, we examined whether the CSF levels of interleukin-10 (IL-10), IL-6, soluble IL-2 receptor (sIL-2R), and beta-2 microglobulin (β2-Mg) can be used to distinguish PCNSL from other focal brain lesions that were radiographically similar to PCNSLs. In case-control study, we analyzed 66 patients with focal brain lesions (PCNSLs: 26 cases; other brain tumors: 40 cases). The CSF IL-10, sIL-2R and β2-Mg levels were significantly higher in PCNSLs than in the other brain tumors. Our results indicated that the CSF IL-10 levels had the highest sensitivity and specificity. Next, we prospectively examined 108 patients with suspected brain PCNSL to validate the

* Corresponding author: Takashi Sasayama. Department of Neurosurgery, Kobe University Graduate School of Medicine, 7-5-1, Kusunoki-cho, Chuo-ku, Kobe, 650-0017 Japan.Tel.: (81) 78-382-5966, fax: (81) 78-382-5979, email: takasasa@med.kobe-u.ac.jp.

diagnostic value of CSF IL-10 in PCNSL patients. The patient cohort included 38 PCNSLs and 70 other brain diseases, including primary and metastatic brain tumors and inflammatory diseases. The CSF levels of IL-10, sIL-2R, and β2-Mg were significantly higher in the patients with PCNSLs than in patients with other focal brain lesions ($p < 0.0001$, $p = 0.006$, and $p < 0.0001$, respectively). The receiver-operator characteristic (ROC) curves showed that the discrimination power of CSF IL-10 and β2-Mg were significantly higher than sIL-2R (Areas under the curves (AUC): 0.996, 0.971, 0.837, respectively).

IL-10 and IL-10 receptor proteins are expressed in most lymphoma cells. However, tumor-associated macrophages (TAMs) that diffusely infiltrate PCNSLs also produce IL-10 and TAM infiltration levels are correlated with CSF IL-10 levels. Furthermore, PCNSL cells highly express the IL-10 receptor and high CSF IL-10 activates the JAK-STAT pathway in PCNSL cells. Our survival analysis revealed that elevated CSF IL-10 levels were associated with poorer prognosis. Our results and other recent studies indicate that IL-10 CSF levels are a useful diagnostic biomarker for patients with PCNSLs. In addition, CSF IL-10 levels may be a prognostic marker for PCNSLs.

Keywords: cerebrospinal fluid, interleukin-10, primary CNS lymphoma, biomarker

INTRODUCTION

Primary central nervous system lymphoma (PCNSL) is an aggressive extra-nodal non-Hodgkin lymphoma (NHL) that involves the brain, spinal cord, and eyes. PCNSL occurs in both immunocompetent and immunocompromised patients and is found in approximately 4% of all brain tumors [1]. The incidence of PCNSLs has increased over the past 3 decades, especially in immunocompetent patients [2]. Treatments using high-dose methotrexate have produced acceptable responses in PCNSL patients, and combined modality therapy has led to response rates of 80 to 90% and a median overall survival of up to 4 years. However, PCNSL has a worse prognosis than other extranodal NHLs [1].

PCNSL is currently diagnosed by performing a histological examination of a brain biopsy specimen. The preoperative diagnosis is often suggested by its radiographic appearance [3]. There are multiple lesions observed in approximately 30% of patients. These lesions frequently occur within the cerebral white matter near the corpus callosum, in the basal ganglia and thalamus, and in the cerebellum. MRI is a sensitive method of detecting PCNSLs. The tumors are highly cellular and have decreased water content due their high nucleus-to-cytoplasm ratio in cells. Therefore, the T2 images show shortening and have a relatively low signal intensity [3]. Diffusion-weighted imaging has also been helpful in distinguishing these masses from other lesions [3]. However, PCNSLs may be associated with a variety of radiological presentations and can simulate other brain diseases, such as glioblastoma, metastatic brain tumors, and multiple sclerosis. Thus, the preoperative diagnosis of PCNSL by radiographic appearance alone may be misleading.

Cerebrospinal fluid (CSF) has various functions, such as protecting the brain, transporting biological substances, and excreting toxins and waste substances. CSF directly contacts the extracellular fluid of the brain. Although the CSF composition reflects the blood plasma, active transport from the blood and secretions from the brain contribute to the CSF composition. Therefore, the CSF composition can indicate biological brain processes, and CSF analysis is indispensable for diagnosing and understanding central nervous system

(CNS) disorders [4, 5]. Thus, chemical examination of CSF is an important tool for the diagnosis of several types of brain tumors [6, 7]. For example, high CSF concentrations of β-human chorionic gonadotropin or a-fetoprotein in conjunction with concordant features on brain MRI are used to diagnose CNS germ cell tumors and can eliminate the need for craniotomy [8].

Several proteins in the CSF are reported to aid in the diagnosis of PCNSL. Jeffery et al. found that the CSF β2-microglobulin (β2-Mg) level is a useful adjunct to the cytological diagnosis of CNS lymphoma [9]. In addition, Kersten et al. reported that soluble CD27 levels in the CSF are elevated in patients with meningeal lymphoid malignancies involving PCNSLs [10]. Moreover, the soluble IL-2 receptor (sIL-2R) in CSF is a valuable marker of CNS involvement in patients with NHL or acute lymphocytic leukemia [11, 12]. Roy et al. proposed that an elevated CSF level of antithrombin III was associated with the presence of CNS lymphoma [13].

IL-10 has broad anti-inflammatory properties because it suppresses both macrophage and dendritic cell function [14, 15]. Conversely, IL-6 is a potent lymphoid growth and differentiation cytokine that is produced by various cell types, such as benign and malignant B and T lymphocytes, monocytes, macrophages, fibroblasts, and hepatocytes [16, 17]. Previous studies demonstrated that the serum IL-6 and IL-10 levels were high in patients with aggressive systemic NHL [18, 19]. Serum IL-10 levels are also elevated in approximately half of patients with HL and the levels are strongly correlated with prognosis independent of other factors [20]. In addition, high IL-10 levels were found in the vitreous fluid of most patients with primary intraocular lymphoma [21]. Thus, IL-10 levels may further confirm the diagnosis of primary intraocular lymphoma [21, 22].

The presence of high IL-10 CSF levels in patients with PCNSL was first reported by Whitcup in 1997 [23]. The authors found that elevated IL-10 levels in CSF were associated with the presentation of malignant cells in CSF [23]. Salmaggi et al. subsequently analyzed the CSF levels of IL-10 in various brain tumors, including PCNSLs [24]. The CSF IL-10 level in PCNSL (mean, 14.8 + 23 pg/mL) was significantly higher than in other CNS tumors (mean, 0.23 + 0.26 pg/mL). However, a limited number of patients were analyzed in their study. In 2012, we reported that the IL-10 levels in CSF are potentially useful biomarker in immunocompetent PCNSL patients [7] In this study, we re-evaluated the diagnostic value of the IL-10, IL-6, sIL-2R, and β2-Mg levels in the CSF samples from patients with PCNSL and other brain diseases in a larger patient cohort.

IL-10 Is a Useful Diagnostic Marker for PCNSL

1. Case-Control Study

The IL-10, IL-6, β2-Mg, and sIL-2R concentrations in CSF were measured in 66 patients with brain lesions [7]. There were 26 patients with PCNSLs (20 cases of DLBCL, 3 cases of intraocular lymphomas, 2 cases of T-cell lymphoma, and 1 case of unclassified lymphoma). The remaining 40 patients had other brain diseases. The pathologies of the patients are summarized in Table 1. The CSF IL-10 levels were undetectable in five PCNSL patients and all patients with other brain diseases. There were two PCNSL patients who had received steroid therapy before CSF examination and had undetectable levels of CSF IL-10. In addition, all of the patients with T cell lymphoma had undetectable levels of CSF IL-10. The median CSF levels of IL-10, IL-6, β2-Mg, and sIL-2R were 27 pg/mL (range, <2 to 1610 pg/ml), 5.4 pg/ml (range, 1.2–264 pg/ml), 4084 mg/l (range, 970–11239 mg/L), and 100 U/ml (range, <50 to 978 U/ml), respectively (Table 1). Conversely, the patients with other brain tumor types had median CSF levels of IL-10, IL-6, β2-Mg, and sIL-2R of <2.0 pg/ml, 2.7 pg/ml (range, 0.8–4780 pg/ml), 1200 mg/l (range, 172–2600 mg/L), and <50 U/mL (range, <50 to 87 U/mL), respectively. The median CSF levels of IL-10, β2-Mg, and sIL-2R were significantly higher in the patients with PCNSL than in other brain tumors ($P < .001$, $P < .001$, and $P < .001$, respectively; calculated using the Mann-Whitney U test).

Table 1. Pathology of the patients

Study	Pathology	Number of patients
Case-control study (January 2004 ~ November 2010)	PCNSL	26
	Diffuse large B-cell lymphoma (DLBCL)	20
	Intraocular lymphoma	3
	T-cell lymphoma	2
	unclassified	1
	Other brain tumor	40
	Glioblastoma,	16
	Grade III glioma	6
	Low-grade glioma	4
	Brain stem glioma	1
	Ependymoma	2
	Germ cell tumor	4
	Metastatic tumor	7
Validation study (December 2010 ~ June 2015)	PCNSL	38
	Diffuse large B-cell lymphoma (DLBCL)	37
	Intraocular lymphoma	1
	Other brain lesions	70
	Glioblastoma	29
	Grade III glioma	7
	Low-grade glioma	9
	Germ cell tumor	3
	Metastatic tumor	8
	Multiple sclerosis	5
	Encephalitis	3
	Meningioma	1
	Cavernous angioma	1
	Cerebral infarction	1
	Chordoma	1
	Cystic lesion	1
	Meningitis	1

2. Validation Study

We performed a prospective study to validate the results of case-control study. One hundred eight patients, who were suspected as PCNSL in MRI study, were enrolled in this study. The pathology of the patients is summarized in Table 1. The patients treated with steroids prior to CSF examination were excluded because steroids may change the immunological microenvironment of the tumor. There were 41 patients with detectable CSF levels of IL-10 (≥2 pg/ml) and 67 patients had undetectable levels (<2 pg/ml). There were 38 patients with PCNSL and 3 patients with other brain lesions (glioma; 2, encephalitis; 1) in the population of patients with detectable IL-10. All patients with undetectable IL-10 were non-PCNSL cases. In patients with PCNSLs, the median CSF levels of IL-10, IL-6, β2-Mg, and sIL-2R were 63 pg/ml, 7.4 pg/ml, 4338 mg/l, and 160 U/ml, respectively. In the patients with other brain lesions, the median CSF levels of IL-10, IL-6, β2-Mg, and sIL-2R were <2.0 pg/ml, 3.5 pg/ml, 1231 mg/l, and <50 U/ml, respectively. The median CSF levels of IL-10, IL-6, β2-Mg, and sIL-2R were significantly higher in patients with PCNSLs than in patients with other brain lesions ($P < .001$, $P = .0023$, $P < .001$, and $P < .001$, respectively; calculated using the Mann-Whitney U test) (Figure 1A).

The ROC curves showed that the discrimination power of CSF IL-10 and β2-Mg were significantly higher than sIL-2R and IL-6. The areas under the curves (AUC) were 0.996, 0.971, 0.837, and 0.316 for IL-10, β2-Mg, sIL-2R, and IL-6, respectively (Figure 1B). Using an IL-10 cutoff level of 5.0 pg/ml, the sensitivity and specificity were 97% and 97%, respectively. Similarly, a cutoff of 2303 mg/l in β2-Mg yielded a specificity of 92% and a sensitivity of 97%. Furthermore, a cutoff of 56 U/mL for sIL-2R yielded a specificity of 91% and a sensitivity of 76%.

The preoperative CSF measurement of IL-10 was useful for clinical decision-making, especially for determining appropriate surgical planning. For example, a patient who had a right parietal lobe tumor and a quite low concentration of CSF IL-10 was treated by craniotomy and gross total tumor resection. The final tumor diagnosis was GBM. Conversely, a patient with a right parietal tumor who had high level of CSF IL-10 was treated by stereotactic biopsy. The final tumor diagnosis was PCNSL and post-operative chemo-radiotherapy was initiated.

CSF IL-10 as a Surrogate Marker for the PCNSL Tumor Status

The CSF levels of IL-10 were examined after completion of therapy in 34 patients. We found that all patients had significantly decreased IL-10 levels compared with the pretreatment levels. The CSF IL-10 levels decreased to undetectable levels (<2 pg/mL) in 26 patients (72%). At the time of CNS relapse the CSF IL-10 levels were elevated. There were high levels of IL-10 in 2 patients with a high CSF lymphoma cell burden. These patients were diagnosed with CSF dissemination. We used serial CSF IL-10 measurements to confirm the tumor status determined by neuroimaging in each of the patients with PCNSL. One example case is depicted in Figure 1C.

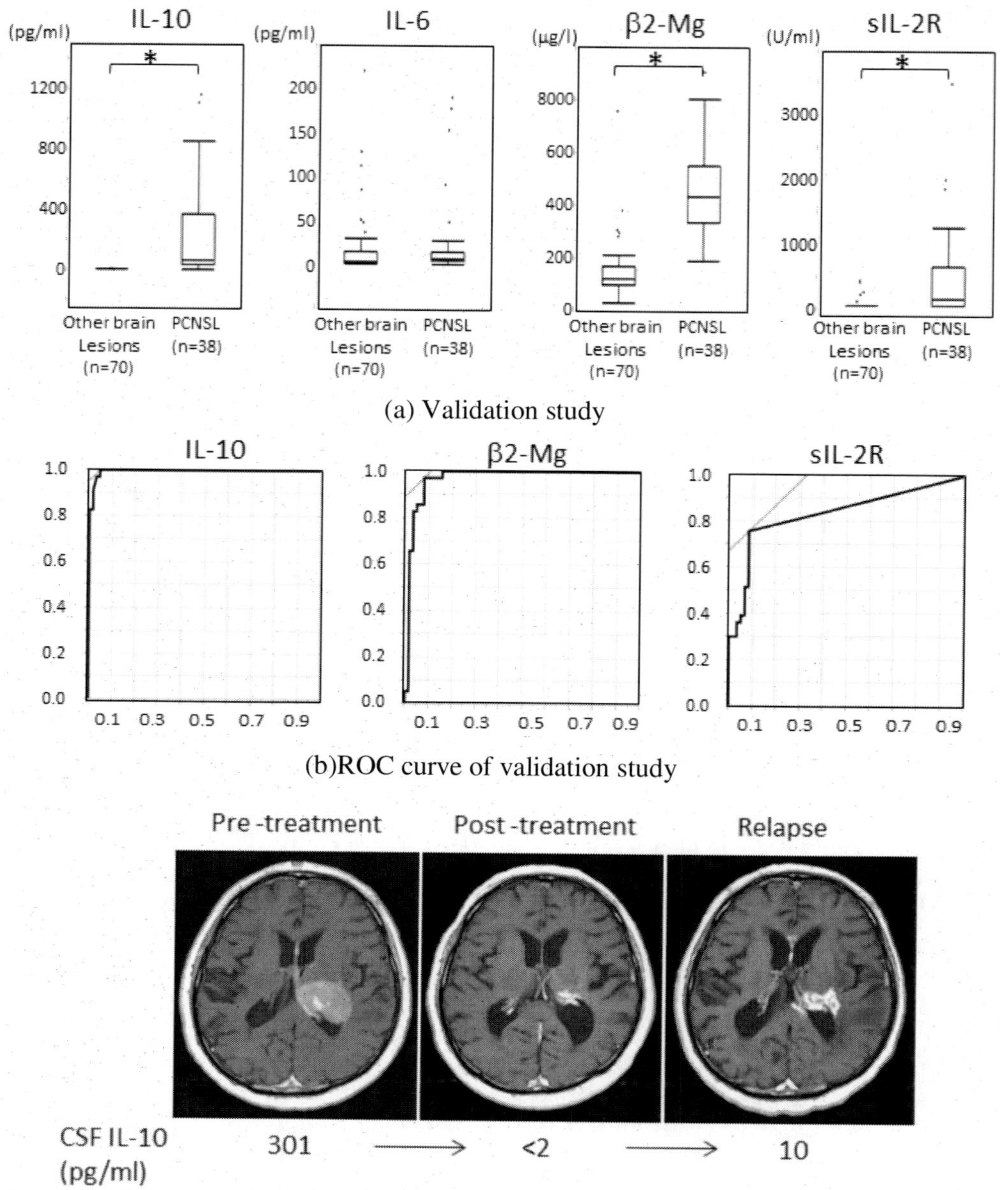

(a) Validation study

(b)ROC curve of validation study

(c) CSF IL-10 as a surrogate marker for the PCNSL tumor status

Figure 1. (A) Pretreatment CSF levels of IL-10, IL-6, β2-Mg, and sIL-2R in PCNSL and other brain lesions. The difference between PCNSL and other brain tumor types was statistically significant (* $P < .001$, Mann–Whitney U test). PCNSL; primary CNS lymphoma. (B) Receiver-operator characteristic (ROC) curves of the CSF IL-10, β2-Mg, and sIL-2R levels. AUC are 0.996, 0.971, and 0.837 for IL-10, β2-Mg, and sIL-2R, respectively. (C) The relationship between the state of the tumor and the CSF concentrations of IL-10. Pre-treatment. Pre-treatment brain MRI revealed enhanced lesions in the left thalamus and IL-10 concentration in CSF were 301 pg/ml. Post-treatment brain MRI revealed a tumor shrinkage and CSF IL-10 fell to <2 pg/ml. At the time of the relapse, the tumor appeared around the lateral ventricles and CSF IL-10 level increased at 10 pg/ml.

Expression and Secretion of IL-10 in PCNSLs

We performed immunohistochemical examinations to determine whether PCNSL tumor cells express IL-10 protein. The results showed that the majority of tumor cells were positive for IL-10 (Figure 2A). Patients with high levels of CSF IL-10 had a tendency to express high IL-10 levels in the tumor cells [7]. In addition, most of the tumor cells were positive for both IL-10RA and IL-10 (Figure 2A) [7]. To examine whether PCNSLs secrete IL-10, we cultured resected PCNSL tissues from 4 patients for 5 days. We then harvested the supernatant and examined the IL-10 levels. The supernatant of PCNSL cells had significantly higher levels of IL-10 (mean 87.3 pg/ml) than control medium (<2 pg/ml) (data not shown). These results indicate that IL-10 is produced and secreted from the PCNSL tissue and acts on the lymphoma cells in an autocrine or paracrine manner.

There are numerous macrophages present in PCNSL tissues, which are termed tumor-associated macrophages (TAMs) [25]. The role of TAMs has been controversial. However, several studies suggested that TAMs contribute to tumor progression, angiogenesis, invasion, and immunosuppression [26]. TAMs produce various cytokines, including IL-10. We found that CD68-positve(+) and CD163+ TAMs had highly infiltrated PCNSL tissue (Figure 2B) and that increased TAM infiltration was associated with high levels of CSF IL-10 (Figure 2C). In addition, we confirmed that TAMs in PCNSL tissue expressed IL-10 protein using double immunofluorescence staining (data not shown). Cumulatively, our results indicate IL-10 is secreted from infiltrated TAMs in PCNSLs and can stimulate the activity of lymphoma cells in a paracrine manner.

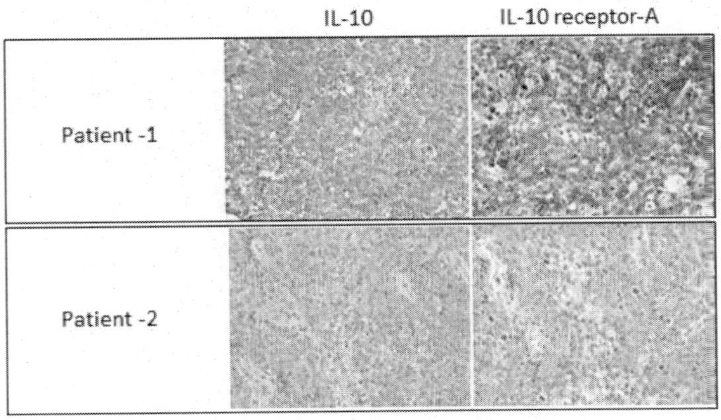

(a) IL-10 and IL-10 receptor-A-expression.

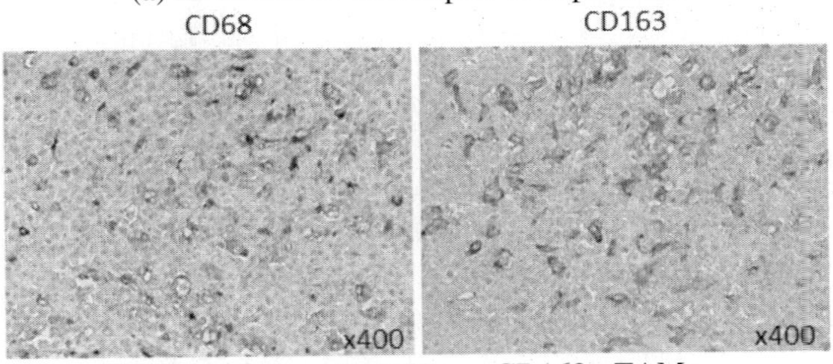

(b) Infiltration of CD68+ or CD163+ TAMs

Figure 2. (Continued)

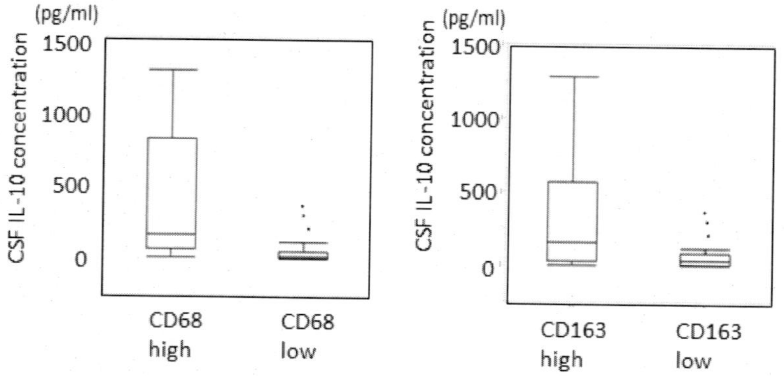

(c) Relationship between CSF IL-10 and TAMs

Figure 2. (A) Immunohistochemistry of IL-10, IL-10 receptor-A (IL-10RA) in 2 PCNSL specimens. IL-10 and IL-10RA are highly expressed in PCNSL specimens. (Original magnification; ×400). Reproduced and modified with permission from Sasayama et al. (2012). (B) Immunohistochemical staining for CD68 and CD163 in PCNSL specimens. (Original magnification; ×400). Reproduced and modified with permission from Sasayama et al. (2015). (C) Relationship between infiltration levels of CD68+ and CD163+ tumor-associated macrophages (TAMs) and CSF IL-10 concentration. High infiltration groups of CD68+ and CD163+ TAM have significantly higher CSF IL-10 concentration compared to low infiltration groups.

CSF IL-10 Activates STAT3 Signaling

IL-10 is known to activate the JAK-STAT signaling pathway via the IL-10 receptor [27]. Activated STAT proteins trigger the transcription of target genes involved in cell proliferation, survival, angiogenesis, and immunity [27]. Therefore, we analyzed the association between STAT3 activity and CSF IL-10 because STAT3 is most frequently activated in tumors. The results showed that the CSF IL-10 levels were statistically associated with STAT3 activation in PCNSLs in immunohistochemical and western blot analyses [28]. In addition, the CSF from PCNSL patients with high IL-10 concentrations could activate STAT3 signaling in PCNSL cells *in vitro* and the addition of a neutralizing anti-IL-10 antibody decreased the CSF-induced activation of STAT3 (Figure 3) [28]. Interestingly, higher levels of CSF IL-10 induced stronger activation of STAT3 (Figure 3). These data indicate that IL-10 in CSF is likely to activate STAT3 signaling in PCNSL.

Association of CSF IL-10 Levels with Prognosis

We previously reported an association of CSF IL-10 levels with the clinical outcome in PCNSL patients [7]. The CSF levels of IL-10 after therapy were not associated with the treatment response. We used a univariate analysis with Cox's proportional hazards model and the log-rank test to determine if elevated CSF levels of IL-10 were significantly associated with a shorter progression-free survival (PFS) (hazard ratio [HR], 3.37; 95% confidence interval [CI], 0.985–11.528; log-rank, $p = 0.038$). There was no statistically significant association identified between the CSF IL-10 levels and overall survival (OS). However, there were trends observed between elevated CSF IL-10 levels and shorter OS (HR, 3.58; 95% CI, 0.918–13.94; log-rank, $p = 0.05$).

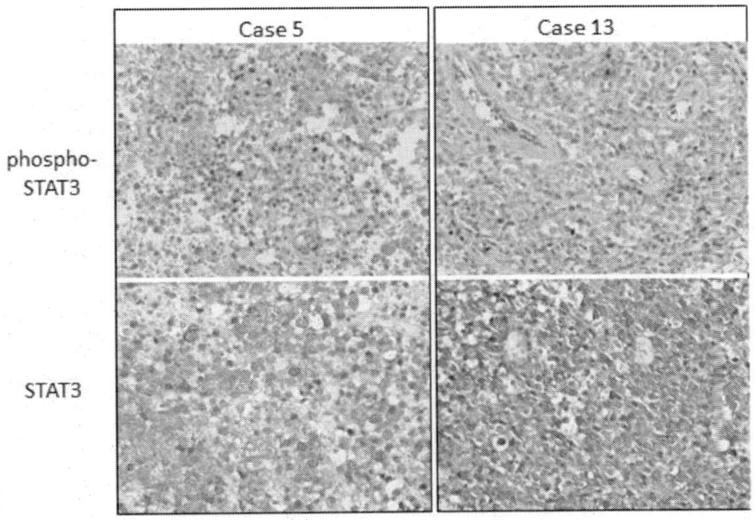

(a) STAT3 expression in PCNSLs

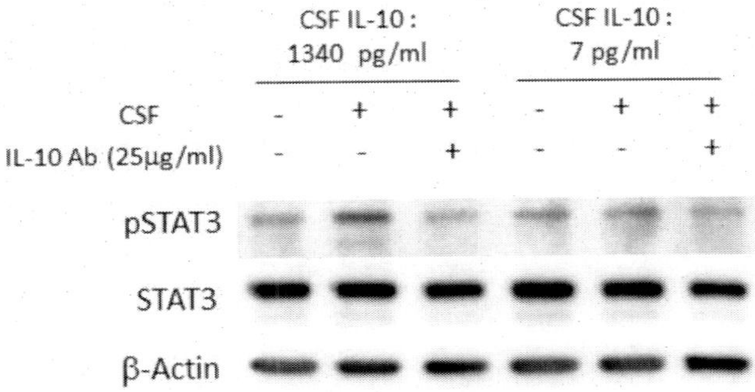

(b) STAT3 activation by CSF-IL-10

Figure 3. (A) Immunohistochemistry of phospho-STAT3 and STAT3 in 2 PCNSL cases with high CSF IL-10 concentrations. Majority of tumor cells express phospho-STAT3. (Original magnification: x200). Reproduced and modified with permission from Mizowaki et al. (2015). (B) Serum-starved lymphoma cells (HKBML) were treated with CSF from a patient containing 1340 pg/ml or 7 pg/ml of IL-10 with/without neutralizing IL-10 antibody (Ab), and the pSTAT3 expression was analyzed. Notably, CSF from a patient containing higher levels of IL-10 induced a higher expression of pSTAT3. Reproduced and modified with permission from Mizowaki et al. (2015).

We recently reported the association between CSF IL-10 levels and prognosis in patients with diffuse large B-cell lymphoma of the CNS [28]. The results of this study were similar, and increased CSF IL-10 was significantly associated with shorter PFS (HR, 2.78; 95% CI, 1.276–6.278; $p = 0.010$). Additionally, there was a trend towards shorter OS in patients with higher CSF IL-10 ($p = 0.08$). These results indicated that the CSF IL-10 levels may be a predictive marker of clinical outcome for PCNSL patients.

DISCUSSION

Diagnostic Biomarker for PCNSL

Several potential CSF diagnostic biomarkers for PCNSL have been reported. The CSF levels of the following biomarkers have been shown to be elevated in PCNSL: sCD27 [10, 29], sCD19 [30], β2-Mg [31], anti-thrombin III [13], free light chain immunoglobulins [32], a specific set of microRNAs [33, 34], IL-10 [7, 35] sIL2-R [7], CXCL13 [36, 37], and neopterin [38]. The CSF levels of sCD27, sCD19, β 2-Mg, IL-10, CXCL13, and neopterin are higher in PCNSL patients than in patients with other types of brain tumors. Although their routine use in clinical practice of lymphoma diagnosis still remains to be established, IL-10 and/or CXCL13 may be the most promising biomarkers.

Kersten et al. reported that the sCD27 levels in the CSF are increased in patients with meningeal spreading of lymphoid malignancies involving PCNSL [10]. The authors revealed a remarkable sensitivity of 100% and specificity of 82% for sCD27 in acute lymphoblastic leukemia and NHLs. However, van den Bent et al. showed there was a low positive predictive value of sCD27 for leptomeningeal involvement in B-cell malignancies. The authors stated that sCD27 was increased in a variety of other predominantly inflammatory neurological disorders, including herpes simplex and zoster infections.

Muniz et al. analyzed the CSF levels of various B-cell–associated markers in 40 B-NHL patients at risk for CNS disease. The authors concluded that higher sCD19 levels in CSF were associated with parenchymal CNS lymphoma in DLBCL. They stated that the utility of the combined FCM detection of lymphoma cells and sCD19 levels in CSF led to a more accurate identification of CNS lymphoma.

Fischer et al. reported that CXCL13 in CSF was a biomarker for CNS lymphoma [39]. CXCL13 is a small cytokine that is selectively chemotactic for B lymphocytes. The authors evaluated CXCL13 concentrations in the CSF of 30 patients with CNS lymphoma, 40 patients with other brain tumors, and 30 patients without malignancy or inflammatory disease. The results show that the CXCL13 levels were significantly increased in patients with CNS lymphoma and were correlated with a response to chemotherapy.

Viaccoz et al. examined the neopterin concentration in the CSF of 124 patients with brain tumors or inflammatory CNS disease. The results showed that the CSF neopterin levels were significantly higher in PCNSL patients than in patients with other brain tumors, pseudotumoral inflammatory brain lesions, and non-tumefactive inflammatory CNS disorders.

Whitcup first reported high levels of IL-10 in the CSF of PCNSL patients in 1997 [23]. The study showed that an IL-10/IL-6 ratio greater than 1 is associated with CNS lymphoma. Subsequently, Salmaggi et al. described that the CSF IL-10 levels in PCNSLs was significantly higher than in other CNS tumors (14.8 ± 23 vs. 0.23 ± 0.26 pg/ml). In 2012, we reported that the CSF IL-10 level is a potentially useful biomarker in immunocompetent PCNSL [7]. We measured the concentration in CSF IL-10 in 26 PCNSL patients and 40 patients with other brain tumors. Our findings showed the sensitivity was 71% and the specificity was 100% at the cut-off value of 9.5 pg/ml [7]. More recently, a study by Sasagawa et al. analyzed the CSF IL-10 concentration in 19 PCNSL patients and 26 non-PCNSL patients. The authors concluded that CSF IL-10 is a useful biomarker for the initial screening of patients with CNS lymphoma [35]. Hashiguchi et al. reported that CSF IL-10 is a possible biomarker for lymphomatosis cerebri [40].

The elevation of both CXCL13 and IL-10 was shown to be highly specific for PCNSL diagnosis. Rubenstein et al. conducted a multicenter study containing 220 patients with various CNS diseases. They showed that bivariate elevated CXCL13 plus IL-10 was 99.3% specific for primary and secondary CNS lymphoma and had significantly greater sensitivity than reference standard CSF tests.

In our prospective study, we examined CSF IL-10 in 38 PCNSL patients and 70 patients with other CNS diseases. The results demonstrated that at an IL-10 cutoff level of 5.0 pg/ml had a sensitivity and specificity of 97.0% and 97%, respectively. It is important to note that patients receiving corticosteroid therapy before CSF examination were excluded because corticosteroids affect cytokine production in lymphoma cells and in other infiltrating immune cells. Although the CSF level of IL-10 is a useful diagnostic marker for patients with PCNSL, it might be improved by combining the analysis of CSF IL-10 with other CSF biomarkers or neuroimaging techniques, such as MR spectroscopy or Positron Emission Tomography.

CSF IL-10 and STAT3

Recent studies have identified STAT3 as an important molecule that mediates tumor-induced immunosuppression [41]. STAT3 is a potent negative regulator of T helper 1 (Th1)-cell-mediated inflammation and is an important activator of many genes that are crucial for immunosuppression [41, 42]. IL-10 acts as an immunosuppressive cytokine. Thus, STAT3 is strongly associated with IL-10. There are many reports investigating the expression of STAT3 in cancer [43]. However, there are a limited number of studies examining PCNSLs. Komohara et al. demonstrated that the majority of PCNSLs expressed pSTAT3 and that the phosphorylation levels of STAT3 were significantly higher in patients with a high infiltration of CD163-positive tumor associated macrophages [25]. Interestingly, in vitro co-culture experiments investigating cell-cell interactions between macrophages and lymphoma cells found that Stat3 in lymphoma cells was strongly activated by co-culture with macrophages [25]. In our study, most of the lymphoma cells were positive for STAT3 activation. Additionally, we found that increased active STAT3 was significantly positively correlated with higher CSF IL-10 levels. Rubenstein et al. also reported that the IL-10 concentration in CSF was associated with JAK-1 activation. JAK-1 is downstream of the IL-10 receptor and activates STAT3. We demonstrated that the CSF from PCNSL patients activates STAT3 in lymphoma cells in vitro. These results indicate that the JAK-STAT3 signaling pathway in PCNSL tumor cells is activated by the CSF IL-10 produced in both lymphoma cells and infiltrated macrophages.

CSF IL-10 and Prognosis

Several reports have shown that elevated IL-10 plasma levels are correlated with poor prognosis in systemic DLBCL [19, 44, 45]. Gupta et al. analyzed the survival of untreated systemic DLBCL patients in the North Center Cancer Treatment Group Trial ND489 by pretreatment serum IL-10 levels. The results showed that the patients with high serum IL-10 had shorter event-free survival than patients with low levels [44]. Based on these results, Nacinović-Duletić and coworkers proposed that evaluating serum IL-10 levels before treatment of systemic DLBCL patients may provide insight into the prognosis and facilitate decision-making regarding therapeutic approaches for individual patients [19]. In addition to DLBCL, high levels of serum IL-10 were reported to be an unfavorable prognostic factor for patients with Hodgkin's lymphoma [20] and adult T-cell leukemia/lymphoma (ATLL) [46]. We previously reported that there was a significant correlation between the clinical outcome and the CSF level of IL-10 in PCNSL patients [7, 28]. Rubinstein et al. also showed that patients with non-HIV–associated PCNSL and SCNSL with elevated CSF concentrations of IL-10 at diagnosis exhibited a significantly shorter time to progression (TTP) compared to patients with low CSF IL-10 [37]. However, larger prospective studies are necessary because these studies evaluated relatively small patient cohorts and were retrospective.

CONCLUSION

The CSF IL-10 concentration is a useful diagnostic marker for PCNSL patients. In our prospective study, we found that the sensitivity was 97% and the specificity was 97% at the cutoff value of 5 pg/m. IL-10 is produced by both lymphoma cells and TAMs, and the JAK-STAT pathway is activated by secreted IL-10 in an autocrine and paracrine manner. Although several reports have shown that an elevated IL-10 level in serum is correlated with poor prognosis in systemic DLBCL, there were only two reports describing the correlation between IL-10 levels in CSF and clinical outcome. We previously showed that high CSF IL-10 levels were associated with poorer prognoses in PCNSL patients. However, larger patient cohorts are required to determine whether an elevated CSF IL-10 concentration is associated with poor prognosis and outcome.

REFERENCES

[1] Prodduturi P, Bierman PJ: Current and emerging pharmacotherapies for primary CNS lymphoma. *Clinical Medicine Insights Oncology* 2012, 6:219-231.

[2] Olson JE, Janney CA, Rao RD, Cerhan JR, Kurtin PJ, Schiff D, Kaplan RS, O'Neill BP: The continuing increase in the incidence of primary central nervous system non-Hodgkin lymphoma: a surveillance, epidemiology, and end results analysis. *Cancer* 2002, 95(7):1504-1510.

[3] Bataille B, Delwail V, Menet E, Vandermarcq P, Ingrand P, Wager M, Guy G, Lapierre F: Primary intracerebral malignant lymphoma: report of 248 cases. *Journal of neurosurgery* 2000, 92(2):261-266.

[4] Frankfort SV, Tulner LR, van Campen JP, Verbeek MM, Jansen RW, Beijnen JH: Amyloid beta protein and tau in cerebrospinal fluid and plasma as biomarkers for dementia: a review of recent literature. *Current clinical pharmacology* 2008, 3(2):123-131.

[5] Helbok R, Broessner G, Pfausler B, Schmutzhard E: Chronic meningitis. *Journal of neurology* 2009, 256(2):168-175.

[6] Diez B, Balmaceda C, Matsutani M, Weiner HL: Germ cell tumors of the CNS in children: recent advances in therapy. *Child's nervous system: ChNS: official journal of the International Society for Pediatric Neurosurgery* 1999, 15(10):578-585.

[7] Sasayama T, Nakamizo S, Nishihara M, Kawamura A, Tanaka H, Mizukawa K, Miyake S, Taniguchi M, Hosoda K, Kohmura E: Cerebrospinal fluid interleukin-10 is a potentially useful biomarker in immunocompetent primary central nervous system lymphoma (PCNSL). *Neuro-oncology* 2012, 14(3):368-380.

[8] Romeo MJ, Espina V, Lowenthal M, Espina BH, Petricoin EF, 3rd, Liotta LA: CSF proteome: a protein repository for potential biomarker identification. *Expert review of proteomics* 2005, 2(1):57-70.

[9] Jeffery GM, Frampton CM, Legge HM, Hart DN: Cerebrospinal fluid B2-microglobulin levels in meningeal involvement by malignancy. *Pathology* 1990, 22(1): 20-23.

[10] Kersten MJ, Evers LM, Dellemijn PL, van den Berg H, Portegies P, Hintzen RQ, van Lier RA, von dem Borne AE, van Oers RH: Elevation of cerebrospinal fluid soluble CD27 levels in patients with meningeal localization of lymphoid malignancies. *Blood* 1996, 87(5):1985-1989.

[11] Chang CS, Liu HW, Lin SF, Chen TP: Soluble interleukin-2 receptor levels in cerebrospinal fluid of patients with acute lymphocytic leukemia or with non-Hodgkin's lymphoma. *Zhonghua Minguo wei sheng wu ji mian yi xue za zhi = Chinese journal of microbiology and immunology* 1989, 22(2):132-137.

[12] Lee W, Kim SJ, Lee S, Kim J, Kim M, Lim J, Kim Y, Cho B, Lee EJ, Han K: Significance of cerebrospinal fluid sIL-2R level as a marker of CNS involvement in acute lymphoblastic leukemia. *Annals of clinical and laboratory science* 2005, 35(4) 407-412.

[13] Roy S, Josephson SA, Fridlyand J, Karch J, Kadoch C, Karrim J, Damon L, Treseler P, Kunwar S, Shuman MA et al.: Protein biomarker identification in the CSF of patients with CNS lymphoma. *Journal of clinical oncology: official journal of the American Society of Clinical Oncology* 2008, 26(1):96-105.

[14] Moore KW, de Waal Malefyt R, Coffman RL, O'Garra A: Interleukin-10 and the interleukin-10 receptor. *Annual review of immunology* 2001, 19:683-765.

[15] Mosser DM, Zhang X: Interleukin-10: new perspectives on an old cytokine. *Immunological reviews* 2008, 226:205-218.

[16] Salles G, Coiffier B: Inherited cytokine response and risk of lymphoma. *The Lancet Oncology* 2006, 7(1):3-4.

[17] Kurzrock R: The role of cytokines in cancer-related fatigue. *Cancer* 2001, 92(6 Suppl.): 1684-1688.

[18] el-Far M, Fouda M, Yahya R, el-Baz H: Serum IL-10 and IL-6 levels at diagnosis as independent predictors of outcome in non-Hodgkin's lymphoma. *Journal of physiology and biochemistry* 2004, 60(4):253-258.

[19] Nacinovic-Duletic A, Stifter S, Dvornik S, Skunca Z, Jonjic N: Correlation of serum IL-6, IL-8 and IL-10 levels with clinicopathological features and prognosis in patients with diffuse large B-cell lymphoma. *International journal of laboratory hematology* 2008, 30(3):230-239.

[20] Vassilakopoulos TP, Nadali G, Angelopoulou MK, Siakantaris MP, Dimopoulou MN, Kontopidou FN, Rassidakis GZ, Doussis-Anagnostopoulou IA, Hatzioannou M, Vaiopoulos G et al.: Serum interleukin-10 levels are an independent prognostic factor for patients with Hodgkin's lymphoma. *Haematologica* 2001, 86(3):274-281.

[21] Cassoux N, Giron A, Bodaghi B, Tran TH, Baudet S, Davy F, Chan CC, Lehoang P, Merle-Beral H: IL-10 measurement in aqueous humor for screening patients with suspicion of primary intraocular lymphoma. *Investigative ophthalmology and visual science* 2007, 48(7):3253-3259.

[22] Chan CC, Buggage RR, Nussenblatt RB: Intraocular lymphoma. *Current opinion in ophthalmology* 2002, 13(6):411-418.

[23] Whitcup SM, Stark-Vancs V, Wittes RE, Solomon D, Podgor MJ, Nussenblatt RB, Chan CC: Association of interleukin 10 in the vitreous and cerebrospinal fluid and primary central nervous system lymphoma. *Archives of ophthalmology* 1997, 115(9): 1157-1160.

[24] Salmaggi A, Eoli M, Corsini E, Gelati M, Frigerio S, Silvani A, Boiardi A: Cerebrospinal fluid interleukin-10 levels in primary central nervous system lymphoma: a possible marker of response to treatment? *Annals of neurology* 2000, 47(1):137-138.

[25] Komohara Y, Horlad H, Ohnishi K, Ohta K, Makino K, Hondo H, Yamanaka R, Kajiwara K, Saito T, Kuratsu J et al.: M2 macrophage/microglial cells induce activation of Stat3 in primary central nervous system lymphoma. *Journal of clinical and experimental hematopathology: JCEH* 2011, 51(2):93-99.

[26] Qian BZ, Pollard JW: Macrophage diversity enhances tumor progression and metastasis. *Cell* 2010, 141(1):39-51.

[27] Yu H, Pardoll D, Jove R: STATs in cancer inflammation and immunity: a leading role for STAT3. *Nature reviews Cancer* 2009, 9(11):798-809.

[28] Mizowaki T, Sasayama T, Tanaka K, Mizukawa K, Takata K, Nakamizo S, Tanaka H, Nagashima H, Nishihara M, Hirose T et al.: STAT3 activation is associated with cerebrospinal fluid interleukin-10 (IL-10) in primary central nervous system diffuse large B cell lymphoma. *Journal of neuro-oncology* 2015.

[29] van den Bent MJ, Lamers CH, van 't Veer MB, Sillevis Smitt PA, Bolhuis RL, Gratama JW: Increased levels of soluble CD27 in the cerebrospinal fluid are not diagnostic for leptomeningeal involvement by lymphoid malignancies. *Annals of hematology* 2002, 81(4):187-191.

[30] Muniz C, Martin-Martin L, Lopez A, Sanchez-Gonzalez B, Salar A, Almeida J, Sancho JM, Ribera JM, Heras C, Penalver FJ et al.: Contribution of cerebrospinal fluid sCD19 levels to the detection of CNS lymphoma and its impact on disease outcome. *Blood* 2014, 123(12):1864-1869.

[31] Caudie C, Bancel J, Dupont M, Matanza D, Poitevin F, Honnorat J: [CSF levels and diagnostic utility of cerebrospinal fluid beta2-microglobulin]. *Annales de biologie clinique* 2005, 63(6):631-637.

[32] Schroers R, Baraniskin A, Heute C, Kuhnhenn J, Alekseyev A, Schmiegel W, Schlegel U, Pels HJ: Detection of free immunoglobulin light chains in cerebrospinal fluids of patients with central nervous system lymphomas. *European journal of haematology* 2010, 85(3):236-242.

[33] Baraniskin A, Kuhnhenn J, Schlegel U, Schmiegel W, Hahn S, Schroers R: MicroRNAs in cerebrospinal fluid as biomarker for disease course monitoring in primary central nervous system lymphoma. *Journal of neuro-oncology* 2012, 109(2):239-244.

[34] Baraniskin A, Kuhnhenn J, Schlegel U, Chan A, Deckert M, Gold R, Maghnouj A, Zollner H, Reinacher-Schick A, Schmiegel W et al.: Identification of microRNAs in the cerebrospinal fluid as marker for primary diffuse large B-cell lymphoma of the central nervous system. *Blood* 2011, 117(11):3140-3146.

[35] Sasagawa Y, Akai T, Tachibana O, Iizuka H: Diagnostic value of interleukin-10 in cerebrospinal fluid for diffuse large B-cell lymphoma of the central nervous system. *Journal of neuro-oncology* 2015, 121(1):177-183.

[36] Krumbholz M, Theil D, Cepok S, Hemmer B, Kivisakk P, Ransohoff RM, Hofbauer M, Farina C, Derfuss T, Hartle C et al.: Chemokines in multiple sclerosis: CXCL12 and CXCL13 up-regulation is differentially linked to CNS immune cell recruitment. *Brain: a journal of neurology* 2006, 129(Pt 1):200-211.

[37] Rubenstein JL, Wong VS, Kadoch C, Gao HX, Barajas R, Chen L, Josephson SA, Scott B, Douglas V, Maiti M et al.: CXCL13 plus interleukin 10 is highly specific for the diagnosis of CNS lymphoma. *Blood* 2013, 121(23):4740-4748.

[38] Viaccoz A, Ducray F, Tholance Y, Barcelos GK, Thomas-Maisonneuve L, Ghesquieres H, Meyronet D, Quadrio I, Cartalat-Carel S, Louis-Tisserand G et al.: CSF neopterin level as a diagnostic marker in primary central nervous system lymphoma. *Neuro-oncology* 2015.

[39] Fischer L, Korfel A, Pfeiffer S, Kiewe P, Volk HD, Cakiroglu H, Widmann T, Thiel E: CXCL13 and CXCL12 in central nervous system lymphoma patients. *Clinical cancer research: an official journal of the American Association for Cancer Research* 2009, 15 (19):5968-5973.

[40] Hashiguchi S, Momoo T, Murohashi Y, Endo M, Shimamura M, Kawasaki T, Kanada S, Nozawa A, Tada M, Koyano S et al.: Interleukin 10 Level in the Cerebrospinal Fluid as a Possible Biomarker for Lymphomatosis Cerebri. *Internal medicine* 2015, 54(12): 1547-1552.

[41] Yu H, Kortylewski M, Pardoll D: Crosstalk between cancer and immune cells: role of STAT3 in the tumour microenvironment. *Nature reviews Immunology* 2007, 7(1):41-51.

[42] Williams LM, Ricchetti G, Sarma U, Smallie T, Foxwell BM: Interleukin-10 suppression of myeloid cell activation--a continuing puzzle. *Immunology* 2004, 113(3): 281-292.

[43] Morikawa T, Baba Y, Yamauchi M, Kuchiba A, Nosho K, Shima K, Tanaka N, Huttenhower C, Frank DA, Fuchs CS et al.: STAT3 expression, molecular features, inflammation patterns, and prognosis in a database of 724 colorectal cancers. *Clinical cancer research: an official journal of the American Association for Cancer Research* 2011, 17(6):1452-1462.

[44] Gupta M, Han JJ, Stenson M, Maurer M, Wellik L, Hu G, Ziesmer S, Dogan A, Witzig TE: Elevated serum IL-10 levels in diffuse large B-cell lymphoma: a mechanism of aberrant JAK2 activation. *Blood* 2012, 119(12):2844-2853.

[45] Lech-Maranda E, Bienvenu J, Broussais-Guillaumot F, Warzocha K, Michallet AS, Robak T, Coiffier B, Salles G: Plasma TNF-alpha and IL-10 level-based prognostic model predicts outcome of patients with diffuse large B-Cell lymphoma in different risk groups defined by the International Prognostic Index. *Archivum immunologiae et therapiae experimentalis* 2010, 58(2):131-141.

[46] Inagaki A, Ishida T, Ishii T, Komatsu H, Iida S, Ding J, Yonekura K, Takeuchi S, Takatsuka Y, Utsunomiya A et al.: Clinical significance of serum Th1-, Th2- and regulatory T cells-associated cytokines in adult T-cell leukemia/lymphoma: high interleukin-5 and -10 levels are significant unfavorable prognostic factors. *International journal of cancer Journal international du cancer* 2006, 118(12):3054-3061.

In: Primary Central Nervous System Lymphoma (PCNSL) ISBN: 978-1-63485-322-4
Editor: Ryuya Yamanaka

Chapter 7

GENE EXPRESSION SIGNATURE-BASED PROGNOSTIC RISK SCORE WITH NETWORK STRUCTURE

Atsushi Kawaguchi*
Center for Comprehensive Community Medicine,
Faculty of Medicine, Saga University, Saga, Japan

ABSTRACT

This article describes the statistical construction of a prognostic risk score (PRS) based on gene expression data. The proposed score has a hieratical structure with subnetworks of genes at lower levels. We also propose the incoporation of supervised learning to obtain a more predictive score. The proposed method is applied to a primary central nervous system lymphoma (PCNSL) study. We show that the proposed method offers PRS with reasonable prediction accuracy as evaluated by the resampling technique.

Keywords: dimension reduction, gene expression data, prognosis, multiblock principal component analysis, network clustering, sparse

INTRODUCTION

The prognostic risk score (PRS) is useful to predict disease development and to decide an appropriate treatment strategy. Early detection of a disease can often lead to an effective cure and a risk score based on genomic information, such as gene expression signature, would yield a subjective diagnosis with converting the prognosis probability or the binary result with its cutoff point. The risk score of each patient is often derived from the sum of multiplied (weighted) gene expression signatures by its corresponding coefficient, which is based on

* Corresponding author: Atsushi Kawaguchi. 5-1-1 Nabeshima, Saga 849-8501, Japan. Email: akawa@cc.saga-u.ac.jp.

statistical modeling, such as the Cox propositional hazards model for a time to event outcome (Chen et al., 2007, Cho et al., 2011) and a logistic regression model for a binary outcome. This method would be relatively easy to construct statistically and use clinically because of the simple formula representation; however, it makes a strong assumption that all predictors have a single additive effect, nevertheless gene information has a complex structure. In addition, it is necessary to select appropriate gene signatures from a large number of candidates, and requres high dimensional data analysis with the number of variables exceeding the number of observations (patients). In this analysis, many classical statistical methods cannot be applied to analyze this kind of data and new techniques are needed to address the high-dimensionality. In earlier studies, the screening of genes, which was less associated with the outcome, was conducted based on the univariate model, and methods have been developed to capture the complex structure (correlation and interaction) of genes. Kawaguchi et al. (2012) used the random survival forests (RSF) method to select genes. It is a machine learning method and is suitable to model the complex structure of genes. Their PRS was constructed by principal components analysis with selected genes. See Libbrecht et al. (2015) for the review of the machine learning. Moreover, Wei (2015) reviewed several advanced approaches including penalized regression methods for survival analysis in genomic studies within the framework of integrative analysis.

Regression-based screening approaches, including the RSF and the univariate method such as the universal t-tests, detect only associated genes with the outcome. In order to detect genes that have an indirect association with the outcome through the association with other genes, pathway (gene network) information is useful and is deposited in the database such as Kyoto Encyclopedia of Genes and Genomes (KEGG) (Kanehisa and Goto, 2000). For exploratory purpose, the network modeling is also developed (Zhao et al., 2012). Zhang et al. (2013) and Sun et al. (2014) developed a method to incorporate the network information into the Cox's proportional hazard model which were compared by Iuliano et al. (2015). Recently, Peterson et al. (2015) proposed the simultaneous construction of linear predictors and the network structure. In this article, we propose a method to establish the PRS as the weighted sum of representative variables of the (sub) networks and to identify the effective parts of a network instead of individual genes. In this study, to elucidate the variations in genes as well as the relationship with the outcome, the entire network was divided into sub networks via the network clustering method and the supervised sparse multiblock principal component analysis was then employed to estimate the coefficients (weights) of the representative variables and theirs.The final PRS was constructed by the Cox propositional hazards model.

This paper is organized as follows: Section 2 describes the proposed method; in Section 3, the proposed method is applied to real data from our previous work, and Section 4 summarizes the study with a final conclusion.

METHODS

In the case of genomic data the number of the candidate predictors is huge and hence a dimension reduction step is necessary for the statistical construction of the PRS. Note that "dimension" here means the number of variables (probe sets or genes). A two-step dimension reduction has been employed here. The first step is to incorporate the network structure into the genes. In addition to reduction of dimension, another critical aspect is that the network structure should also represent (easily visualized) the role of genes that indirectly contribute to the PRS. In order to understand the characteristics of networks, the effective method is to identify communities. Clustering analysis can be used to divide the entire network into subnetworks and the typical number of clusters would be approximately 5000, as in our study. In the case of a study with a small sample size, the dimension may not be suffiecntly reduced and hence in the second step supervised sparse multiblock principal component analysis (SSM-PCA) is applied to further reduce the dimension. The resulting score is used to construct the PRS by the Cox proportional hazards regression model. The summary of the proposed method is displayed in Figure 1.

Network Clustering

First, the entire network with each variable being a node is determined via graphical modeling of data with all possible variables. The extended version of the Chow–Liu algorithm was implemented in the minForest function in the gRapHD package (Edwards et al., 2010). Second, the nodes of the estimated network are clustered based on similarity (within the framework of graph theory). This is referred to as network clustering. Considerations for overlapping clustering have been recently developed with Ahn et al. (2010) performing the pioneering study, and Becker et al. (2012) extended it with a new algorithm based on their proposed modularity. We used the R package linkcomm developed by Kalinka and Tomancak (2011) to implement the method proposed by Becker et al. (2012).

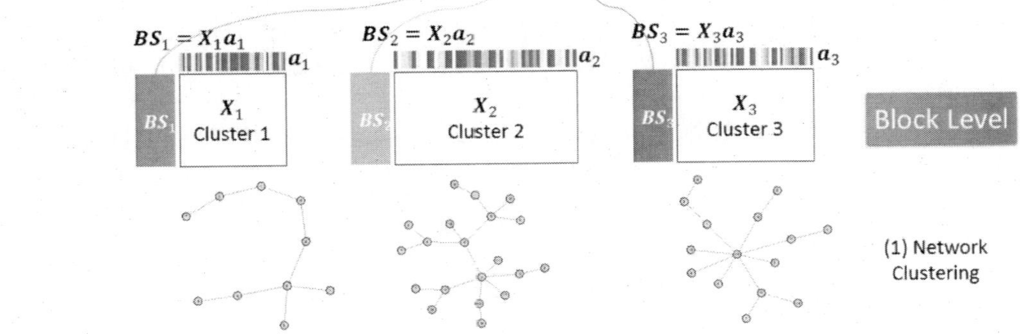

Figure 1. Schematic explanation of the analysis method. (1) network clustering is applied to make clusters of variables (probe sets or genes); (2) SSM-PCA is applied to compute the score; (3) multiple scores are considered to be new variables for the common statistical multivariate analysis based on the cox proportional hazards regression model, which yields the final prognostic risk score.

SSM-PCA

Traditional PCA provides a linear combination of variables (gene expression signatures; GESs), which is referred to as a score. This is the summation of GESs with the each GES weighted by some value (e.g., a1, a2,… corresponding to GES1, GES2,…); that is, the score can be represented by the following equation:

$$\text{Score} = \text{a1} \times \text{GES1} + \text{a2} \times \text{GES2} + \cdots \tag{1}$$

Note that a1, a2,… are referred to weights or loadings and are estimated by maximizing the variance of the score. This is one method to construct the prognostic risk score. Once the score (namely, the weights) is computed, another score can be computed from the residual data. Each score is referred to a component. Thus, we could obtain multiple components from a data set.

Multiblock PCA was used in this study. Each block corresponds to the sub network derived from the network clustering. These are summarized as block scores as in equation (1). Then, the super score SS, which is the linear combination of the block scores, can be obtained by

$$SS = \text{b1} \times BS1 + \text{b2} \times BS2 + \cdots \tag{2}$$

where BS's are block scores, which are the linear combinations of GES within the cluster as in (1). Note that the super weights b1, b2,… are estimated by maximizing the variance of the super score. Traditional PCA would be also applicable but it requires representative variables for each cluster, for which have possible representations, for example, the mean value of GESs for each cluster, or the separately calculated PCA score for each cluster as in Ma et al. (2011). The multiblock PCA can simultaneously decide the weights for the block and super levels by optimizing the one criteria, the variance of the super score.

Since traditional PCA has to use all variables (GSEs or their clusters) in estimating the score, researchers cannot know which variables are important. Thus, sparse modeling has been developed, which is the regularized estimation procedure that imposes small value weights into zero controlled by the regularized parameter. The variables with their weight not equaling to 0 are interpreted as the selected variables. Li et al. (2012) developed the sparse multiblock PCA and applied it to multi genomic data sets. These methods are based on the regularized maximization of the variance. The original idea of maximizing variance comes from that the variance is a measure of the variation of variables. Thus, the PCA score represents a new variable that has the highest data variation. This method is useful for an exploratory analysis, and is referred to as the unsupervised method. On the other hand, if the outcome variable, such as the patient's prognosis is available, the supervised method would be more useful. The score maximizing the variance might not be related with the outcome and it would be hard to interpret through the weights or selected predictors. Thus, we proposed the SSM-PCA, in which the weighted values are estimated by not only maximizing the variance of the score but by also correlating the score and the outcome variable. The details are shown in the Appendix.

Prognostic Risk Score Based on a Statistical Regression Model

The score computed in the previous section can also be the PRS, however, as in traditional PCA, multiple components can be obtained from SSM-PCA and a linear combination of these scores would yield a more predictive PRS than the one component. Since the number of components is smaller than the number of patients, the regression model would be more suitable in terms of statistics and it also requires the outcome, thus allowing for the aformenetioned linear combination. The regression coefficient vector is a measure of how much each of score in is contained within a risk and is estimated by maximizing the likelihood function in the established way of the statistical inference. For a binary outcome, the logistic regression model can be applied and it provides the probability that represents the uncertainty of individual status. This would enable us to implement the probability prediction approach, which is useful for medical studies. For a time-to-event outcome, the Cox proportional hazards regression model, which is one of the most popular survival analytical approaches, provides the time-dependent survival probability, such as one year survival, and the obtained linear combination of predictors (scores) can be binarized by an appropriate cut-off point as good or poor prognosis, as in the logistic regression model.

Evaluation

The constructed risk score should be evaluated the predictive accuracy for the practical usage. The Brier score (Brier, 1950) is a measure of prediction ability and the survival version of the mean squared loss between the estimated survival function and the individual status (for example, dead or alive) at some time t. The integrated version of the Brier score is also available and can evaluate the overall observation time. The C-index (Harrel et al., 1982) is another measure and a time-to-event version of the discriminant measure, which is close to the area under the receiver operating characteristic (ROC) curve (AUC) for a binary outcome. For a fixed time, the time-dependent ROC analysis has been developed (Heagerty et al. 2010, Blanche et al. 2012, Lambert and Chevret 2014, Rodríguez-Álvarez et al. 2015).

Ideally, the accuracy of prediction is independent of data used in constructing the PRS because of the overfit problem; however, its applicability is reduced in some cases, such as rare diseases. In that case, the resampling technique, such as the cross-validation technique (Simon et al., 2011), would be useful. Bin et al. (2014) evaluated the prediction ability of several survival models and the resampling technique within the framework of an omics data study. Collins et al. (2015) introduced other measures in addition to these and suggested a 100 to 200-event requirement for appropriate evaluation. We used R package pec (Mogensen et al., 2012) for the computation of resampling-based estimation of prediction error as described in Schumacher et al. (2007) and the bootstrap cross-validation Brier score.

Application

Data used here to test the applicability were obtained from Gene Expression Omnibus (accession number GSE34771). Kawaguchi et al. (2012) constructed the gene expression signature–based prognostic risk score for patients with primary central nervous system lymphoma (PCNSL) with genes that are predictive of overall survival (OS) by using the random survival forests model.

Data

There were 32 PCNSL patients with the median age of 64.1 years (range, 44-76 years); 17 patients (53%) were male and 15 (47%) were female. Note that two patients "PCNSL RY 4" and "PCNSL RY 22" were excluded from the GSE34771. The outcome OS was defined as the time from first diagnosis to death or last follow-up. Tissues from each tumor were subjected to total RNA extraction. One milligram of RNA was processed for hybridization to a GeneChip Human Genome U133 Plus 2.0 Expression Array (Affymetrix Inc.), which contained approximately 47,000 genes. See Kawaguchi et al. (2012) for the details.

The preprocessing of gene expression data was conducted by the using the R software and Bioconductor. The Affymetrix GeneChip probe-level data were preprocessed using MAS 5.0 (Affymetrix Inc.) for background adjustment and log-transformation (base 2). Each array was normalized by applying a quantile normalization to impose the same empirical distribution of intensities to each array. For probe sets mapped to the same Entrez Gene ID, only the probe with the largest variant based on the interquartile range was retained. The probe sets with the low variant were also removed. This filtering was implemented by the nsFilter function of the genefilter package. In total, 10,273 genes that passed the above filter criteria were considered for further analysis. For the supervision, the formula based on 21 genes identified in Kawaguchi et al. (2012) was used.

Results

The first fitted graph had 10,080 nodes and 10,079 edges, and the clustering yielded 4,984 communities (sub-networks) with the largest cluster having 42 nodes; that is, the results of fitting the proposed method without the regularization were as follows: the number of blocks was 4,984 for the one component and the maximum number of variables (genes) within the block was 42. The three super scores obtained as the result of the SSM-PCA were used to construct PRS by fitting the cox regression model as the covariate.

$$\mathrm{PRS} = 0.0039 \times \mathrm{SS1} - 0.3658 \times \mathrm{SS2} + 0.6702 \times \mathrm{SS3}$$

where SS1, SS2, and SS3 are the super scores for the first, second, and third component. The numbers of selected blocks (networks) were 3, 1, and 1 for the first, second, and third component, respectively and networks and the corresponding block weights were displayed in Figure 2 to Figure 6.

The BRCA1 gene was included in the first component network. The KIAA0226L had the smallest weight or least contribution to the OS in this component; however, this gene was connected the BRCA1 through the EHHADH.

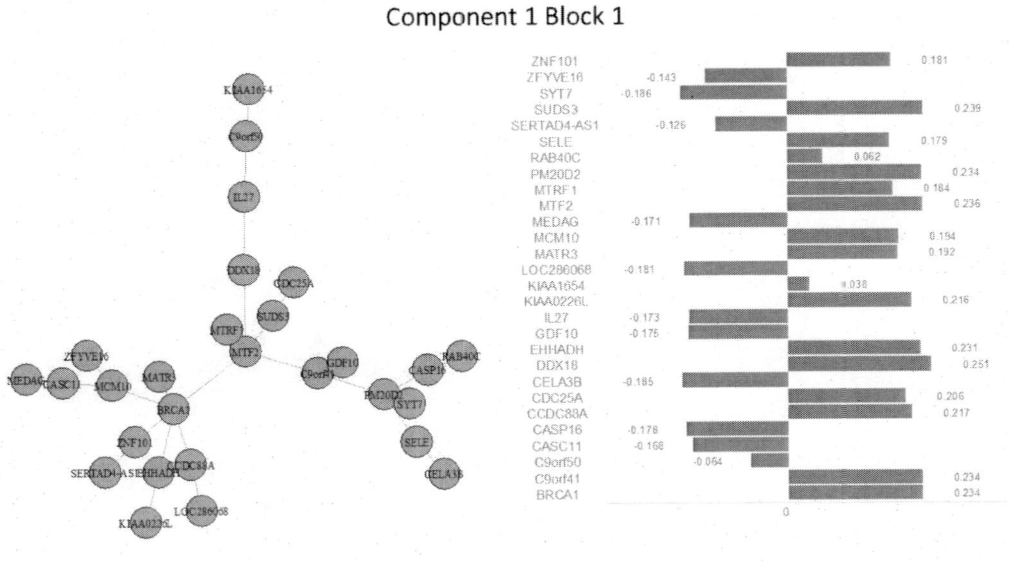

Figure 2. Selected networks and block weights (Component 1 Block 1).

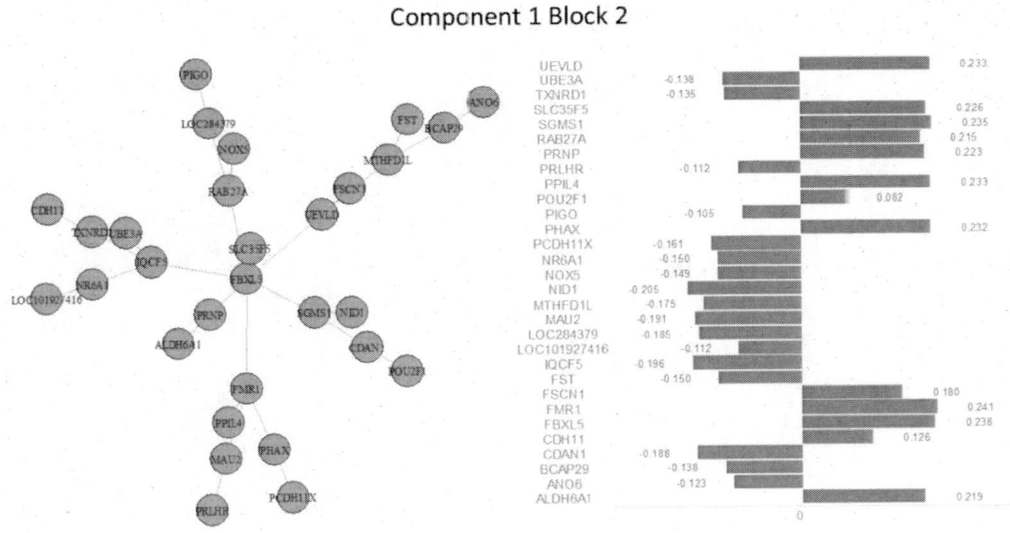

Figure 3. Selected networks and block weights (Component 1 Block 2).

The PRS's were binarized by the minimum p-value method, and patients were grouped based on the following: high group if PRS ≥ 0.35 and low group if PRS < 0.35. The Kaplan-Meier curves for each group are displayed in Figure 7.

The hazard ratio was 0.120 (95% Confidence Interval, 0.041-0.354) and the logrank p-value was $p < 0.0001$, indicating significant difference between survival curves at the 5% level.

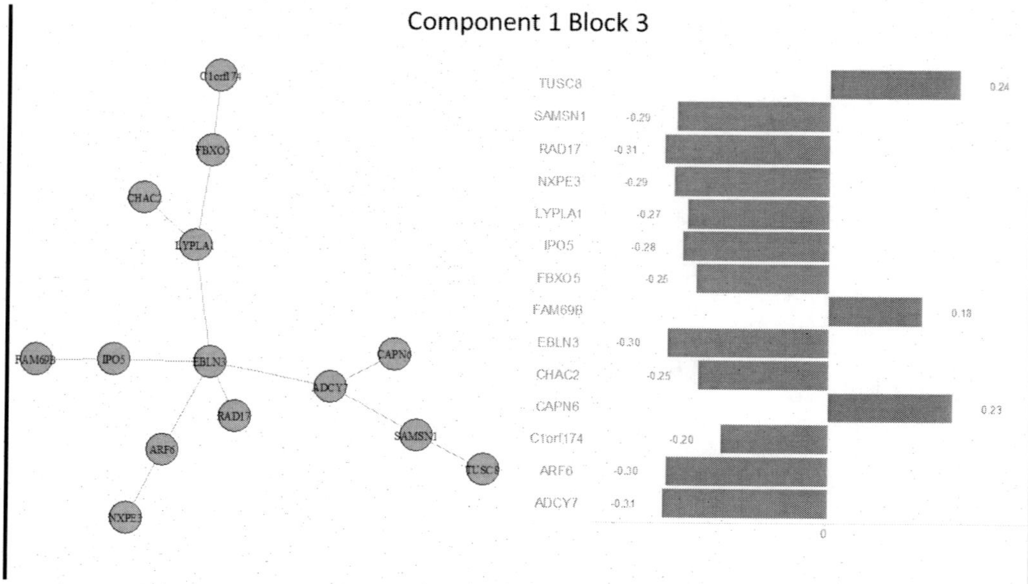

Figure 4. Selected networks and block weights (Component 1 Block 3).

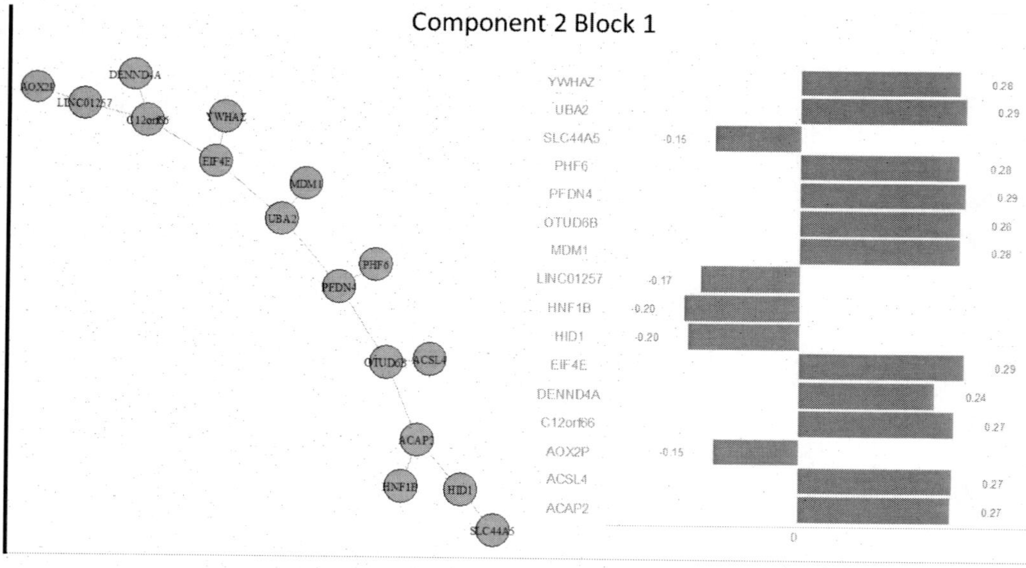

Figure 5. Selected networks and block weights (Component 2 Block1).

Next step was to determine prediction errors for the constructed PRS through comparison of the un- and supervised version of the suparse multiblock PCA. Figure 8 shows the result of the evaluation with the number of iteration of B = 10,000.

The entire curve based on the SSM-PCA was below that of the unsupervised. Acutually, the integrated Brier score between 0 and 2.5 years for the bootstrap cross-validation estimate of the prediction error was the lowest for the supervised method. Thus, the effectiveness of the prediction of the supervised feature was demonstrated.

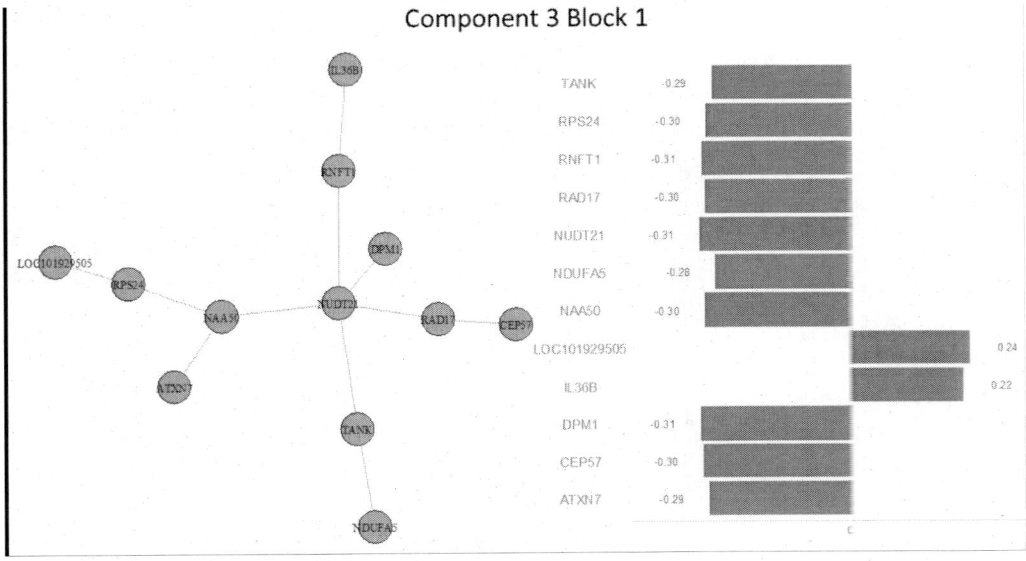

Figure 6. Selected networks and block weights (Component 3 Block1).

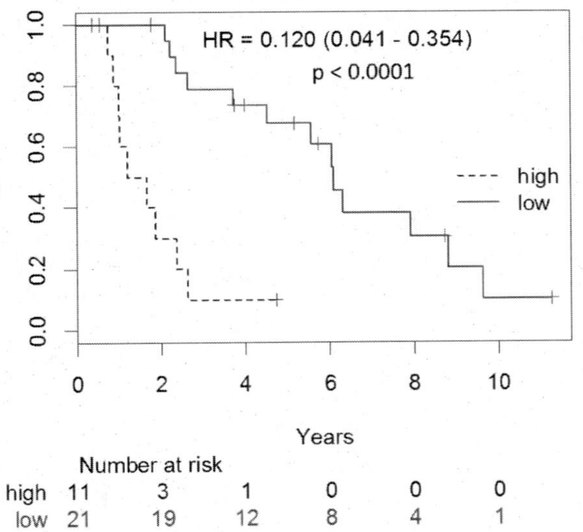

Figure 7. The Kaplan-Meier curves for two groups divided by the PRS.

DISCUSSION

We developed the method to construct a PRS with three key features: (1) Data driven (sub) network construction; (2) Effective network identification; (3) Supervised dimension reduction. There are several methods to construct the PRS on the basis of time to event outcomes, and several softwares are available (Moni et al., 2014 and Chen et al., 2014).

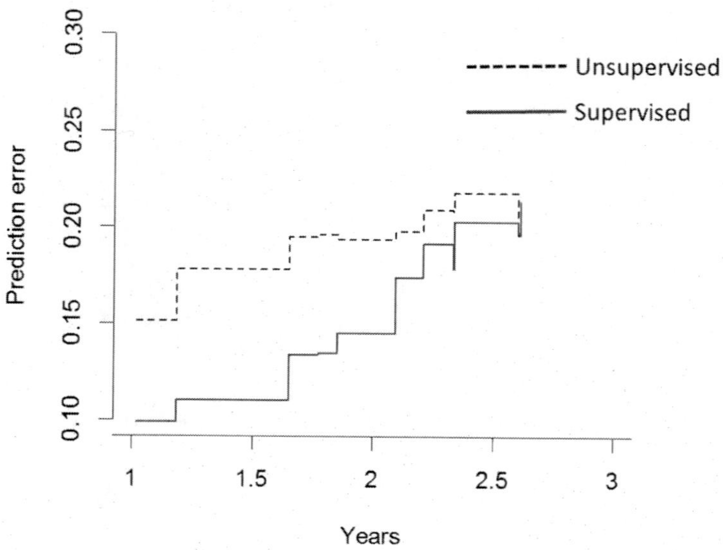

Figure 8. Prediction error curves for unsupervised and supervised method.

The main difference in the proposed method from the existing methods is that the resulting score can be interpreted as the gene structure through the representative variable of a sub network provided as the block score. Although this study showed that the supervised dimension reduction was effective for prediction, further investigation about the performance in the other types of cancers affecting a large number of patients (for example data from TCGA (http://cancergenome.nih.gov/)) might be required. The software is being developed as a new version of the mama R package.

Database details on the gene related networks, such as the biological pathways in KEGG, are available (Klingström and Plewczynski, 2011 for review), and they can be also used in the proposed method; however, graphical modeling and the Bayesian network model would be reasonable for an exploratory analysis (Yu et al., 2013). In addition, the estimated and selected networks would be characterized by its structure (Salter-Townshend et al, 2012) or network component analysis (Jayavelu et al., 2015).

Besides GWAS data, there are other forms of genetic data such as SNPs, copy number variation, microRNA, DNA methylation, and proteomics. The integration of several types of data would provide complementary and more comprehensive genetic information. Kim et al. (2012) proposed a data integration framework for different levels of genomic data by employing graph-based semi-supervised learning. Kristensen et al., (2014) and Ritchie et al. (2015) provided the review. As an extension of our proposed method, the hierarchical block structure with more than two levels would be applicable for the integration of multiple omic datasets.

In conclusion, our method will help to establish a diagnostic procedure for cancer based on genomic data.

APPENDIX

We provide the brief mathematical explanation for the SSM-PCA method. Consider n subjects and M clusters obtained by the network clustering. X_m is the $n \times p_n$ gene signature matrix for the m-th block (cluster). Subjects also have a univariate outcome, with the n-dimensional outcome vector denoted by Z. We consider super score SS with multiblock structure as follows:

$$\boldsymbol{SS} = \sum_{m=1}^{M} b_m \boldsymbol{X}_m \boldsymbol{a}_m \tag{A1}$$

where $\boldsymbol{a}_m$ is the weight vector for the m-th sub-blocks $\boldsymbol{X}_m$. $\boldsymbol{b} = (b_1, b_2, \ldots, b_M)^{\mathsf{T}}$ is the weight vector for the super-block. Note that let $\boldsymbol{BS}_m = \boldsymbol{X}_m \boldsymbol{a}_m$, which is referred to the block score.

When matrices $\boldsymbol{X}_m$ are normalized by its column, the weights are estimated by maximizing the following function.

$$\mathrm{L}(\boldsymbol{a}, \boldsymbol{b}) = (1 - \mu)\, \boldsymbol{SS}^{\mathsf{T}} \boldsymbol{SS} + \mu \boldsymbol{SS}^{\mathsf{T}} \boldsymbol{Z} - \mathrm{P}_\lambda(\boldsymbol{b}) \tag{A2}$$

subject to $\|\boldsymbol{a}_m\|^2 = 1$, $\|\boldsymbol{b}\|^2 = 1$ where $\boldsymbol{a} = (\boldsymbol{a}_1, \boldsymbol{a}_2, \ldots, \boldsymbol{a}_M)^{\mathsf{T}}$ and $0 \le \mu \le 1$ is the proportion of the supervision. Note that when $\mu = 0$ the regularized PCA is induced and when μ is closed to 1 the strong supervision to the outcome. In our experience, the moderate value of μ is adequate and $\mu = 0.75$ was used in this article. $\mathrm{P}_\lambda(x)$ is the penalty function $\mathrm{P}_\lambda(x) = 2\lambda|x|$. λ is the regularized parameter that is used to control the sparsity. The larger value of the regularization parameter λ has many non-zero elements in $\boldsymbol{b}$ values from which its optimal value is selected by minimizing the Bayesian information criterion (BIC).

$$\mathrm{BIC}(\lambda) = \log\left(\frac{\sum_{m=1}^{k} \left\|\widehat{\boldsymbol{X}}_m^{(k)} - \boldsymbol{X}_m\right\|^2}{n \sum_{m=1}^{k} p_m}\right) + \frac{\log\left(n \sum_{m=1}^{k} p_m\right)}{n \sum_{m=1}^{k} p_m} \mathrm{df}(\lambda)$$

where $\widehat{\boldsymbol{X}}_m^{(k)} = \boldsymbol{U}_m \boldsymbol{P}_m^{\mathsf{T}}$ with $\boldsymbol{U}_m = \left[\boldsymbol{BS}_m^{(1)}, \ldots, \boldsymbol{BS}_m^{(k)}\right]$ and $\boldsymbol{P}_m = \left[\boldsymbol{p}_m^{(1)}, \ldots, \boldsymbol{p}_m^{(k)}\right]$, $\boldsymbol{p}_m = \boldsymbol{X}_m^{\mathsf{T}} \boldsymbol{BS}_m / \boldsymbol{BS}_m^{\mathsf{T}} \boldsymbol{BS}_m$ is the projection of $\boldsymbol{Y}_m$ onto the k-dimensional subspace spanned by the k weight vectors. df is the number of effective parameters, which depend on the value of λ.

The algorithm for maximizing the equation (A2) is given as follows.

1. Initialize $\boldsymbol{SS}$.
2. Repeat until convergence.
3. $\tilde{\boldsymbol{a}}_m = b_m \boldsymbol{X}_m^{\mathsf{T}} \{(1 - \mu)\boldsymbol{SS} + \mu \boldsymbol{Z}\}$ and normalize $\widehat{\boldsymbol{a}}_m = \tilde{\boldsymbol{a}}_m / \|\tilde{\boldsymbol{a}}_m\|_2$ $(m = 1, 2, \ldots, p)$.
4. Putting $\boldsymbol{BS}_m = \boldsymbol{X}_m \widehat{\boldsymbol{a}}_m$, $\tilde{b}_m = h_\lambda(\boldsymbol{BS}_m^{\mathsf{T}} \{(1 - \mu)\boldsymbol{SS} + \mu \boldsymbol{Z}\})$ where $h_\lambda(y) = \mathrm{sign}(y)(|y| > \lambda)_+$ then putting $\tilde{\boldsymbol{b}} = \left(\tilde{b}_1, \tilde{b}_2, \ldots, \tilde{b}_M\right)^{\mathsf{T}}$ and normalize as $\widehat{\boldsymbol{b}} = \tilde{\boldsymbol{b}} / \left\|\tilde{\boldsymbol{b}}\right\|_2$.
5. Set $\boldsymbol{SS} = \sum_{m=1}^{M} \widehat{b}_m \boldsymbol{BS}_m$.
6. (Deflation step) Set $\boldsymbol{p}_m = \boldsymbol{X}_m^{\mathsf{T}} \boldsymbol{BS}_m / \boldsymbol{BS}_m^{\mathsf{T}} \boldsymbol{BS}_m$, $\boldsymbol{X}_m \leftarrow \boldsymbol{X}_m - \boldsymbol{BS}_m \boldsymbol{p}_m^{\mathsf{T}}$.

Note that the deflation step yield the multiple components and several alternatives and the formulation of $\tilde{\boldsymbol{a}}_m$ can be incorporate the sparse function $h_\lambda(y)$ as well as $\tilde{b}_m$. In our experience, the predictive accuracy was lost when the sparsity considered in $\tilde{\boldsymbol{a}}_m$.

ACKNOWLEDGMENTS

This study was supported in part by a Grants-in-Aid from the Ministry of Education, Culture, Sport, Science and Technology of Japan (24700286). For this research work we used the supercomputer of ACCMS, Kyoto University.

REFERENCES

Ahn, Y.Y., Bagrow, J.P., and Lehmann, S., (2010). Link communities reveal multiscale complexity in networks. *Nature*, 466(7307), 761-764.

Blanche, P, Latouche, A., and Viallon V (2012). Time-dependent AUC in the presence of censored data: A survey study. *arXiv preprint arXiv*:1210.6805.

Becker, E., Robisson, B., Chapple, C.E., Guénoche, A., and Brun, C. (2011). Multifunctional proteins revealed by overlapping clustering in protein interaction network. *Bioinformatics* 1, 28(1), 84-90.

Chen, H.-Y., S.-L. Yu, C.-H. Chen, G.-C. Chang, C.-Y. Chen, A. Yuan, C.-L. Cheng, C.-H. Wang, H.-J. Terng, S.-F. Kao, W.-K. Chan, H.-N. Li, C.-C. Liu, S. Singh, W. J. Chen, J. J. W. Chen and P.-C. Yang (2007). A five-gene signature and clinical outcome in non–small-cell lung cancer. *New England J. Med.* 356(1), 11-20.

Chen, X., Sun, X., and Hoshida, Y. (2014). Survival analysis tools in genomics research. *Human genomics*, 8(1), 21.

Cho, J. Y., Lim, J. Y., Cheong, J. H., Park, Y. Y., Yoon, S. L., Kim, S. M., Kim, S. B., Kim, H., Hong, S. W., Park, Y. N., Noh, S. H., Park, E. S., Chu, I. S., Hong, W. K., Ajani, J. A., and Lee, J. S. (2011). Gene expression signature–based prognostic risk score in gastric cancer. *Clinical Cancer Res.* 17(7), 1850-1857.

Collins, G. S., Ogundimu, E. O., and Altman, D. G. (2015). Sample size considerations for the external validation of a multivariable prognostic model: a resampling study. *Stats. in Med.* in press.

De Bin, R., Sauerbrei, W., and Boulesteix, A. L. (2014). Investigating the prediction ability of survival models based on both clinical and omics data: two case studies. *Stats. in Med.* 33 (30), 5310-5329.

Edwards, D., de Abreu, G.C.G., ad Labouriau, R. (2010). Selecting high- dimensional mixed graphical models using minimal AIC or BIC forests. *BMC Bioinformatics*, 11, 8.

Harrell, F. E., Califf, R. M., Pryor, D. B., Lee, K. L., and Rosati, R. A. (1982). Evaluating the yield of medical tests. *JAMA*, 247(18), 2543-2546.

Heagerty, P. J., Lumley, T., and Pepe, M. S. (2000). Time-dependent ROC curves for censored survival data and a diagnostic marker. *Biometrics*, 337-344.

Iuliano, A., Occhipinti, A., Angelini, C., De Feis, I., and Lió, P. (2015). Applications of Network-based Survival Analysis Methods for Pathways Detection in Cancer. In:

Computational Intelligence Methods for Bioinformatics and Biostatistics (pp. 76-88). Springer International Publishing.

Jayavelu, N. D., Aasgaard, L. S., and Bar, N. (2015). Iterative sub-network component analysis enables reconstruction of large scale genetic networks. *BMC Bioinformatics*, 16(1), 366.

Kalinka AT, and Tomancak P. (2011). linkcomm: an R package for the generation, visualization, and analysis of link communities in networks of arbitrary size and type. *Bioinformatics.* 15; 27(14), 2011-2012.

Kanehisa, M., and Goto, S. (2000). KEGG: kyoto encyclopedia of genes and genomes. *Nucleic acids research*, 28(1), 27-30.

Kawaguchi, A., Iwadate, Y., Komohara, Y., Sano, M., Kajiwara, K., Yajima, N., Tsuchiya, N., Homma, J., Aoki, H., Kobayashi, T., Sakai, Y., Hondoh, H., Fujii, Y., Kakuma, T., and Yamanaka, R. (2012). Gene Expression Signature–Based Prognostic Risk Score in Patients with Primary Central Nervous System Lymphoma. *Clinical Cancer Res.*, 18(20), 5672-5681.

Kim, D., Shin, H., Song, Y. S., and Kim, J. H. (2012). Synergistic effect of different levels of genomic data for cancer clinical outcome prediction. *J. Biomedical Informatics*, 45(6), 1191-1198.

Klingström, T., and Plewczynski, D. (2011). Protein–protein interaction and pathway databases, a graphical review. *Briefings in bioinformatics*, 12(6), 702-713.

Kristensen, V. N., Lingjærde, O. C., Russnes, H. G., Vollan, H. K. M., Frigessi, A., and Børresen-Dale, A. L. (2014). Principles and methods of integrative genomic analyses in cancer. *Nature Reviews Cancer*, 14(5), 299-313.

Lambert, J., and Chevret, S. (2014). Summary measure of discrimination in survival models based on cumulative/dynamic time-dependent ROC curves. *Statistical methods in medical research*, 0962280213515571.

Libbrecht, M. W., and Noble, W. S. (2015). Machine learning applications in genetics and genomics. *Nature Reviews Genetics.*

Li, W., Zhang, S., Liu, C. C., and Zhou, X. J. (2012). Identifying multi-layer gene regulatory modules from multi-dimensional genomic data. *Bioinformatics*, 28(19), 2458-2466.

Ma, S., Kosorok, M. R., Huang, J., and Dai, Y. (2011). Incorporating higher-order representative features improves prediction in network-based cancer prognosis analysis. *BMC medical genomics*, 4(1), 5.

Mogensen, U. B., Ishwaran, H., and Gerds, T. A. (2012). Evaluating random forests for survival analysis using prediction error curves. *Journal of statistical software*, 50(11), 1.

Moni, M. A., and Liò, P. (2014). comoR: a software for disease comorbidity risk assessment. *Journal of clinical bioinformatics*, 4(1), 1-11.

Paik, S., Shak, S., Tang, G., Kim, C., Baker, J., Cronin, M., Baehner, F. L., Walker, M. G., Watson, D., Park, T., Hiller, W., Fisher, E. R., Wickerham, D. L., Bryant, J., and Wolmark, N. (2004). A multigene assay to predict recurrence of tamoxifen-treated, node-negative breast cancer. *New England Journal of Medicine*, 351(27), 2817-2826.

Peterson, C. B., Stingo, F. C., and Vannucci, M. (2015). Joint Bayesian variable and graph selection for regression models with network-structured predictors. *Statistics in medicine.*

Ritchie, M. D., Holzinger, E. R., Li, R., Pendergrass, S. A., and Kim, D. (2015). Methods of integrating data to uncover genotype-phenotype interactions. *Nature Reviews Genetics*, 16(2), 85-97.

Rodríguez-Álvarez, M. X., Meira-Machado, L., Abu-Assi, E., and Raposeiras-Roubín, S. (2015). Nonparametric estimation of time-dependent ROC curves conditional on a continuous covariate. *Statistics in medicine*.

Schumacher, M., Binder, H., and Gerds, T. (2007). Assessment of survival prediction models based on microarray data. *Bioinformatics*, 23(14), 1768-1774.

Simon, R. M., Subramanian, J., Li, M. C., and Menezes, S. (2011). Using cross-validation to evaluate predictive accuracy of survival risk classifiers based on high-dimensional data. *Briefings in bioinformatics*, 12(3), 203-214.

Sun, H., Lin, W., Feng, R., Li, H. (2014) Network-Regularized high-dimensional cox regression for analysis of genomic data. *Statistica Sinica* 24, 1433-1459.

Salter-Townshend, M., White, A., Gollini, I., and Murphy, T. B. (2012). Review of statistical network analysis: models, algorithms, and software. *Statistical Analysis and Data Mining: The ASA Data Science Journal*, 5(4), 243-264.

Wei, Y. (2015). Integrative Analyses of Cancer Data: A Review from a Statistical Perspective. *Cancer Informatics*, 14(Suppl. 2), 173-181.

Yu, D., Kim, M., Xiao, G., and Hwang, T. H. (2013). Review of biological network data and its applications. *Genomics and informatics*, 11(4), 200-210.

Zhao, T., Liu, H., Roeder, K., Lafferty, J., and Wasserman, L. (2012). The huge package for high-dimensional undirected graph estimation in R. *The Journal of Machine Learning Research*, 13(1), 1059-1062.

In: Primary Central Nervous System Lymphoma (PCNSL)
Editor: Ryuya Yamanaka
ISBN: 978-1-63485-322-4

Chapter 8

MICRORNAS REGULATION AND PRIMARY CENTRAL NERVOUS SYSTEM LYMPHOMA

Tomohiko Kanayama[1,*], Azusa Hayano[2] and Ryuya Yamanaka[1,2]
[1]Laboratory of Molecular Target Therapy for Cancer,
Graduate School of Medical Science,
Kyoto Prefectural University of Medicine, Kyoto, Japan
[2]Department of Medical Science, Graduate School for Health Care Science,
Kyoto Prefectural University of Medicine, Kyoto, Japan

ABSTRACT

MicroRNAs (miRNAs) are non-coding regulatory RNAs, consisting of 19–25 nucleotides. Small miRNAs act through RNA interference mechanisms to regulate various cellular processes, including cell proliferation, differentiation, angiogenesis, and apoptosis in various organs and tissues, and require two RNase III complexes for activation. Unlike exogenous small interfering RNAs (siRNAs), miRNA can inhibit the translation of many mRNA sequences through the RNA-induced silencing complex, when its sequence is imperfectly matched with the target mRNA sequence. The general miRNA biogenesis pathway has been well established over a decade of intensive research in during which increases and decreases in miRNA expression have been reported in various organ samples from patients with a range of diseases, including cancer. Regarding cancer, in an early study, Calin and colleagues reported a link between miRNA dysregulation and tumor malignancy in chronic lymphocytic leukemia. Recently, Fischer and colleagues reported differential miRNA expression in nodal and non-nodal lymphomas, such as primary central nervous system lymphoma (PCNSL).

Among various miRNAs, miR-21, the most abundant miRNA in patients with PCNSL, has been well characterized as an oncogenic miRNA. In addition, several groups reported miR-21 as a strong candidate biomarker in the serum and cerebrospinal fluid (CSF) from patients with PCNSL. This chapter focuses on miRNA biology in cancer and the studies about miRNA expression and regulation in PCNSL.

* Corresponding Author address: Laboratory of Molecular Target Therapy for Cancer, Graduate School of Medical Science, Kyoto Prefectural University of Medicine, Kyoto, Japan. Email: tomokana@koto.kpu-m.ac.jp.

Keywords: microRNA, PCNSL, biomarker

INTRODUCTION

Primary central nervous system lymphoma (PCNSL) is a rare subtype of extra-nodal non-Hodgkin's lymphoma (NHL). It most commonly occurs in the brain, and though it accounts for only 2%–3% of NHL cases, its incidence has been increasing. More than 90% of PCNSLs are diffuse large B-cell lymphomas (DLBCLs). PCNSL is usually an aggressive lymphoma, and is characterized by a poorer prognosis than other systemic lymphomas with similar histological features [1].

The central nervous system (CNS) normally lacks a lymphatic system, and therefore, the mechanisms underlying DLBCL development in the CNS remain unclear. Recent studies have revealed the dysregulation of microRNA (miRNA) expression in cancer cells [2-5]. The mature miRNAs, which are 19–25 nucleotides long, non-coding RNAs, can regulate gene expression by binding to partially complementary target sites in the 3′ untranslated regions (UTRs) of target mRNAs, resulting in the degradation of target mRNAs or translational repression of the encoded proteins via several mechanisms [6-8].

Some specific miRNAs downregulate the expression of tumor suppressor genes such as *P53* and *PTEN*, thus promoting tumorigenesis (onco-miRNA [9-13]), while others downregulate the expression of oncogenes such as *MYC* and *BCL2*, thus exerting tumor suppressor effects in cancer cells (tumor suppressor-miRNA [9, 14-17]). To understand the cancer-specific miRNA signature, the characteristics of miRNA expression have been compared between cancer cells and other diseased cells or normal control cells by using overall miRNA expression analyses such as microarray analysis and miRNA sequencing analysis [18-20]. In the span of a decade, numerous miRNAs have been identified through the development of several detection techniques. From miRBase (http://www.mirbase.org/ release 21, updated June 2014) information, over 2500 human mature miRNAs have been registered so far. Many of these have not been characterized completely and their functions in human organs, including the brain, remain unclear. Several studies have focused on the well-known and well-characterized miRNAs and their roles in disease and cell development, their target genes, and expression patterns [21]. In this chapter, recent studies on miRNA expression and function in lymphomas, mainly DLBCL and PCNSL, are discussed. To develop a novel diagnostic biomarker for PCNSL, recent studies focused on miRNA expression analysis in cerebrospinal fluid (CSF) and serum are also discussed.

1. REGULATION OF MIRNA EXPRESSION IN CANCER

1.1. miRNA Biogenesis in Cancer

miRNAs are generally transcribed by RNA polymerase II (RNA pol II) as long primary transcripts from various genomic regions, including genes (exons and introns) and other non-coding regions (Figure 1a) [6, 22]. Primary miRNAs (pri-miRNAs) (>1 kbp in length) have characteristic hairpin structures and are converted to precursor miRNAs (pre-miRNAs; 70–

100 bp) by Drosha/DiGeorge syndrome critical region gene 8 (DGCR8) RNase III complex (Figure 1 b) [6, 22]. The pre-miRNAs are exported from the nucleus into the cytoplasm via an exportin 5-mediated mechanism (Figure 1c) [6, 22], where the action of another RNase III, Dicer, generates short mature miRNAs (19–25 bp) (Figure 1d). The mature miRNAs are incorporated into a large protein complex termed the RNA-induced silencing complex (RISC) [6, 22]. The mature miRNA duplex is recognized by the Argonaute (Ago) protein-containing RISC-loading complex (RLC) and is unwound into two single-stranded RNAs, the guide strand and the passenger strand (Figure 1e). The passenger strand (designated as miRNA* in Figure 1) is degraded, and the guide strand RNA is incorporated into the RISC. The binding of the miRNA guide strand with target mRNAs occurs via approximately 7 nucleotide-long stretches, the so-called "seed sequence," present in the 5′ region of the miRNA. The mature single-stranded miRNA regulates the expression of target genes via imperfect binding with the 3′ UTR of target mRNAs through the Ago-containing RISC (Figure 1f) [6, 22]. Besides this canonical mechanism of miRNA-mediated gene regulation, non-canonical pathways such as Drosha/ DGCR8-independent miRNA biogenesis have been reported [7] RISC-mediated target mRNA silencing is promoted by mRNA degradation through the recruitment of decapping and deadenylation enzymes to the miRNA-bound mRNA, or is performed by translation initiation and elongation inhibition by inhibition of ribosomal subunit recruitment into the translational 80S ribosomal complex [7, 22].

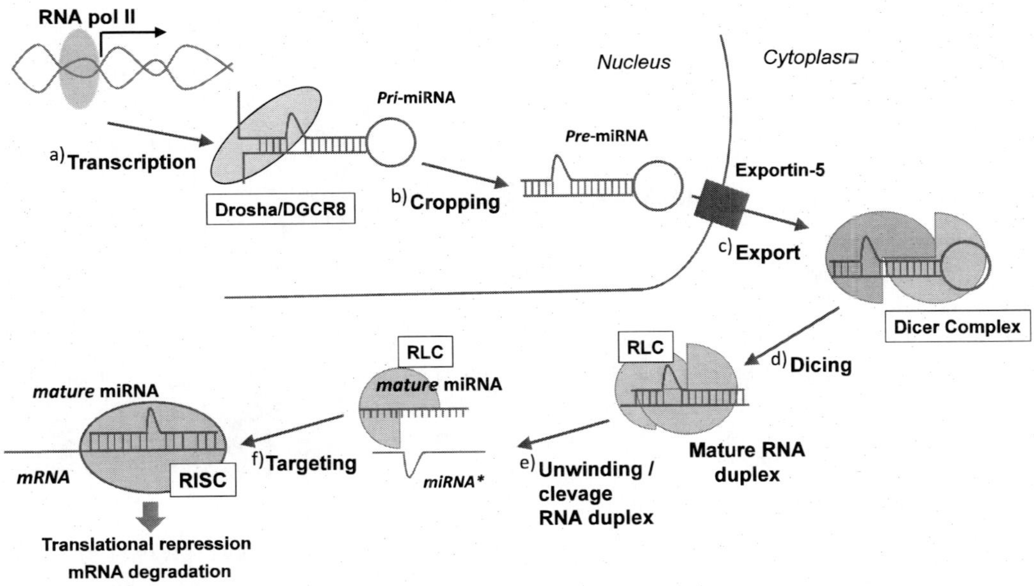

Figure 1. General mechanism of miRNA biogenesis.

1.2. Genome Amplification and Deletion

miRNA transcripts are derived from various genomic regions (e.g., introns and exons of genes, non-coding regions), and most miRNAs are transcribed by RNA pol II. Therefore, miRNA expression is affected by chromosomal alterations such as loss of heterozygosity (LOH) and amplifications such as translocations and single-nucleotide polymorphisms [23,

24]. Calin et al. [25] first reported that LOH in 13q14, where miR-15a/miR-16-1 is located, constitutes the most frequent chromosomal deletion in chronic lymphocytic leukemia (CLL). The most common chromosomal abnormalities in CLL detectable by cytogenetics include deletions in 13q (55%), 11q (18%), and 17p (8%), and trisomy 12 (12%–16%) [23, 26]. Further investigation revealed that miR-15a/miR-16-1 and miR-34 families (miR-34b/c located in 11q23) are transcriptionally inducible by p53 (located in 17p13). Fabbri et al. showed that miR-15a/miR-16-1 binds to the 3′ UTR of *P53* mRNA to suppress p53 activity; on the other hand, they also reported that the miR-34 family binds to the coding region of *ZAP70* to suppress ZAP70 [26], and the high expression of ZAP70 serves as a poor prognostic factor of CLL [27]. In this way, 11q/13q/17p linkage-derived miRNA/p53 feedback circuitry is associated with the pathogenesis and prognosis of CLL. These findings may explain the model for the indolent form of CLL involving 13q deletions, in which increased p53 levels are associated with transactivation of miR-34b/c and reduced levels of ZAP70 [26].

Tagawa et al. reported genome amplification at 13q31-32 in malignant DLBLC [28, 29]. Six miRNA genes (miR-17, miR-18, miR-19a/b, miR-20a, and miR-92-1) are clustered within the non-protein-coding gene C13orf25 (13q31). With a 13q31 gain/amplification, the higher expressions of these miRNAs are comparable with their expressions without 13q31 amplification [30].

Calin et al. pointed out that many miRNA genes are located in cancer-associated genomic regions or in fragile sites in which sister chromatid exchange, translocation, deletion, and amplification is frequent [31]. These regions include the chromosomal regions mentioned above.

1.3. miRNA Clusters and miRNA Transcription

Several miRNA clusters, such as C13orf25 (miR-17-92 cluster) in 13q31, and their association with diseases including cancer, have been the subjects of extensive research [30-36]. Previous studies have found that a substantial fraction of miRNAs is located in polycistronic transcripts, implying a common phenomenon of miRNA clustering. Clustered miRNAs are generally similar in sequence (e.g., miR-222/221, miR-29a/29b, miR-15a/16-1 clusters), but can sometimes differ (e.g., miR-17-92, miR-106b/93/25, miR-106a-363 clusters) [37-40].

The expression of the miR-17-92 cluster—a well-studied miRNA cluster—is regulated by the transcription factor (TF) Myc [12, 40]. In patients with CLL, the expression of some miRNAs in this cluster is different from that of others, depending on *P53* expression [41]. For example, a loss of p53 results in high expression of miR-19/miR-92a (onco-miRNA) and low expression of miR-17/miR-20 (tumor suppressor-miRNA). The normal expression of *P53* leads to a high miR-17/miR-20 expression. The relationship between p53 and imbalanced miR-17-92 expression suggests that increased expression of oncogenic miR-17-92 members and decreased expression of tumor suppressive members probably accelerates disease progression [41]. Considering that miR-18 expression remains unchanged in patients with CLL compared with that in normal controls, another speculation is that miR-18 may be subjected to modification during its maturation process to induce specific miRNA degradation [29, 42].

On one hand, while Myc regulates the transcription of several miRNA clusters, tumor-suppressor miRNAs directly targeting *MYC* have also been well-studied [40, 43-46]. Interestingly, the tumor suppressor gene *P53* regulates miRNA expression, and onco-miRNAs that directly target *P53* have also been reported [47]. In this manner, the TF-miRNA circuit can influence diverse oncogenesis-related processes, such as cell cycle regulation, apoptosis, metabolism, angiogenesis, epithelial to mesenchymal transition, and metastasis. Therefore, miRNA dysregulation has been suggested as an important mechanism for the aberrant expression of a list of oncogenes and/or tumor suppressor genes that are not affected directly by genetic mutations or transcriptional regulation in tumorigenesis.

1.4. Epigenetic Regulation of miRNA Expression

Aberrant epigenetic changes are a well-known feature of cancer cells, such as DNA hypermethylation of tumor suppressor genes involving DNA methyltransferases (DNMT1 or DNMT3A and DNMT3B), extensive genomic DNA hypomethylation, and alteration of histone modification patterns such as acetylation, methylation, and phosphorylation [48-50]. Similar to protein coding genes, miRNA genes are also subject to epigenetic changes in cancer. A large proportion of miRNA loci are associated with CpG islands giving a strong basis to their regulation by DNA methylation. Most studies have used treatment with chromatin remodeling drugs (e.g., DNMT inhibitors such as 5-aza-2′-deoxycytidine) to reveal epigenetically silenced miRNAs. Global DNA methylation analysis further revealed an extensive influence of DNA hypermethylation and hypomethylation on the regulation of miRNA expression. Most studies on the epigenetic silencing of miRNA genes in cancer have focused on CpG island hypermethylation [48-50]. By contrast, Dudziec et al. demonstrated that the methylation of CpG island shores, which are regions located within 2 kb of CpG islands, strongly affects gene expression and is frequently associated with the downregulation of miRNA expression in bladder cancer [51].

In a study by Baer et al. on the epigenetic regulation of miRNAs in CLL, promoters for 781 miRNAs were identified by upstream H3K4 me3 enrichment by using a panel of leukemic cell lines, primary CLL cells, and healthy B cells. Over 100 miRNAs were found to be the targets of recurrent aberrant methylation in CLL cells. Hypomethylation accounted for more than 60% of differential methylation [50]. Moreover, while DNA hypermethylation occurred preferentially in CpG islands, hypomethylation was almost exclusively found adjacent to the CpG islands or in the CpG-free promoters [50]. The patterns of hypomethylation are in concordance with the observations of extensive genome-wide DNA hypomethylation in CLL [52]. Inverse correlations between DNA methylation and the expression of miRNAs, such as mir-129-2, mir-551b, and mir-708 (hypermethylated miRNAs) and mir-21, mir-34a, mir-135a, mir-155, mir-574, mir-664, mir-1204, and the cluster mir-29a/29b-1 (hypomethylated miRNAs) were found to be DNA methylation-dependent in CLL [50].

Other than DNA methylation, histone acetylation represents another dysregulated epigenetic phenomenon in cancer. A decrease in the level of acetylated histones can downregulate the expression of anti-oncogenic miRNAs, as evidenced by studies utilizing histone deacetylase inhibitors (e.g., 4-phenylbutyric acid) [53].

Meanwhile, DNA or histone modification enzymes are also targets of dysregulated miRNAs in cancer. Fabbri et al. first reported that the miR-29 family, whose expression is downregulated in cancer, can target DNMT3 [54], and that the ectopic expression of miR-29 family in lung cancer could restore methylation at loci containing tumor suppressor genes (e.g., those encoding WWOX and FHIT), which are aberrantly methylated in lung cancer [54]. A study by Fabbri et al. showed that DNMT3A is a prognostic factor in lung cancer, and the overexpression of miR-29 suppressed tumorigenicity [54]. Moreover, further studies revealed that miR-29 downregulates the expression of oncogenes such as *TCL1*, *MCL1*, and *BCL2L2* and indirectly activates the p53 pathway through p85a (PI3K subunit) targeting [55]. It also became apparent that in cancer, DNMTs are regulated by several miRNAs (e.g., miR-148a, miR-143) [56-58].

Some miRNAs (e.g., miR-101, miR-26a) affect chromatin modification by targeting EZH2, another important epigenetic factor. EZH2 is a member of the polycomb group of proteins, which are key regulators that silence numerous developmental genes. EZH2 is the catalytic subunit of polycomb repressive complex 2, and trimethylates H3K27 [58].

1.5. Alterations in miRNA Processing

The expression of miRNA can also be modified as a result of defects in the miRNA biogenesis pathway (Figure 1). Dysregulation of the enzymes and cofactors involved in these post-transcriptional pathways can affect the levels of mature miRNAs and have important biological effects. In the canonical pathway, two RNase III enzyme complexes—the Drosha/DGCR8 complex and the Dicer complex—are important for the complete maturation of miRNA [59]. Analysis of mature and pri-miRNA expression in tumor and normal samples revealed that the correlation between pri-miRNA and mature miRNA was disrupted in tumor samples [59]. Available evidence suggests global alteration in miRNA processing in cancer. Knockdown of Drosha, DGCR8, or Dicer increased tumorigenicity in mouse lung adenocarcinoma [60, 61], while knockout of p68 or p72, other Drosha/DGCR8 microprocessor complex components, in mice resulted in embryonic lethality. Studies focused on proteins interacting with p68 have revealed that several TFs, such as p53, Smads, and estrogen receptor-α, positively regulate microprocessor activity [62-64]. Similarly, hippo tumor suppressor signaling related Yes-associated protein 1 negatively regulates microprocessor activity by interfering with the association of p72 with the microprocessor complex [65].

Recent studies have contributed toward elucidating the mechanism of expression of the key regulators involved in miRNA processing. The expression of the key components of miRNA biogenesis, including Dicer, is regulated by tumor-derived miRNAs such as the miR-103/107 family, miR-221/222 family, miR-29a, and miR-15a/16-1 [66-70]. In addition, the expression of Dicer is upregulated by miR-200c, which is associated with decreased migration and invasion in breast cancer [67].

2. MIRNA IN PCNSL

The molecular biology of PCNSL is not well understood. Two groups have published the "CNS" signatures of PCNSL, or the unique gene expression and pathway signatures, by comparing PCNSL with non-CNS DLBCL [71-74]. Considering the architecture of CNS lymphoma, there are at least two major growth patterns of PCNSL, which are characterized by low or high tumor cell density. High-density tumors that express activated STAT-6 are associated with a worse prognosis after treatment with standard methotrexate-based regimens than are tumors of low cell density, independent of STAT-6 activation status [71].

These observations coincided with previous studies in which PCNSL was found to share characteristics with systemic DLBCL with respect to the activated B cells (ABCs; e.g., immunoglobulin [Ig] M expression, lack of class switch recombination, NF-kB pathway activation) and the germinal center B cell (GCB) subtypes (high Ig gene mutation frequency with ongoing somatic hypermutation, BCL6 expression) [75-77]. This section will discuss the miRNA expression in DLBCL, including PCNSL.

In the later sections, the advancements in the investigation of biomarkers from patient samples brought about by a decade of developments in detection technologies are discussed.

2.1. miRNA Expression in PCNSL Tissue

In DLBCL, miRNAs are well characterized in terms of their roles in hematopoiesis and lymphomagenesis [78-81]. Roehle et al. reported altered miRNA expression in DLBCL compared with that in normal lymph nodes (upregulated: miR-155, miR-210, miR-17-5p, and miR-106a; downregulated: miR-150, miR-145, miR-328, miR-139, miR-99a, miR-10a, miR-95, miR-149, miR-320, miR-151, and let-7e) [82]. Malumbres et al. identified DLBCL subtype-specific miRNA signatures (i.e., specific to ABC-like-DLBCL or GCB-like-DLBCL) [83]. High expression of nine miRNAs in ABC-like-DLBCL has been identified (miR-146b, miR-146a, miR-21, miR-155, miR-500, miR-222, miR-363, miR-574-3p, and miR-574-5p).

With respect to the relationship between the expression of single miRNAs and survival in patients with DLBCL, Roehle et al. showed that a reduction in miR-127 levels significantly correlates with poor event-free survival (EFS) and overall survival (OS). MiR-127 was previously reported to be methylated in tumor cells, and the expression level was inversely proportional to the expression of BCL6, a known proto-oncogene [53]. Moreover, reduced expression of four miRNAs (miR-21, miR-23a, miR-27a, and miR-34a) was found to be associated with poor OS. Reduced miR-19 expression is correlated with poor EFS, whereas reduced expression of miR-195 and let-7g is associated with good EFS [82].

Malumbres et al. reported the correlation between the differential expression of miRNAs between GCB-like and ABC-like cell lines and the outcome of DLBCL patients treated with rituximab-CHOP (R-CHOP). The high expression of miR-222, characteristically expressed in ABC-like cell lines, was associated with inferior OS and progression-free survival (PFS). No correlations between the expression of miR-21 or miR-155 and OS or PFS were observed [83]. Meanwhile, Iqbal et al. reported that high expression of three miRNAs (miR-16, miR-155, and miR-363) was significantly associated with R-CHOP therapy failure in DLBCL, whereas high expression of miR-24 was associated with a favorable treatment response.

According to this report, the low expression of three genes—KLHL5, PSIP1, and CHD9—regulated by miR-155 had a significant correlation with poor EFS in ABC-like DLBCL, but not in GCB-DLBCL [84].

Fischer et al. reported that the expression of 13 miRNAs (miR-9, miR-20b, miR-155, miR-340, miR-17-5p, miR-148a, miR-30b, miR-27b, miR-26b, miR-146b, miR-20a, miR-30c, and let-7g) was significantly higher in PCNSL than in nodal DLBCL [84]. Meanwhile, the expression of five miRNAs (miR-199a, miR-214, miR-432, miR-193b, and miR-145) was reduced in PCNSL compared with that in nodal DLBCL. Of the 13 miRNAs whose expression was upregulated in PCNSL, miR-9, miR-20b, miR-155, miR-340, miR-17-5p, and miR-148a showed the highest expression [85].

Fischer's study also showed that miR-155 and miR-92, members of the miR-17-92 cluster, were highly expressed in both PCNSL and nodal DLBCL. Other than miR-92, other members of the mir-17-92 family (miR-17-5p, miR-20a, and miR-20b) were also upregulated in PCNSL. The expression of miR-17-92 family members is upregulated via the Myc pathway, thus accelerating Myc-induced lymphoma development [85]. In PCNSL, downregulation of miR-145 expression, which directly suppress the expression of Myc, also suggests Myc pathway activation.

Moreover, upregulation of the expression of miR-9 and miR-30 families in PCNSL might cause a Myc activation-mediated block in B cell terminal differentiation through the inhibition of PRDM-1-mediated Myc repression. In GCBs, miR-9 and miR-30 are overexpressed, leading to the downregulation of PRDM-1, a regulator of plasma cell differentiation [86, 87]. These results could shed light on the stronger Myc expression observed in PCNSL than in nodal DLBCL [73].

In addition, miR-17-92 [88, 89] and miR-155 [90-92] have been reported to exhibit oncogenic properties in lymphoma [21]. Notably, miR-155 upregulation has been reported in response to immune stimuli such as tumor necrosis factor-α, and this miRNA has been demonstrated to attenuate TGF-β-mediated activation by retinoblastoma protein [92].

Here, miR-21 overexpression has been observed in many types of cancers including lymphomas [8]. The role of miR-21 in cancer has been characterized by using *in vitro* and *in vivo* models [10-11]. These studies have identified miR-21 as an onco-miRNA to which some tumors including lymphoma are "addicted" [11]. MiR-21 expression is significantly elevated in both DLBCL and PCNSL [93]. Interestingly, miR-21 higher expression is observed in activated B cells response to IL-4, helper T-cell produced cytokine [94]. These results suggested miR-21 may help maintain B cell hyperactivation in lymphomagenesis [5]. As mentioned above, miR-21 is robustly expressed in DLBCLs, miR-21 has been regarded as a candidate of most potent biomarker from biomaterials (e.g., serum, CSF) in patient with DLBCLs.

Robertus et al. reported the expression of 15 miRNAs by using qRT-PCR (miR-21, miR-19, miR-15b, miR-92a, miR-20a, miR-15a, miR-19a, miR-17-5p, miR-181a, miR-155, miR-18a, miR-221, miR-17-3p, miR-127, and miR-16). In DLBCL, miR-21 and miR-19b are highly expressed; in particular, miR-21 has a 100-fold higher expression level and miR-19b has a 10-fold higher expression level compared with other miRNAs [92]. Robertus' study especially showed that miR-17-5p and miR-127 are candidates for markers that can distinguish between PCNSL and other extra-nodal testicular DLBCLs [93].

2.2. miRNA as a Biomarker in Patients with PCNSL

Identification of the origin of a disease is critical to successful treatment. Therefore, if miRNAs could distinguish tumor origins, subtypes, oncogenic mutations, and cancer predispositions, and regulate the most important cellular processes, it is logical to hypothesize that these elements can help predict cancer prognosis and/or responses to specific therapies. Particularly, the development of non-invasive techniques is crucial for facilitating diagnostic analysis. For this, blood samples from patients are most convenient for the detection of cancer-specific biomarkers. CSF is also suitable for detection, follow-up, and prognostication in CNS diseases such as PCNSL and brain cancer [95-98].

The use of non-coding RNAs (miRNAs in particular) has gained significant attention since the discovery that these RNA species could be detected both extra-and intracellularly in peripheral tissues and as free or exosomal RNAs in culture medium from tumor cells. Regarding the tumor-derived RNAs in culture medium, these RNAs have also been detected as circulating free or exosomal RNAs in blood and CSF [98]. The increasing use of powerful detection techniques such as massive sequencing has significantly boosted the search for minimally invasive disease indicators [96]. This technology is rapidly evolving and promises great advances in the field of biomarker discovery, particularly in the area of nervous system pathology. The CNS is the least accessible of all tissues; therefore, advances in this field will be of great benefit. Similar to detection technologies, several advanced methods for extraction and preparation of RNAs from tissue samples have been developed.

These strategies accelerate the exploration of miRNA profiles in the serum and CSF of patients with various cancers [94, 99-103].

As mentioned above, in various cancers, increased miR-21 expression is an indicator of poor outcome. However, in DLBCL, decreased miR-21 expression indicates poor prognosis. A recent study showed higher expression of miR-21, miR-155, and miR-210 in the serum of patients with DLBLC than in normal controls [104]. Thus, high miR-21 levels in serum are associated with a more favorable clinical outcome in DLBCL [104]. Fang et al. also reported a higher expression of miR-21 in the serum of patients with DLBCL. Elevated levels of miR-155, miR-15, miR-16, and miR-29c and low levels of miR-34a have been detected in the serum of patients with DLBCL [105].

Baraniskin et al. reported the expression of six miRNAs (miR-21, miR-19b, miR-92a, miR-15b, miR-106b, and miR-204) and control miRNA (miR-24) in the CSF taken from patients with PCNSL and healthy controls. A higher expression of three candidate miRNAs (miR-21, miR-19b, and miR-92) was observed in the CSF of patients with PCNSL than in healthy controls. The expression of these three miRNAs in the CSF also distinguishes PCNSL from other diseases derived from the CNS. Hence, these miRNAs are potential candidates for biomarkers [106]. Baraniskin et al. also reported miRNA expression in the CSF of patients diagnosed with PCNSL [107]. The expression of miR-21, miR-19b, and miR-92 was monitored in patients with different clinical statuses. The difference in patient status (e.g., complete remission, recurrence after initial partial remission, disease recurrence following complete remission) was reflected in the differences in miRNA expression. In the case of complete remission, these three miRNAs were undetectable in the CSF [107]. Another study by Baraniskin showed that the expression of miR-15b and miR-21 in CSF could be used to distinguish between PCNSL and glioma [108]. Moreover, in other tumors, such as classical Hodgkin lymphoma, serum miRNA levels were observed to change after therapy [99, 109].

Mao et al. reported conflicting data about the correlation between serum and CSF miR-21 levels and prognosis in patients with PCNSL [110]. These conflicting results need to be confirmed through additional analyses by using different datasets.

Roth et al. recently reported an analysis of serum miRNA expression patterns in PCNSL patients by using next-generation sequencing and qRT-PCR. In that study, distinctions between PCNSL patients with long-term and short-term survival were validated by using miRNA. Twelve miRNAs (miR-151-a, miR-151-b, miR-106a-5p, miR-219-5p, miR-17-5p, miR-6130, miR-183-3p, miR-30d-5p, miR-181c-3p, miR-96-5p, miR-194-5p, and miR-503-5p) were found to differ significantly between the two groups [111].

From these results, despite available data regarding miRNA expression in rare CNS disease subtypes, datasets specific to PCNSL remain few in number, and the characteristics of PCNSL remain unclear. However, a large-data, comprehensive analysis on DLBCL was published in 2015 [19]. Similar future research concerning PCNSL will facilitate the understanding of characteristics associated with an improved prognosis.

In a previous report, microarray profiling in combination with real-time RT-PCR and locked nucleic acid-based in situ hybridization, uncovered 44 miRNAs expressed in the adult mouse brain network. Interestingly, >3-fold enrichment of this miRNA profile was detected in the spinal cord, cerebellum, medulla oblongata, pons, hypothalamus, hippocampus, neocortex, olfactory bulb, eye, and pituitary gland [112]. Various expression patterns in different areas of the brain indicate the complexity of brain development. Such studies might clarify the etiologies of brain diseases through the analysis of miRNA expression in the human brain.

Conclusion

The past decade yielded an explosion of research focused on small non-coding RNAs, such as exogenous siRNAs and endogenous miRNAs. Progressive improvements in analytical techniques have revealed patterns of miRNA dysregulation in various cancers.

Currently, researchers continue to encounter difficulties in the sampling and preparation of materials suitable for diagnostic procedures. To improve the detection of small molecules such as miRNAs in blood and CSF samples, we must distinguish between the normal tissue microenvironment and disease-derived molecules. After another decade of research and the use of advanced miRNA-RNA network tools, we expect that the functions of most of the poorly-understood miRNAs will be elucidated.

References

[1] Ferreri AJ, Marturano E. (2012) Primary CNS lymphoma. *Best Pract Res Clin Haematol.*, 25, 119-30.

[2] Lawrie CH. (2013) MicroRNAs and lymphomagenesis: a functional review. *Br J Haematol.*, 160, 571-81.

[3] Tagawa H, Ikeda S, Sawada K. (2013) Role of microRNA in the pathogenesis of malignant lymphoma. *Cancer Sci.*, 104, 801-9.

[4] Lawrie CH, Saunders NJ, Soneji S, Palazzo S, Dunlop HM, Cooper CD, Brown PJ, Troussard X, Mossafa H, Enver T, Pezzella F, Boultwood J, Wainscoat JS, Hatton CS. (2008) MicroRNA expression in lymphocyte development and maligrancy. *Leukemia,* 22, 1440-6.

[5] Jardin F, Figeac M. (2013) MicroRNAs in lymphoma, from diagrosis to targeted therapy. *Curr Opin Oncol.*, 25, 480-6.

[6] Davis-Dusenbery BN, Hata A. (2010) MicroRNA in Cancer: The Involvement of Aberrant MicroRNA Biogenesis Regulatory Pathways. *Genes Cancer.*, 1, 1100-14.

[7] Li Z, Rana TM. (2014) Therapeutic targeting of microRNAs: current status and future challenges. *Nat Rev Drug Discov.*, 13, 622-38.

[8] Iorio MV, Croce CM. (2012) MicroRNA dysregulation in cancer: diagnostics, monitoring and therapeutics. A comprehensive review. *EMBO Mol Med.*, 4, 143-59.

[9] Zhang B, Pan X, Cobb GP, Anderson TA. (2007) microRNAs as oncogenes and tumor suppressors. *Dev Biol.*, 302, 1-12.

[10] Yang CH, Pfeffer SR, Sims M, Yue J, Wang Y, Linga VG, Paulus E, Davidoff AM, Pfeffer LM. (2015) The oncogenic microRNA-21 inhibits the tumor suppressive activity of FBXO11 to promote tumorigenesis. *J Biol Chem.*, 290, 6037-46.

[11] Medina PP, Nolde M, Slack FJ. (2010) OncomiR addiction in an in vivo model of microRNA-21-induced pre-B-cell lymphoma. *Nature,* 467, 86-90.

[12] Dal Bo M, Bomben R, Hernández L, Gattei V. (2015) The MYC/miR-17-92 axis in lymphoproliferative disorders: A common pathway with therapeutic potential. *Oncotarget,* 6, 19381-92.

[13] Babar IA, Cheng CJ, Booth CJ, Liang X, Weidhaas JB, Saltzman WM, Slack FJ. (2012) Nanoparticle-based therapy in an in vivo microRNA-155 (miR-155)-dependent mouse model of lymphoma. *Proc Natl Acad Sci U S A.,* 109, E1695-704.

[14] Saito Y, Nakaoka T, Saito H. (2015) microRNA-34a as a Therapeutic Agent against Human Cancer. *J Clin Med.*, 4, 1951-9.

[15] Yamakuchi M, Ferlito M, Lowenstein CJ. (2008) miR-34a repression of SIRT1 regulates apoptosis. *Proc Natl Acad Sci U S A.*, 105, 13421-6.

[16] He L, He X, Lim LP, de Stanchina E, Xuan Z, Liang Y, Xue W, Zender L, Magnus J, Ridzon D, Jackson AL, Linsley PS, Chen C, Lowe SW, Cleary MA, Hannon GJ. (2007) A microRNA component of the p53 tumour suppressor network. *Nature,* 447, 1130-4.

[17] Calin GA, Cimmino A, Fabbri M, Ferracin M, Wojcik SE, Shimizu M, Taccioli C, Zanesi N, Garzon R, Aqeilan RI, Alder H, Volinia S, Rassenti L, Liu X, Liu CG, Kipps TJ, Negrini M, Croce CM. (2008) MiR-15a and miR-16-1 cluster functions in human leukemia. *Proc Natl Acad Sci U S A., 105*, 5166-71.

[18] Gattolliat CH, Uguen A, Pesson M, Trillet K, Simon B, Doucet L, Robaszkiewicz M, Corcos L. (2015) MicroRNA and targeted mRNA expression profiling analysis in human colorectal adenomas and adenocarcinomas. *Eur J Cancer*, 51, 409-20.

[19] Lim EL, Trinh DL, Scott DW, Chu A, Krzywinski M, Zhao Y, Robertson AG, Mungall AJ, Schein J, Boyle M, Mottok A, Ennishi D, Johnson NA, Steidl C, Connors JM, Morin RD, Gascoyne RD, Marra MA. (2015) Comprehensive miRNA sequence analysis reveals survival differences in diffuse large B-cell lymphoma patients. *Genome Biol.,* 16:18.

[20] Iorio MV, Ferracin M, Liu CG, Veronese A, Spizzo R, Sabbioni S, Magri E, Pedriali M, Fabbri M, Campiglio M, Ménard S, Palazzo JP, Rosenberg A, Musiani P, Volinia S,

Nenci I, Calin GA, Querzoli P, Negrini M, Croce CM. (2005) MicroRNA gene expression deregulation in human breast cancer. *Cancer Res.*, 65, 7065-70.
[21] Calin GA, Croce CM. (2006) MicroRNA signatures in human cancers. *Nat Rev Cancer.*, 6, 857-66.
[22] Jansson MD, Lund AH. (2012) MicroRNA and cancer. *Mol Oncol.*, 6, 590-610.
[23] Döhner H, Stilgenbauer S, Benner A, Leupolt E, Kröber A, Bullinger L, Döhner K, Bentz M, Lichter P. (2000) Genomic aberrations and survival in chronic lymphocytic leukemia. *N Engl J Med.*, 343, 1910-6.
[24] Gong J, Tong Y, Zhang HM, Wang K, Hu T, Shan G, Sun J, Guo AY. (2012) Genome-wide identification of SNPs in microRNA genes and the SNP effects on microRNA target binding and biogenesis. *Hum Mutat.*, 33, 254-63.
[25] Calin GA, Dumitru CD, Shimizu M, Bichi R, Zupo S, Noch E, Aldler H, Rattan S, Keating M, Rai K, Rassenti L, Kipps T, Negrini M, Bullrich F, Croce CM. (2002) Frequent deletions and down-regulation of micro- RNA genes miR15 and miR16 at 13q14 in chronic lymphocytic leukemia. *Proc Natl Acad Sci U S A.,* 99, 15524-9.
[26] Fabbri M, Bottoni A, Shimizu M, Spizzo R, Nicoloso MS, Rossi S, Barbarotto E, Cimmino A, Adair B, Wojcik SE, Valeri N, Calore F, Sampath D, Fanini F, Vannini I, Musuraca G, Dell'Aquila M, Alder H, Davuluri RV, Rassenti LZ, Negrini M, Nakamura T, Amadori D, Kay NE, Rai KR, Keating MJ, Kipps TJ, Calin GA, Croce CM. (2011) Association of a microRNA/TP53 feedback circuitry with pathogenesis and outcome of B-cell chronic lymphocytic leukemia. *JAMA.,* 305, 59-67.
[27] Dürig J, Nückel H, Cremer M, Führer A, Halfmeyer K, Fandrey J, Möröy T, Klein-Hitpass L, Dührsen U. (2003) ZAP-70 expression is a prognostic factor in chronic lymphocytic leukemia. *Leukemia,* 17, 2426-34.
[28] Tagawa H, Tsuzuki S, Suzuki R, Karnan S, Ota A, Kameoka Y, Suguro M, Matsuo K, Yamaguchi M, Okamoto M, Morishima Y, Nakamura S, Seto M. (2004) Genome-wide array-based comparative genomic hybridization of diffuse large B-cell lymphoma: comparison between CD5-positive and CD5-negative cases. *Cancer Res.,* 64, 5948-55.
[29] Tagawa H, Seto M. (2005) A microRNA cluster as a target of genomic amplification in malignant lymphoma. *Leukemia,* 19, 2013-6.
[30] Mogilyansky E, Rigoutsos I. (2013) The miR-17/92 cluster: a comprehensive update on its genomics, genetics, functions and increasingly important and numerous roles in health and disease. *Cell Death Differ.,* 20, 1603-14.
[31] Calin GA, Sevignani C, Dumitru CD, Hyslop T, Noch E, Yendamuri S, Shimizu M, Rattan S, Bullrich F, Negrini M, Croce CM. (2004) Human microRNA genes are frequently located at fragile sites and genomic regions involved in cancers. *Proc Natl Acad Sci U S A.,* 101, 2999-3004.
[32] Navarro A, Gaya A, Martinez A, Urbano-Ispizua A, Pons A, Balagué O, Gel B, Abrisqueta P, Lopez-Guillermo A, Artells R, Montserrat E, Monzo M. (2008) MicroRNA expression profiling in classic Hodgkin lymphoma. *Blood,* 111, 2825-32.
[33] Li C, Kim SW, Rai D, Bolla AR, Adhvaryu S, Kinney MC, Robetorye RS, Aguiar RC. (2009) Copy number abnormalities, MYC activity, and the genetic fingerprint of normal B cells mechanistically define the microRNA profile of diffuse large B-cell lymphoma. *Blood,* 113, 6681-90.

[34] Troppan K, Wenzl K, Deutsch A, Ling H, Neumeister P, Pichler M. (2014) MicroRNAs in diffuse large B-cell lymphoma: implications for pathogenesis, diagnosis, prognosis and therapy. *Anticancer Res.*, 34, 557-64.

[35] Lu TX, Young KH, Xu W, Li JY. (2016) TP53 dysfunction in diffuse large B-cell lymphoma. *Crit Rev Oncol Hematol.*, 97, 47–55.

[36] Yu J, Wang F, Yang GH, Wang FL, Ma YN, Du ZW, Zhang JW. (2006) Human microRNA clusters: genomic organization and expression profile in leukemia cell lines. *Biochem Biophys Res Commun.*, 349, 59-68.

[37] Wu HL, Heneidi S, Chuang TY, Diamond MP, Layman LC, Azziz R, Chen YH. (2014) The expression of the miR-25/93/106b family of micro-RNAs in the adipose tissue of women with polycystic ovary syndrome. *J Clin Endocrinol Metab.*, 99, E2754-61.

[38] Dylla L, Jedlicka P. (2013) Growth-promoting role of the miR-106a~363 cluster in Ewing sarcoma. *PLoS One,* 8, e63032.

[39] Welten SM, Bastiaansen AJ, de Jong RC, de Vries MR, Peters EA, Boonstra MC, Sheikh SP, La Monica N, Kandimalla ER, Quax PH, Nossent AY. (2014) Inhibition of 14q32 MicroRNAs miR-329, miR-487b, miR-494, and miR-495 increases neovascularization and blood flow recovery after ischemia. *Circ Res.*, 115, 696-708.

[40] Olive V, Jiang I, He L. (2010) mir-17-92, a cluster of miRNAs in the midst of the cancer network. *Int J Biochem Cell Biol.*, 42, 1348-54.

[41] Li Y, Vecchiarelli-Federico LM, Li YJ, Egan SE, Spaner D, Hough MR, Ben-David Y. (2012) The miR-17-92 cluster expands multipotent hematopoietic progenitors whereas imbalanced expression of its individual oncogenic miRNAs promotes leukemia in mice. *Blood,* 119, 4486-98.

[42] Michlewski G, Guil S, Semple CA, Cáceres JF. (2008) Posttranscriptional regulation of miRNAs harboring conserved terminal loops. *Mol Cell*, 32, 383-93.

[43] Kumar P, Luo Y, Tudela C, Alexander JM, Mendelson CR. (2013) The c-Myc-regulated microRNA-17~92 (miR-17~92) and miR-106a~363 clusters target hCYP19A1 and hGCM1 to inhibit human trophoblast differentiation. *Mol Cell Biol.*, 33, 1782-96.

[44] Zhao ZN, Bai JX, Zhou Q, Yan B, Qin WW, Jia LT, Meng YL, Jin BQ, Yao LB, Wang T, Yang AG. (2012) TSA suppresses miR-106b-93-25 cluster expression through downregulation of MYC and inhibits proliferation and induces apoptosis in human EMC. *PLoS One*, 7, e45133.

[45] Alencar AJ, Malumbres R, Kozloski GA, Advani R, Talreja N, Chinichian S, Briones J, Natkunam Y, Sehn LH, Gascoyne RD, Tibshirani R, Lossos IS. (2011) MicroRNAs are independent predictors of outcome in diffuse large B-cell lymphoma patients treated with R-CHOP. *Clin Cancer Res.*, 17, 4125-35.

[46] Jackstadt R, Hermeking H. (2015) MicroRNAs as regulators and mediators of c-MYC function. *Biochim Biophys Acta.*, 1849, 544-53.

[47] Rokavec M, Li H, Jiang L, Hermeking H. (2014) The p53/microRNA connection in gastrointestinal cancer. *Clin Exp Gastroenterol.*, 7, 395-413.

[48] Baer C, Claus R, Plass C. (2013) Genome-wide epigenetic regulation of miRNAs in cancer. *Cancer Res.*, 73, 473-7.

[49] Lopez-Serra P, Esteller M. (2012) DNA methylation-associated silencing of tumor-suppressor microRNAs in cancer. *Oncogene,* 31, 1609-22.

[50] Baer C, Claus R, Frenzel LP, Zucknick M, Park YJ, Gu L, Weichenhan D, Fischer M, Pallasch CP, Herpel E, Rehli M, Byrd JC, Wendtner CM, Plass C. (2012) Extensive promoter DNA hypermethylation and hypomethylation is associated with aberrant microRNA expression in chronic lymphocytic leukemia. *Cancer Res.*, 72, 3775-85.

[51] Dudziec E, Miah S, Choudhry HM, Owen HC, Blizard S, Glover M, Hamdy FC, Catto JW. (2011) Hypermethylation of CpG islands and shores around specific microRNAs and mirtrons is associated with the phenotype and presence of bladder cancer. *Clin Cancer Res.*, 17, 1287-96.

[52] Kulis M, Heath S, Bibikova M, Queirós AC, Navarro A, Clot G, Martínez-Trillos A, Castellano G, Brun-Heath I, Pinyol M, Barberán-Soler S, Papasaikas P, Jares P, Beà S, Rico D, Ecker S, Rubio M, Royo R, Ho V, Klotzle B, Hernández L, Conde L, López-Guerra M, Colomer D, Villamor N, Aymerich M, Rozman M, Bayes M, Gut M, Gelpí JL, Orozco M, Fan JB, Quesada V, Puente XS, Pisano DG, Valencia A, López-Guillermo A, Gut I, López-Otín C, Campo E, Martín-Subero JI. (2012) Epigenomic analysis detects widespread gene-body DNA hypomethylation in chronic lymphocytic leukemia. *Nat Genet.*, 44, 1236-42.

[53] Saito Y, Liang G, Egger G, Friedman JM, Chuang JC, Coetzee GA, Jones PA. (2006) Specific activation of microRNA-127 with downregulation of the proto-oncogene BCL6 by chromatin-modifying drugs in human cancer cells. *Cancer Cell*, 9, 435-43.

[54] Fabbri M, Garzon R, Cimmino A, Liu Z, Zanesi N, Callegari E, Liu S, Alder H, Costinean S, Fernandez-Cymering C, Volinia S, Guler G, Morrison CD, Chan KK, Marcucci G, Calin GA, Huebner K, Croce CM. (2007) MicroRNA-29 family reverts aberrant methylation in lung cancer by targeting DNA methyltransferases 3A and 3B. *Proc Natl Acad Sci U S A.*, 104, 15805-10.

[55] Chung HJ, Choi YE, Kim ES, Han YH, Park MJ, Bae IH. (2015) miR-29b attenuates tumorigenicity and stemness maintenance in human glioblastoma multiforme by directly targeting BCL2L2. *Oncotarget*, 6, 18429-44.

[56] Ng EK, Tsang WP, Ng SS, Jin HC, Yu J, Li JJ, Röcken C, Ebert MP, Kwok TT, Sung JJ. (2009) MicroRNA-143 targets DNA methyltransferases 3A in colorectal cancer. *Br J Cancer*, 101, 699-706.

[57] Braconi C, Huang N, Patel T. (2010) MicroRNA-dependent regulation of DNA methyltransferase-1 and tumor suppressor gene expression by interleukin-6 in human malignant cholangiocytes. *Hepatology*, 51, 881-90.

[58] Suzuki H, Maruyama R, Yamamoto E, Kai M. (2013) Epigenetic alteration and microRNA dysregulation in cancer. *Front Genet.*, 4, 258.

[59] Thomson JM, Newman M, Parker JS, Morin-Kensicki EM, Wright T, Hammond SM. (2006) Extensive post-transcriptional regulation of microRNAs and its implications for cancer. *Genes Dev.*, 20, 2202-7.

[60] Han J, Lee Y, Yeom KH, Kim YK, Jin H, Kim VN. (2004) The Drosha-DGCR8 complex in primary microRNA processing. *Genes Dev.,* 18, 3016-27.

[61] Fukuda T, Yamagata K, Fujiyama S, Matsumoto T, Koshida I, Yoshimura K, Mihara M, Naitou M, Endoh H, Nakamura T, Akimoto C, Yamamoto Y, Katagiri T, Foulds C, Takezawa S, Kitagawa H, Takeyama K, O'Malley BW, Kato S. (2007) DEAD-box RNA helicase subunits of the Drosha complex are required for processing of rRNA and a subset of microRNAs. *Nat Cell Biol.*, 9, 604-11.

[62] Fuller-Pace FV, Ali S. (2008) The DEAD box RNA helicases p68 (Ddx5) and p72 (Ddx17): novel transcriptional co-regulators. *Biochem Soc Trans.*, 36, 609-12.

[63] Kumar MS, Lu J, Mercer KL, Golub TR, Jacks T. (2007) Impaired microRNA processing enhances cellular transformation and tumorigenesis. *Nat Genet.*, 39, 673-7.

[64] Musilova K, Mraz M. (2015) MicroRNAs in B-cell lymphomas: how a complex biology gets more complex. *Leukemia,* 29, 1004-17.

[65] Mori M, Triboulet R, Mohseni M, Schlegelmilch K, Shrestha K, Camargo FD, Gregory RI. (2014) Hippo signaling regulates microprocessor and links cell-density-dependent miRNA biogenesis to cancer. *Cell,* 156, 893-906.

[66] Kang W, Tong JH, Lung RW, Dong Y, Zhao J, Liang Q, Zhang L, Pan Y, Yang W, Pang JC, Cheng AS, Yu J, To KF (2015) Targeting of YAP1 by microRNA-15a and microRNA-16-1 exerts tumor suppressor function in gastric adenocarcinoma. *Mol Cancer*, 14, 52.

[67] Cochrane DR, Cittelly DM, Howe EN, Spoelstra NS, McKinsey EL, LaPara K, Elias A, Yee D, Richer JK. (2010) MicroRNAs link estrogen receptor alpha status and Dicer levels in breast cancer. *Horm Cancer*, 1, 306-19.

[68] Martello G, Rosato A, Ferrari F, Manfrin A, Cordenonsi M, Dupont S, Enzo E, Guzzardo V, Rondina M, Spruce T, Parenti AR, Daidone MG, Bicciato S, Piccolo S. (2010) A MicroRNA targeting dicer for metastasis control. *Cell,* 141, 1195-207.

[69] Inoue T, Iinuma H, Ogawa E, Inaba T, Fukushima R. (2012) Clinicopathological and prognostic significance of microRNA-107 and its relationship to DICER1 mRNA expression in gastric cancer. *Oncol Rep.*, 27, 1759-64.

[70] Luo Z, Dai Y, Zhang L, Jiang C, Li Z, Yang J, McCarthy JB, She X, Zhang W, Ma J, Xiong W, Wu M, Lu J, Li X, Li X, Xiang J, Li G. (2013) miR-18a promotes malignant progression by impairing microRNA biogenesis in nasopharyngeal carcinoma. *Carcinogenesis,* 34, 415-25.

[71] Rubenstein JL, Shen A, Batchelor TT, Kadoch C, Treseler P, Shuman MA. (2009) Differential gene expression in central nervous system lymphoma. *Blood*, 113, 266-7.

[72] Montesinos-Rongen M, Brunn A, Bentink S, Basso K, Lim WK, Klapper W, Schaller C, Reifenberger G, Rubenstein J, Wiestler OD, Spang R, Dalla-Favera R, Siebert R, Deckert M. (2008) Gene expression profiling suggests primary central nervous system lymphomas to be derived from a late germinal center B cell. *Leukemia,* 22, 400-5.

[73] Rubenstein JL, Fridlyand J, Shen A, Aldape K, Ginzinger D, Batchelor T, Treseler P, Berger M, McDermott M, Prados M, Karch J, Okada C, Hyun W, Parikh S, Haqq C, Shuman M. (2006) Gene expression and angiotropism in primary CNS lymphoma. *Blood*, 107, 3716-23.

[74] Tun HW, Personett D, Baskerville KA, Menke DM, Jaeckle KA, Kreinest P, Edenfield B, Zubair AC, O'Neill BP, Lai WR, Park PJ, McKinney M. (2008) Pathway analysis of primary central nervous system lymphoma. *Blood*, 111, 3200-10.

[75] Camilleri-Broët S, Crinière E, Broët P, Delwail V, Mokhtari K, Moreau A, Kujas M, Raphaël M, Iraqi W, Sautès-Fridman C, Colombat P, Hoang-Xuan K, Martin A. (2006) A uniform activated B-cell-like immunophenotype might explain the poor prognosis of primary central nervous system lymphomas: analysis of 83 cases. *Blood*, 107, 190-6.

[76] Braaten KM, Betensky RA, de Leval L, Okada Y, Hochberg FH, Louis DN, Harris NL, Batchelor TT. (2003) BCL-6 expression predicts improved survival in patients with primary central nervous system lymphoma. *Clin Cancer Res.*, 9, 1063-9.

[77] Jiang L, Marlow LA, Cooper SJ, Roemeling CV, Menke DM, Copland JA, Tun HW. (2010) Selective central nervous system tropism of primary central nervous system lymphoma. *Int J Clin Exp Pathol.* 3, 763-7.

[78] Visani M, Acquaviva G, Marucci G, Ragazzi M, Fraceschi E, Brandes A, Tallini G, Pession A, Biase D. (2015) MicroRNA in Brain Neoplasia: A Review. *Int J Brain Disord Treat.,* 1:002.

[79] Mazan-Mamczarz K, Gartenhaus RB. (2013) Role of microRNA deregulation in the pathogenesis of diffuse large B-cell lymphoma (DLBCL). *Leuk Res.,* 37, 1420-8.

[80] Zheng J, Xu J, Ma S, Sun X, Geng M, Wang L. (2013) Clinicopathological study of gene rearrangement and microRNA expression of primary central nervous system diffuse large B-cell lymphomas. *Int J Clin Exp Pathol.*, 6, 2048-55.

[81] Eis PS, Tam W, Sun L, Chadburn A, Li Z, Gomez MF, Lund E, Dahlberg JE. (2005) Accumulation of miR-155 and BIC RNA in human B cell lymphomas. *Proc Natl Acad Sci U S A.*, 102, 3627-32.

[82] Roehle A, Hoefig KP, Repsilber D, Thorns C, Ziepert M, Wesche KO, Thiere M, Loeffler M, Klapper W, Pfreundschuh M, Matolcsy A, Bernd HW, Reiniger L, Merz H, Feller AC. (2008) MicroRNA signatures characterize diffuse large B-cell lymphomas and follicular lymphomas. *Br J Haematol.*, 142, 732-44.

[83] Malumbres R, Sarosiek KA, Cubedo E, Ruiz JW, Jiang X, Gascoyne RD, Tibshirani R, Lossos IS. (2009) Differentiation stage-specific expression of microRNAs in B lymphocytes and diffuse large B-cell lymphomas. *Blood,* 113, 3754-64.

[84] Iqbal J, Shen Y, Huang X, Liu Y, Wake L, Liu C, Deffenbacher K, Lachel CM, Wang C, Rohr J, Guo S, Smith LM, Wright G, Bhagavathi S, Dybkaer K, Fu K, Greiner TC, Vose JM, Jaffe E, Rimsza L, Rosenwald A, Ott G, Delabie J, Campo E, Braziel RM, Cook JR, Tubbs RR, Armitage JO, Weisenburger DD, Staudt LM, Gascoyne RD, McKeithan TW, Chan WC. (2015) Global microRNA expression profiling uncovers molecular markers for classification and prognosis in aggressive B-cell lymphoma. *Blood,* 125, 1137-45.

[85] Fischer L, Hummel M, Korfel A, Lenze D, Joehrens K, Thiel E. (2011) Differential micro-RNA expression in primary CNS and nodal diffuse large B-cell lymphomas. *Neuro Oncol.*, 13, 1090-8.

[86] Zhang J, Jima DD, Jacobs C, Fischer R, Gottwein E, Huang G, Lugar PL, Lagoo AS, Rizzieri DA, Friedman DR, Weinberg JB, Lipsky PE, Dave SS. (2009) Patterns of microRNA expression characterize stages of human B-cell differentiation. *Blood,* 113, 4586-94.

[87] Lawrie CH, Soneji S, Marafioti T, Cooper CD, Palazzo S, Paterson JC, Cattan H, Enver T, Mager R, Boultwood J, Wainscoat JS, Hatton CS. (2007) MicroRNA expression distinguishes between germinal center B cell-like and activated B cell-like subtypes of diffuse large B cell lymphoma. *Int J Cancer*, 121, 1156-61.

[88] Hayashita Y, Osada H, Tatematsu Y, Yamada H, Yanagisawa K, Tomida S, Yatabe Y, Kawahara K, Sekido Y, Takahashi T. (2005) A polycistronic microRNA cluster, miR-17-92, is overexpressed in human lung cancers and enhances cell proliferation. *Cancer Res.*, 65, 9628-32.

[89] Rinaldi A, Poretti G, Kwee I, Zucca E, Catapano CV, Tibiletti MG, Bertoni F. (2007) Concomitant MYC and microRNA cluster miR-17-92 (C13orf25) amplification in human mantle cell lymphoma. *Leuk Lymphoma,* 48, 410-2.

[90] Mashima R. (2015) Physiological roles of miR-155. *Immunology,* 145, 323-33.

[91] Faraoni I, Antonetti FR, Cardone J, Bonmassar E. (2009) miR-155 gene: a typical multifunctional microRNA. *Biochim Biophys Acta*, 1792, 497-505.

[92] Jiang D, Aguiar RC. (2014) MicroRNA-155 controls RB phosphorylation in normal and malignant B lymphocytes via the noncanonical TGF-β1/SMAD5 signaling module. *Blood,* 123, 86-93.

[93] Robertus JL, Harms G, Blokzijl T, Booman M, de Jong D, van Imhoff G, Rosati S, Schuuring E, Kluin P, van den Berg A. (2009) Specific expression of miR-17-5p and miR-127 in testicular and central nervous system diffuse large B-cell lymphoma. *Mod Pathol.*, 22, 547-55.

[94] Thapa DR, Bhatia K, Bream JH, D'Souza G, Rinaldo CR, Wolinsky S, Detels R, Martínez-Maza O. (2012) B-cell activation induced microRNA-21 is elevated in circulating B cells preceding the diagnosis of AIDS-related non-Hodgkin lymphomas., *AIDS*, 26, 1177-80.

[95] Jørgensen LK, Poulsen MØ, Laursen MB, Marques SC, Johnsen HE, Bøgsted M, Dybkær K. (2015) MicroRNAs as novel biomarkers in diffuse large B-cell lymphoma--a systematic review. *Dan Med J.,* 62, A5048.

[96] Shalaby T, Grotzer MA. (2015) Tumor-Associated CSF MicroRNAs for the Prediction and Evaluation of CNS Malignancies. *Int J Mol Sci.*, 16, 29103-19.

[97] Wei D, Wan Q, Li L, Jin H, Liu Y, Wang Y, Zhang G. (2015) MicroRNAs as Potential Biomarkers for Diagnosing Cancers of Central Nervous System: a Meta-analysis. *Mol Neurobiol.*, 51, 1452-61.

[98] Rao P, Benito E, Fischer A. (2013) MicroRNAs as biomarkers for CNS disease. *Front Mol Neurosci.*, 6, 39.

[99] Jones K, Nourse JP, Keane C, Bhatnagar A, Gandhi MK. (2014) Plasma microRNA are disease response biomarkers in classical Hodgkin lymphoma. *Clin Cancer Res.,* 20, 253-64.

[100] Drusco A, Bottoni A, Laganà A, Acunzo M, Fassan M, Cascione L, Antenucci A, Kumchala P, Vicentini C, Gardiman MP, Alder H, Carosi MA, Ammirati M, Gherardi S, Luscrì M, Carapella C, Zanesi N, Croce CM. (2015) A differentially expressed set of microRNAs in cerebro-spinal fluid (CSF) can diagnose CNS malignancies. *Oncotarget*, 6, 20829-39.

[101] Akers JC, Ramakrishnan V, Kim R, Phillips S, Kaimal V, Mao Y, Hua W, Yang I, Fu CC, Nolan J, Nakano I, Yang Y, Beaulieu M, Carter BS, Chen CC. (2015) miRNA contents of cerebrospinal fluid extracellular vesicles in glioblastoma patients. *J Neurooncol.*, 123, 205-16.

[102] Mitchell PS, Parkin RK, Kroh EM, Fritz BR, Wyman SK, Pogosova-Agadjanyan EL, Peterson A, Noteboom J, O'Briant KC, Allen A, Lin DW, Urban N, Drescher CW, Knudsen BS, Stirewalt DL, Gentleman R, Vessella RL, Nelson PS, Martin DB, Tewari M. (2008) Circulating microRNAs as stable blood-based markers for cancer detection. *Proc Natl Acad Sci U S A.,* 105, 10513-8.

[103] Shi R, Wang PY, Li XY, Chen JX, Li Y, Zhang XZ, Zhang CG, Jiang T, Li WB, Ding W, Cheng SJ. (2015) Exosomal levels of miRNA-21 from cerebrospinal fluids associated with poor prognosis and tumor recurrence of glioma patients. *Oncotarget,* 6, 26971-81.

[104] Lawrie CH, Gal S, Dunlop HM, Pushkaran B, Liggins AP, Pulford K, Banham AH, Pezzella F, Boultwood J, Wainscoat JS, Hatton CS, Harris AL. (2008) Detection of elevated levels of tumour-associated microRNAs in serum of patients with diffuse large B-cell lymphoma. *Br J Haematol.*, 141, 672-5.

[105] Fang C, Zhu DX, Dong HJ, Zhou ZJ, Wang YH, Liu L, Fan L, Miao KR, Liu P, Xu W, Li JY. (2012) Serum microRNAs are promising novel biomarkers for diffuse large B cell lymphoma. *Ann Hematol.*, 91, 553-9.

[106] Baraniskin A, Kuhnhenn J, Schlegel U, Chan A, Deckert M, Gold R, Maghnouj A, Zöllner H, Reinacher-Schick A, Schmiegel W, Hahn SA, Schroers R. (2011) Identification of microRNAs in the cerebrospinal fluid as marker for primary diffuse large B-cell lymphoma of the central nervous system. *Blood*, 117, 3140-6.

[107] Baraniskin A, Kuhnhenn J, Schlegel U, Schmiegel W, Hahn S, Schroers R. (2012) MicroRNAs in cerebrospinal fluid as biomarker for disease course monitoring in primary central nervous system lymphoma. *J Neurooncol.*, 109, 239-44.

[108] Baraniskin A, Kuhnhenn J, Schlegel U, Maghnouj A, Zöllner H, Schmiegel W, Hahn S, Schroers R. (2012) Identification of microRNAs in the cerebrospinal fluid as biomarker for the diagnosis of glioma. *Neuro Oncol.*, 14, 29-33.

[109] Teplyuk NM, Mollenhauer B, Gabriely G, Giese A, Kim E, Smolsky M, Kim RY, Saria MG, Pastorino S, Kesari S, Krichevsky AM. (2012) MicroRNAs in cerebrospinal fluid identify glioblastoma and metastatic brain cancers and reflect disease activity. *Neuro Oncol.*, 14, 689-700.

[110] Mao X, Sun Y, Tang J. (2014) Serum miR-21 is a diagnostic and prognostic marker of primary central nervous system lymphoma. *Neurol Sci.*, 35, 233-8.

[111] Roth P, Keller A, Hoheisel JD, Codo P, Bauer AS, Backes C, Leidinger P, Meese E, Thiel E, Korfel A, Weller M. (2015) Differentially regulated miRNAs as prognostic biomarkers in the blood of primary CNS lymphoma patients. *Eur J Cancer*, 51, 382-90.

[112] Bak M, Silahtaroglu A, Møller M, Christensen M, Rath MF, Skryabin B, Tommerup N, Kauppinen S. (2008) MicroRNA expression in the adult mouse central nervous system. *RNA*, 14, 432-44.

In: Primary Central Nervous System Lymphoma (PCNSL) ISBN: 978-1-63485-322-4
Editor: Ryuya Yamanaka

Chapter 9

A CROSS PATIENT IMAGE ANALYSIS OF PCNSL USING VOXEL-BASED LESION MAPPING WITH SIGNIFICANT FOCUS ON GCB AND NON-GCB CLASSIFICATION

Manabu Kinoshita**, MD, PhD
Department of Neurosurgery, Osaka Medical Center for Cancer and Cardiovascular Diseases, Osaka, Japan

ABSTRACT

MRI group analysis is a powerful tool to elucidate pathological conditions in the brain that are challenging to reveal from single subject analysis. This chapter aims to focus on the special distribution characteristics of primary central nervous system lymphoma (PCNSL) within the brain with respect to GCB and non-GCB classification of diffuse large B-cell lymphoma (DLBCL) using voxel-based MRI group analysis. MR images of PCNSL patients are registered onto averaged standard anatomical MRI (MNI152) and gadolinium-enhanced lesions are extracted and a lesion frequency map created. Lymphoma subtypes are classified as GCB or non-GCB by immunohistochemistry. PCNSL frequency map showed that these tumors tended to occur around the lateral, 3rd and 4th ventricles. Furthermore, GCB lymphomas located at the upper tegmentum and cerebellum around the 4th ventricle, while non-GCB lymphomas tended to occupy the anterior fornix.

Keywords: voxel-based MRI group analysis, GCB and non-GCB

---

* Corresponding Author address: Manabu Kinoshita, Department of Neurosurgery, Osaka Medical Center for Cancer and Cardiovascular Diseases, 1-3-3 Nakamichi, Higashinari-ku, Osaka 537-8511, Japan. Email: mail@manabukinoshita.com.

Introduction

It is well kown that Primary central nervous system lymphomas (PCNSLs) are mostly diffuse large B-cell lymphomas (DLBCLs). DLBCL can then be sub-classified according to its cell surface expressing markers especially by B-cell differentiation markers. B-cells can be divided into germinal center B-cells (GCBs) and non-GCBs, according to expression patterns of CD10, BCL-6, MUM-1 and CD138 [1, 2]. CD10 and BCL-6 are markers considered to express in germinal center B-cells. It is also known that BCL-6 is essential for germinal center formation itself in normal B-cells [3, 4]. On the other hand, MUM-1 and CD138 are considered to represent markers of B-cell activation [1], and CD138 expression in particular is considered to be present in B-cell activation to plasma cells [5]. In normal B-cells, BCL-6 and MUM-1 are exclusive in their expressions [6]. Expression patterns of these B-cell markers reportedly differ between PCNSL and systemic peripheral nodal (NL) DLBCL [7, 8], making PCNSL a unique entity of DLBCL. The clinical impact of categorizing DLBCL into GCB and non-GCB DLBCL was once persued under the hope that this classification could lead to identifying prognostic factors in PCNSL. Although this classification worked well for NL DLBCL in the pre-rituximab era, controversial results have been publishted as to the prognostic value of this classification of PCNSL. In fact, patient prognoses between GCB and non-GCB lymphomas differ when treated by cyclophosphamide, doxorubicin, vincristine, prednisone (CHOP)-based chemotherapy with or without rituximab. [9, 10] Likewiase, some studies have shown that cases of GCB or BCL-6-positive PCNSL show better prognosis compared to non-GCB or BCL-6-negative cases in both PCNSL and NL [8, 11-13], while other reports have questioned these findings [14-17]. Significance of this classificaitoin from a biological point of view, however, should not be underestimated and pursued. Conventional analysis may have been overlooking differences in biological properties between these two groups of PCNSL. In this chapter, difference of special distribution between GCB and non-GCB PCNSL is discussed in order to elucidate that subclasification of PCNSL into GCB and non-GCB PCNSL is sifnificant to better understand the tumor biology of PCNSL, along with detailed introduction of the techniques used for analysis.

Methods for Analysis and Results

Immunohistochemistry for GCB and Non-GCB Classification

Standard hematoxylin and eosin (HE) staining and immunohistochemical study of CD-79α and CD-45RO should be performed. CD-79α can be used as a B-cell marker [18], while CD-45RO as a T-cell marker [19]. In our institution antibody for CD-79α staining is provide from DAKO (Tokyo, Japan) and CD-45RO from Nichirei (Tokyo, Japan). All stainings can be performed with formalin-fixed paraffin-embedded tissue. In addition, immunostaining of CD10 (clone 56C6), BCL-6 (clone PG-B6P), MUM-1 (clone MUM1p) and CD138 (clone BC/B-B4) is necessary for GCB and non-GCB classification. All 4 antibodies are avaliable from abcam (Cambridge, MA).

As to detailed procedures, tissue samples are fixed in 10% neutral-buffered formalin and 6 μm thick paraffin-embedded sections are stained with hematoxylin and eosin. To enhance immunostaining, 15-min autoclave treatment should be performed before staining. After washing with Tris buffer, sections are reacted with each of the primary antibodies at 4°C overnight. After another wash, sections stained with each antibody are reacted for 30 min at room temperature with Simplestain MAX-PO(multi) (Nichirei, Tokyo, Japan). For visualization of immune complexes, sections are immersed in 0.02% 3,3'-diaminobenzidine tetrahydrochloride (DAB Wako Pure Chemical Industries, Osaka, Japan), and 0.01% H_2O_2 in Tris buffer. Finally, slides are counterstained with hematoxylin and embedded in a universal mount. For all antigens, a cut-off of at least 30% is set as positive [2, 14]. This cut-off is validated by comparing immunohistochemistry results and microarray data to classify GCB and non-GCB DLBCL [2, 14].

Classification of GCB and Non-GCB DLBCL

CD10, BCL-6, and MUM-1 are used for classifying DLBCL into either GCB or non-GCB lymphoma, as previously described by Hans et al. [2, 14]. First, CD10 positivity corresponds to GCB DLBCL. For CD10 negative cases, BCL-6 positivity is assessed and BCL-6 negative cases are assigned to non-GCB. Finally, CD10 negative and BCL-6 positve cases are classified into non-GCB when MUM-1 is positive and GCB when MUM-1 is negative. As BCL-6 and MUM-1 expression is considered to be muturally exclusive in normal B-cell development, co-expression of these two markers should be considered abnormal. High percentage of co-expression of BCL-6 and MUM-1 is characteristic of PCNSL. Published reports revealed that co-expression of BCL-6 and MUM-1 can be observed in about 50% of PCNSL while only 15-30% co-expression is observed in NL DLBCL. This fact along with low CD10 positivity in PCNSL suspects that PCNSL derives from a more uniform B-cell population than NL DLBCL [14].

Lesion Localization Analysis within the Brain - The Concept

Previous location analysis investigations mainly relied on individual anatomical identification of the lesions. Due to technical limitations, individual differences in size and shape of the brain hamper cross-patient analysis of lesion location. Now that image registration and 3-dimensional structural deformation algorithms is widely available, it is now possible to deform and register individual brain images onto an averaged standard brain image [20]. This technique allows objective and statistically verifiable cross-patient analyses of lesion locations.

Image Registration to Standard Brain Image

The first step for analysis is to deform and register individual brains to a standard brain image refered to as MNI152, an averaged human brain MRI from 152 healthy volunteer. Digital Imaging and Communications in Medicine (DICOM) format images must be first converted to Neuroimaging Informatics Technology Initiative (NIfTI) format. This can be accomplished using various freely available on-line softwares, most of which can operate on Windows, MacOS and Linux. We tend to use MRIconvert (University of Oregon Lewis Center for Neuroimaging, Eugene, OR) or Multi-image Analysis GUI (Mango: University of Texas Health Science Center, San Antonio, TX). NIfTI data is then registered to a 1.0-mm isotropic, high-resolution T1-weighted brain atlas provided by the Montreal Neurological Institute (MNI152) using a mutual information algorithm with a 12-degree of freedom transformation. The most widely used software for this perpose is FSL (FMRIB, Oxford, UK) using the FLIRT command. FLIRT command can ran either on command line or graphical user interface (GUI) provided by FSL. Image registrations must next be visually confirmed as misregistration occasionally occurs during image demormation. Multi-image Analysis GUI (Mango) will be the best choise when manual adjustment is required.

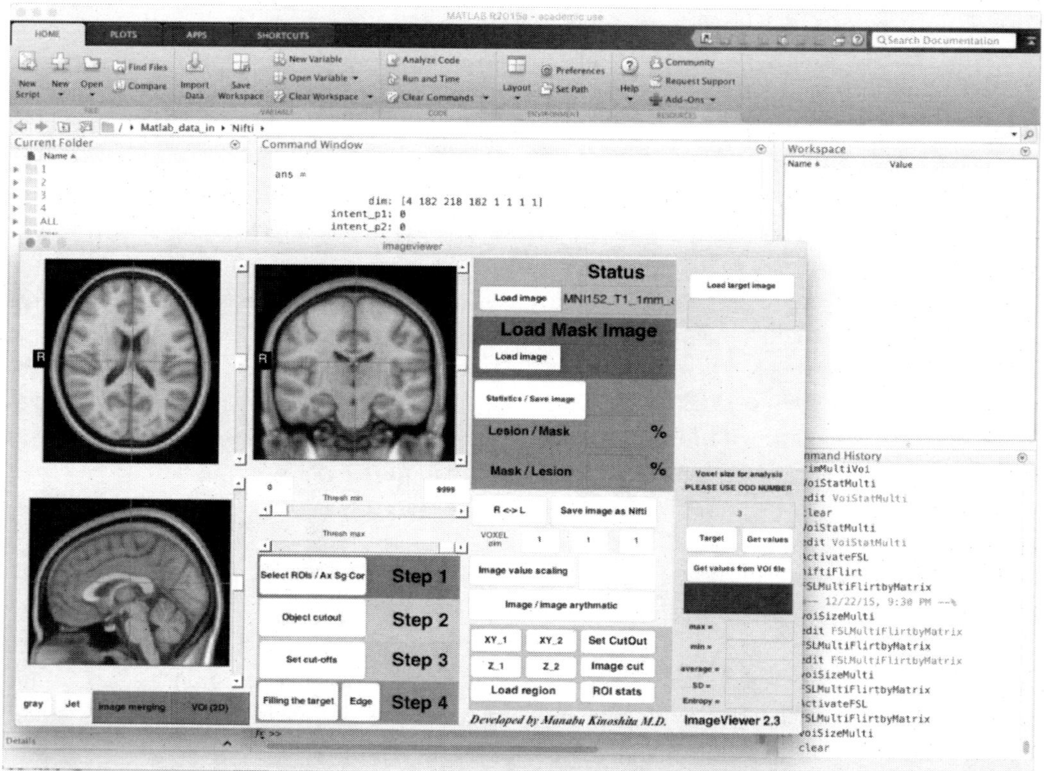

Figure 1. In-house developed image-analyzing software written in Matlab showing MNI152 on screen.

Lesion Extraction and Frequency Map Reconstruction

After image registrations were completed, gadolinium-enhancing lesions should be semi-automatically segmented. We have been using an image editing software developed in-house on Matlab (MathWorks, Natick, MA) (Figure 1). The gadolinium-enhancing lesion is first roughly segmented by manual segmentation performed in three different orientations (axial, coronal and sagittal), followed by threshold-based segmentation of the lesion. The segmented lesion is assigned a value of 1 and the non-segmented lesion a value of 0, saved as 3-

dimensional voxels-of-interest (VOIs). When multiple lesions were present, as is often the case with PCNSL, those lesions must be combined and considered as one VOI per patient.

After all of the VOIs are extracted, all VOIs among the group of interest are summed using the in-house developed software, and averaged by the number of patients, which allows to create a heat-map representing the frequency of lesion occurrence within the brain. This map can be superimposed on the reference MNI152 for better visulalization and interpretation.

Prefferd Location of PCNSL within the Brain

When 100 PCNSLs is collected and a lesion frequency map is reconstructed, it is clearly shown that gadolinium-enhanced lesions accumulated at around the ventricles and basal ganglia as well as the corpus callosum and splenium [21]. Previous studies have analyzed and documented anatomical locations within the brain at which PCNSL tends to arise [22] and suggested that this neoplasm prefers to arise in deep-seated locations, such as the basal ganglia and white matter surrounding the ventricles. Current study [21] shows a more robust and objective spatial distribution, as can be appreciated by the frequency map for PCNSL (Figure 2), an observation in line with previous findings but offering more certainty and objectivity.

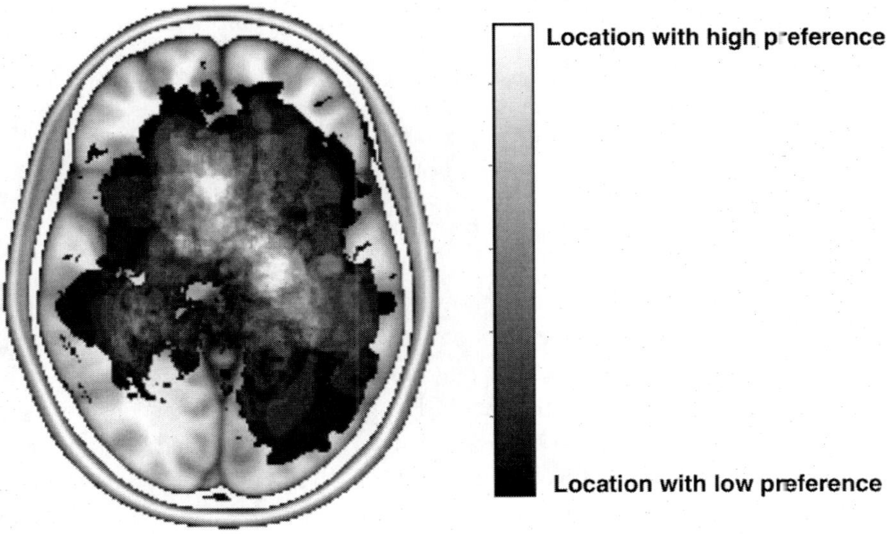

Figure 2. A lesion frequency map of 100 PCNSL. A notabale accumulation of the lesion can be seen at around the ventricles and basal ganglia.

GCB and Non-GCB PCNSL Localize Differently within the Brain

When GCB and non-GCB PCNSL were compared on the lesion frequency map, a significant difference in spatial distribution of the disease is noted. While non-GCB tends to occupy the outer segment of the supratentorial white matter of the brain, GCB tends to occupy midline posterior portion of the supratentorial white matter along with the white matter around the 4th ventricle (Figure 3). Subsequently these differences were statistically challenged. As each voxel has a 2 by 2 contingency table comprising tumor versus non-tumor and GCB versus non-GCB subtype, Fisher's exact test can be applied voxel-wise and setting a p-value less than 0.05 identifies any voxel that showed a significant difference. In addition, correction for cluster-size is performed using random permutation analysis. This technique has already been demonstrated in elucidating spatial distribution difference of glioblastoma according to its MGMT promoter methylation or IDH1 mutation status. [23, 24] This analysis shows hotspots that exhibited significant differences in spatial distribution of the lesion between GCB and non-GCB PCNSL. Those hotspots clustered at specific locations, such as the anterior portion of the fornix, upper tegmentum, and superior medullary velum [21].

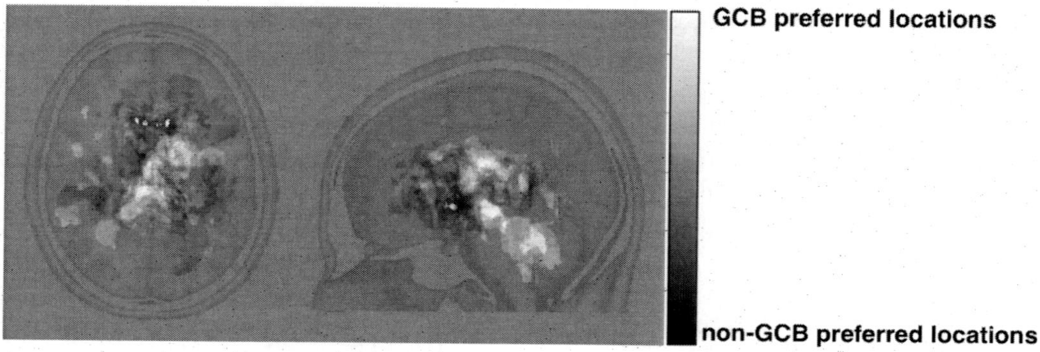

Figure 3. A lesion frequency map of GCB versus non-GCB PCNSL. Non-GCB tends to occupy the outer segment of the supratentorial white matter of the brain while GCB tends to occupy midline posterior portion of the supratentorial white matter along with the white matter around the 4th ventricle.

Summary and Future Direction

Although the above-mentioned observations clearly show that GCB and non-GCB PCNSL entail different biological properties on the locations they arise, prognostic impact of the observed location distribution difference between GCB and non-GCB PCNSL is uncertain. The impact of location distribution of PCNSL on treatment outcome of the disease should be evaluated in future studies in a prospective setting. In general, the correlation of neuroradiological images and histopathology of PCNSL is not well studied compared to gliomas [23, 24] and this type of research should be more widely available among the research community.

References

[1] Chang C-C, McClintock S, Cleveland RP, Trzpuc T, Vesole DH, Logan B, et al. Immunohistochemical expression patterns of germinal center and activation B-cell markers correlate with prognosis in diffuse large B-cell lymphoma. *Am J Surg Pathol.* 2004 Apr;28(4):464–70.

[2] Hans CP, Weisenburger DD, Greiner TC, Gascoyne RD, Delabie J, Ott G, et al. Confirmation of the molecular classification of diffuse large B-cell lymphoma by immunohistochemistry using a tissue microarray. *Blood.* 2004 Jan 1;103(1):275–82.

[3] Barrans SL, Carter I, Owen RG, Davies FE, Patmore RD, Haynes AF, et al. Germinal center phenotype and bcl-2 expression combined with the International Prognostic Index improves patient risk stratification in diffuse large B-cell lymphoma. *Blood.* 2002 Feb 15;99(4):1136–43.

[4] Niu H. The proto-oncogene BCL-6 in normal and malignant B cell development. Hematol Oncol. John Wiley and Sons, Ltd; 2002 Dec;20(4):155–66.

[5] Sanderson RD, Børset M. Syndecan-1 in B lymphoid malignancies. *Ann Hematol.* 2002 Mar;81(3):125–35.

[6] Carbone A, Gloghini A, Larocca LM, Capello D, Pierconti F, Canzonieri V, et al. Expression profile of MUM1/IRF4, BCL-6, and CD138/syndecan-1 defines novel histogenetic subsets of human immunodeficiency virus-related lymphomas. *Blood.* 2001 Feb 1;97(3):744–51.

[7] Shibamoto Y, Ogino H, Suzuki G, Takemoto M, Araki N, Isobe K, et al. Primary central nervous system lymphoma in Japan: changes in clinical features, treatment, and prognosis during 1985-2004. Neuro-Oncology. Oxford University Press; 2008 Aug;10(4):560–8.

[8] Lin C-H, Kuo K-T, Chuang S-S, Kuo S-H, Chang JH, Chang K-C, et al. Comparison of the expression and prognostic significance of differentiation markers between diffuse large B-cell lymphoma of central nervous system origin and peripheral nodal origin. *Clin Cancer Res.* 2006 Feb 15;12(4):1152–6.

[9] Perry AM, Cardesa-Salzmann TM, Meyer PN, Colomo L, Smith LM, Fu K, et al. A new biologic prognostic model based on immunohistochemistry predicts survival in patients with diffuse large B-cell lymphoma. *Blood.* 2012 Sep 13;120(11):2290–6.

[10] Winter JN. Prognostic significance of Bcl-6 protein expression in DLBCL treated with CHOP or R-CHOP: a prospective correlative study. *Blood.* 2006 Jun 1;107(11):4207–13.

[11] Braaten KM, Betensky RA, de Leval L, Okada Y, Hochberg FH, Louis DN, et al. BCL-6 expression predicts improved survival in patients with primary central nervous system lymphoma. *Clin Cancer Res.* 2003 Mar;9(3):1063–9.

[12] Levy O, Deangelis LM, Filippa DA, Panageas KS, Abrey LE. Bcl-6 predicts improved prognosis in primary central nervous system lymphoma. Cancer. Wiley Subscription Services, Inc., A Wiley Company; 2008 Jan 1;112(1):151–6.

[13] Wilson WH, Dunleavy K, Pittaluga S, Hegde U, Grant N, Steinberg SM, et al. Phase II study of dose-adjusted EPOCH and rituximab in untreated diffuse large B-cell lymphoma with analysis of germinal center and post-germinal center biomarkers. *J Clin Oncol. American Society of Clinical Oncology;* 2008 Jun 1;26(16):2717–24.

[14] Camilleri-Broët S, Crinière E, Broët P, Delwail V, Mokhtari K, Moreau A, et al. A uniform activated B-cell-like immunophenotype might explain the poor prognosis of primary central nervous system lymphomas: analysis of 83 cases. *Blood.* 2006 Jan 1;107(1):190–6.

[15] Chang C-C, Kampalath B, Schultz C, Bunyi-Teopengco E, Logan B, Eshoa C, et al. Expression of p53, c-Myc, or Bcl-6 suggests a poor prognosis in primary central

nervous system diffuse large B-cell lymphoma among immunocompetent individuals. *Arch Pathol Lab Med.* 2003 Feb;127(2):208–12.

[16] Kinoshita M, Hashimoto N, Izumoto S, Okita Y, Kagawa N, Maruno M, et al. Immunohistological profiling by B-cell differentiation status of primary central nervous system lymphoma treated by high-dose methotrexate chemotherapy. *J Neurooncol.* 2010 Aug;99(1):95–101.

[17] Momota H, Narita Y, Maeshima AM, Miyakita Y, Shinomiya A, Maruyama T, et al. Prognostic value of immunohistochemical profile and response to high-dose methotrexate therapy in primary CNS lymphoma. *J Neurooncol.* 2010 Jul;98(3):341–8.

[18] Chu PG, Arber DA. CD79: a review. *Appl Immunohistochem Mol Morphol.* 2001 Jun;9(2):97–106.

[19] Weiss LM, Arber DA, Strickler JG. Nasal T-cell lymphoma. *Ann Oncol.* 1994;5 Suppl 1:39–42.

[20] Lancaster JL, Tordesillas-Gutiérrez D, Martinez M, Salinas F, Evans A, Zilles K, et al. Bias between MNI and Talairach coordinates analyzed using the ICBM-152 brain template. *Hum Brain Mapp.* 2007 Nov;28(11):1194–205.

[21] Kinoshita M, Sasayama T, Narita Y, Yamashita F, Kawaguchi A, Chiba Y, et al. Different spatial distribution between germinal center B and non-germinal center B primary central nervous system lymphoma revealed by magnetic resonance group analysis. *Neuro-Oncology.* 2014 May;16(5):728–34.

[22] Bataille B, Delwail V, Menet E, Vandermarcq P, Ingrand P, Wager M, et al. Primary intracerebral malignant lymphoma: report of 248 cases. *J Neurosurg.* 2000 Feb;92(2):261–6.

[23] Ellingson BM, Cloughesy TF, Pope WB, Zaw TM, Phillips H, Lalezari S, et al. Anatomic localization of O6-methylguanine DNA methyltransferase (MGMT) promoter methylated and unmethylated tumors: A radiographic study in 358 de novo human glioblastomas. *NeuroImage.* Elsevier Inc. Elsevier Inc; 2012 Jan 16;59(2):908–16.

[24] Lai A, Kharbanda S, Pope WB, Tran A, Solis OE, Peale F, et al. Evidence for Sequenced Molecular Evolution of IDH1 Mutant Glioblastoma From a Distinct Cell of Origin. *Journal of Clinical Oncology.* 2011 Oct 24;:1–9.

III. Management

In: Primary Central Nervous System Lymphoma (PCNSL)
Editor: Ryuya Yamanaka
ISBN: 978-1-63485-322-4

Chapter 10

RADIOTHERAPY FOR PRIMARY CNS LYMPHOMA

Yuta Shibamoto*
Department of Radiology,
Nagoya City University Graduate School of Medical Sciences, Nagoya, Japan

ABSTRACT

Before the 1980's, radiation therapy played the most important role in the treatment of primary CNS lymphoma (PCNSL), but its role has changed due to the increased use of systemic chemotherapy. In this article, the current status of radiotherapy for PCNSL is reviewed and optimal forms of radiotherapy, including the treatment volume and radiation dose, are discussed. Data from nationwide Japanese surveys of PCNSL patients treated with radiation therapy suggest that the prognosis of PCNSL patients improved in the 1990's, probably owing to the use of high-dose-methotrexate-containing chemotherapy. It was however observed that the prognosis for patients treated with radiation alone also improved in the 1990's. Omission of radiation therapy has been attempted, but recent analyses indicated that radiation therapy plays an important role in the attempt at curing PCNSL. Optimal combination of radiation and chemotherapy seems to be an important issue in the near future.

Keywords: brain neoplasm, lymphoma, central nervous system, radiotherapy, chemotherapy

INTRODUCTION

Primary CNS lymphoma (PCNSL) responds relatively quickly to radiation therapy, like the majority of extra-CNS lymphomas. The complete disappearance of enhancing tumor masses is frequently observed following conventional radiation therapy. Hence, radiation alone after surgical resection or biopsy was the standard treatment for PCNSL before the late

* Correspondence: M.D., Department of Radiology, Nagoya City University Graduate School of Medical Sciences, 1 Kawasumi, Mizuho-cho, Mizuho-ku, Nagoya 467-8601 Japan. Phone: (+81)52-853-8274; Fax: (+81)52-852-5244; E-mail: yshiba@med.nagoya-cu.ac.jp.

1970's. However, the outcome of patients treated by radiation alone was generally poor [1-5]. Particularly, old studies reported 5-year survival rates of less than 10%. This poor outcome was in striking contrast with that reported for other extranodal localized (stage I) lymphomas [6, 7]. Although the initial response of PCNSL to radiation is generally good, local recurrence in the irradiated volume as well as remote CNS recurrence outside of the treatment volume is frequently observed. This led to alteration of the treatment strategy, including the use of systemic chemotherapy since the late 1970's. Combination with chemotherapy regimens used for systemic lymphoma did not yield remarkable results [8-11], but subsequently, high-dose methotrexate (MTX)-containing regimens were found to be effective and have spread worldwide [12-21]. However, a big flaw has been pointed out regarding the routine use of MTX-containing chemotherapy in that it has spread without firm evidence demonstrated by randomized trials. Even without phase III studies, a recent trend is being further developed in Western countries to use the chemotherapy first and reserve radiation therapy until recurrence. However, such approaches have not been generally accepted throughout the world, and there has recently appeared an idea to reevaluate the role of radiation therapy [22]. Thus, it can be concluded that the standard treatment for PCNSL has not yet been established, because of the paucity of reliable randomized clinical trials. In Japan, radiation therapy is still used in the first-line treatment of non-elderly patients with PCNSL in combination with chemotherapy, generally using MTX-containing regimens. In this article, the author summarizes the results of radiation therapy for PCNSL, characterizes its role, and discusses optimal forms of radiation therapy.

STRATEGY FOR DIAGNOSIS

Before discussing radiation therapy, the author would like to present an opinion regarding the management of patients suspected to have PCNSL. CNS lymphoma (CNSL), either primary or secondary, showing typical imaging characteristics is not hard to diagnose using contrast-enhanced MRI (or even CT) [10]. Typically, CNSL shows marked homogenous contrast enhancement surrounded by broad low-intensity areas on T1-weighted MR images, high-intensity areas on T2-weighted images, and low-density areas on CT. The mass effect is, however, relatively small even in a large tumor. It is not difficult to diagnose typical cases from these imaging findings. In addition, if corticosteroids are used and the tumor shrinks in response to it (although steroids are not recommended before biopsy), the clinical diagnosis of CNSL becomes firmly supported. If the patient has extra-CNS lymphoma, biopsy of the CNS tumor possessing these imaging characteristics is unnecessary and should be avoided. Therefore, when imaging findings suggest CNSL, positron emission tomography with 18-fluorodeoxyglucose is highly recommended to evaluate the existence of extra-cranial lymphoma. If there is no extra-CNS lesion, a diagnosis of PCNSL becomes very likely. Nevertheless, the author recommends biopsy of the suspected PCNSL. Extensive resection is not recommended, since it has not been proven to improve the prognosis [22].

Biopsy is recommended for the following reasons. Based on the current classification of lymphoma, most PCNSLs are categorized as diffuse large B-cell lymphoma. However, a small proportion of PCNSLs are of T-cell origin, and there exist other types of B-cell lymphoma in PCNSL [23]. Differentiation among the various histological subtypes of lymphoma is difficult with imaging studies. More importantly, the classification of lymphoma may further change in the future, since the present classification does not necessarily reflect the origin of lymphoma cells. Considering these facts, the author thinks it would be meaningful to obtain a biopsy and establish the histopathological diagnosis, thereafter storing the specimen for the future.

TREATMENT STRATEGY

Considering the poor results obtained by radiation therapy alone, combination with chemotherapy has been investigated since the late 1970's. Most regimens of chemotherapy investigated so far can be classified into the following two groups: one is regimens used for systemic lymphoma, such as CHOP (cyclophosphamide, doxorubicin, vincristine, and prednisolone) +/- rituximab, and the other is high-dose MTX ($\geq$3.5 g/m^2) either alone or in combination with other drugs. The outcome of patients treated by the former regimens was mostly unsatisfactory [9-11]. A small randomized study suggested no benefit of adding CHOP chemotherapy to whole-brain radiation [11]. These unsatisfactory results were attributed to poor penetration of the compounds across the blood-brain barrier, especially given before radiation therapy. However, the author and coworkers [10] suggested that the use of CHOP or CHOP-like chemotherapy after radiation therapy might improve the outcome, since radiation therapy disrupts the blood-brain barrier [24]. The drugs that do not cross the blood-brain barrier may cross it when given after radiation therapy. This hypothesis, however, has yet to be examined extensively.

In contrast, studies investigating high-dose-MTX-containing regimens appear to have been successful [12-21]. Many such studies achieved median survival times of 30-45 months and 5-year survival rates of 30-40%. However, no randomized studies comparing radiation alone with radiation plus high-dose-MTX-based chemotherapy have been carried out. The investigators of chemoradiation trials have generally mentioned that the outcome they obtained is a marked improvement over the results obtained previously by radiotherapy alone (i.e., 5-year survival <10%). Even in the absence of randomized studies, some investigators state that such chemoradiation therapy is definitely superior to radiation alone [25]. This methodology (i.e., to compare with very old data obtained by radiation alone), however, does not seem to be justified in the era of evidence-based medicine.

Nevertheless, attempts to omit radiation therapy in elderly patients and reserve radiation for recurrence after primary chemotherapy in younger patients have steadily spread. Chemotherapy alone is associated with a higher recurrence rate but it has been reported to be associated with less neurotoxicity. A recent randomized trial comparing high-dose MTX alone and in combination with radiation therapy clearly indicated a lower progression-free survival in patients undergoing chemotherapy alone, as stated later [26]. In terms of the cure rate, chemoradiation therapy is superior to chemotherapy alone, and recently many neurooncologists appear to be reconsidering the use of radiation therapy, even with lower doses than previously employed [22]. Thus, the optimal treatment policy still needs to be established in the near future.

Radiation Therapy

Results of Radiotherapy Alone

In Table 1, reported results of radiation monotherapy for PCNSL are summarized. Results of old small-scale studies are included in the two reviews [1, 2]. Relatively old literature indicates a poor outcome for PNCSL patients treated by radiation alone; the reported 5-year survival rates are mostly less than 10%. A considerably high proportion of PCNSLs show local recurrence. Although recurrence within the CNS apart from the primary lesion is also common regardless of the radiation treatment volume [5, 27, 28], in-field local recurrence is often encountered. Therefore, it is argued that the radiosensitivity of PCNSL may be lower than that of other extranodal lymphomas. This relatively low radiosensitivity may be intrinsic to PCNSL cells, but alternatively, it may be owing to the tumor bed (i.e., brain parenchyma). Similarly, CNS germinomas are known to require higher radiation doses for local control than their testicular counterparts (i.e., seminomas) [29]. Nevertheless, the previously reported 5-year survival rates of less than 10% appear to be too low for PCNSL that infrequently metastasizes to extra-CNS organs.

The main reason for the poor results in the past is not clear, but, in the author's experience, the diagnosis of PCNSL was not readily made before 1980, and the treatment policy for PCNSL patients was not well established. Some of our patients received excessive surgery, leading to a poor postoperative performance status and dying soon thereafter. The author's group recently reported that the proportion of good PS patients was significantly higher in more recent years than in preceding years [23]. With the development of a diagnostic strategy and improvement in physicians' recognition of PCNSL, patients may now be diagnosed at an earlier stage than before. We speculate that improvement in general care and an earlier diagnosis may be some of the reasons for improvement in the prognosis.

Table 1. Results of radiation monotherapy for PCNSL

First author (Group)	Publication year	n	Median survival (months)	5-year survival (%)
Littman (Review)	1975	150	-	6
Leibel (Review)	1987	114	24	7
Shibamoto (Kyoto)	1990	16	8	6
Nelson (RTOG)	1992	41	12	28 (at 2 years)
Watne (Norway)	1992	15	19	13
Ishikawa (Gunma)	2003	25	13*	35
Shibamoto (JASTRO)	2005	132	18	18

Kyoto = Kyoto University Hospital; RTOG = Radiation Therapy Oncology Group; Norway = Norwegian Radium Hospital; Gunma = Gunma University Hospital; JASTRO = Japanese Society for Therapeutic Radiology and Oncology CNS Lymphoma Study Group. *For 33 patients including 8 patients undergoing systemic chemotherapy without methotrexate.

On the other hand, the author's group reported a 5-year survival of 18.0% in Japanese patients treated by radiotherapy alone between 1990 and 1999 [30]. The patients were collected through retrospective multi-institutional studies of the Japanese Society for

Radiation Oncology (JASTRO) Lymphoma Study Group and the Chubu Radiation Oncology Group (CROG) [31-33]. It should be noted that combination chemotherapy was gradually increasing during the 1990's, and many of these patients were regarded as not indicated for or refused chemotherapy. Nevertheless, the survival data were better than those reported before 1990. For comparison with chemoradiation studies, 62 patients with ages between 16 and 65 years and PS 0-3 were also analyzed in that study. In terms of the age and PS, these patients are considered eligible for a prospective study of chemoradiation by the European Organization for Research and Treatment of Cancer (EORTC 20962) [20]. For these 62 patients, the median survival time was 26 months, and survival rates were 69% at 1 year, 53% at 2 years, 33% at 3 years, and 24% at 5 years. For comparison, the median survival time was 46 months and 2-year survival rate was 69% in the EORTC 20962 trial. A report by Ishikawa et al. [34] published in 2003 also indicated much better survival rates for PCNSL patients treated by radiation alone, as compared to published older data.

We have continued this survey of PCNSL, and data for patients seen between 2000 and 2004 and those during 2005-2009 have been published [23,35]. In the most recent survey [35], 315 patients were collected; 78% of them received chemotherapy, and 84% of the chemotherapy regimens were high-dose-MTX-based. As a result, 70 patients treated with radiation alone had a 5-year survival rate of only 13%. Similarly, the 5-year survival rates for patients treated with radiation therapy alone were 9.0% for the period of 1995-2004 (*n* = 87) and 15.8% for the period of 1985-1994 (*n* = 208) [35]. Figure 1 shows overall survival curves for patients treated by radiotherapy alone during the periods 1985-1994, 1995-2004, and 2005-2009. The data on radiation therapy alone during the more recent eras do not seem to represent the true outcome obtained by radiation monotherapy. The Japanese data for patients treated between 1990 and 1999 (i.e., 5-year survival of 18%) may be closer to the expected prognosis of PCNSL patients treated by radiation therapy alone.

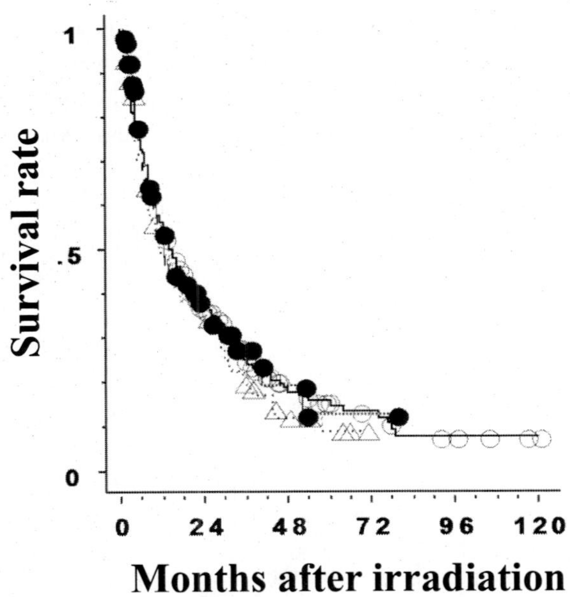

Figure 1. Survival curves for PCNSL patients treated by radiotherapy alone during 1985-1994 (○, n = 208), 1995-2004 (●, n = 87), and 2004-2009 (Δ, n =70).

Optimal Treatment Volume

Whole-brain irradiation has been commonly used to treat PCNSL patients. The rationale for using a whole-brain field is that PCNSL is often multiple and that the boundary of PCNSL lesions is obscure; tumor cells are believed to usually invade the normal brain over a few centimeters from a contrast-enhanced tumor mass. Therefore, whole-brain irradiation is safe in terms of not missing viable tumor cells. This was especially so in the era before MRI or CT. Following the traditional use of whole-brain fields, the majority of PCNSL patients are still being treated with whole-brain radiation. On the other hand, the toxicity of whole-brain radiation has been stressed by medical oncologists. The neurotoxicity includes dementia and a decline in PS. The neurotoxicity is more specific to the treatment of PCNSL patients, since we observed only a little, if any, decline in the mini-mental state examination score after whole-brain irradiation in patients with brain metastases from other cancers [36]. The author speculates that PCNSL grows invasively against normal brain tissue so that such normal cells, even if they retain their function at the diagnosis of PCNSL, are vulnerable to radiation. On the other hand, brain metastases and other tumors invade normal tissue less aggressively and normal cells are considered to be more resistant to the adverse effects of radiation. In the author's experience with Japanese patients, however, this neurotoxicity is not so frequently encountered in those younger than 60 years treated mainly with radiation therapy, and the author thinks this adverse event is also closely related to the use of MTX. The author suggests that neurotoxicity when treated by radiation alone might have been somewhat exaggerated by neurooncologists in Western countries. However, this possible difference in neurotoxicity may be due to a racial difference and our policy of radiation therapy, especially with respect to the treatment volume, as is described later.

Thus, the concern over neurotoxicity seems to be strengthened when chemotherapy, especially high-dose MTX, is used in combination. On the other hand, one may expect high-dose MTX to eradicate microscopic diseases, so the author and coworkers have postulated the use of extended focal radiation field with wide (about 4 cm) margins from a tumor mass when PCNSL lesions are single and solitary. This is especially true when chemotherapy including high-dose MTX is used. After 40 Gy, we reduce the treatment volume and use a localized radiation field with 1-1.5-cm margins. We retrospectively analyzed 43 patients treated by a partial-brain radiation field [27]. When patients were treated with a localized field with less than 4 cm margins, out-of-field recurrences were frequently seen (83% at 3 years). With wider margins ($\geq$ 4 cm), the rate for out-of-field recurrence was 22% at 3 years, and overall survival did not seem to differ from that of patients receiving whole-brain radiation therapy. Therefore, it was concluded that partial-brain irradiation with wide margins may well deserve consideration in patients with a single lesion undergoing high-dose-MTX-containing chemotherapy. We are still continuing to use extended focal radiation fields for patients with a single lesion.

Figure 2 shows survival curves for PCNSL patients after whole-brain or partial-brain irradiation enrolled in the above-mentioned Japanese surveys [37]. All patients treated between 1985 and 2009 were included. Patients treated with partial-brain fields had a 5-year survival rate of 29% (n = 85), while those treated with whole-brain fields had a 5-year survival of 24.8% (n = 969; P = 0.80). Even when whole-brain radiation is employed, the whole-brain should not be irradiated with a full dose. After 40 or 30 Gy depending upon the case, the radiation field should be reduced to only cover regions of macroscopic tumors at the diagnosis with a margin. There is no rationale for using the same dose for macroscopic lesions and prophylaxis for possible microscopic lesions. Using whole-brain fields throughout the treatment should be avoided.

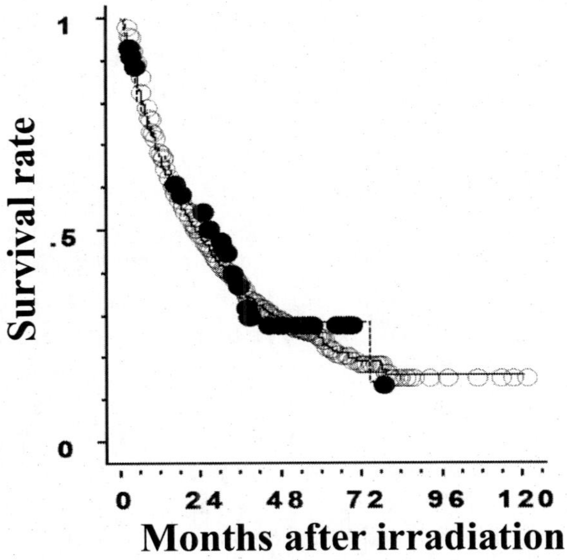

Figure 2. Survival curves for PCNSL patients treated with whole-brain radiation (○, n = 969) and those treated with partial-brain radiation (●, n = 85).

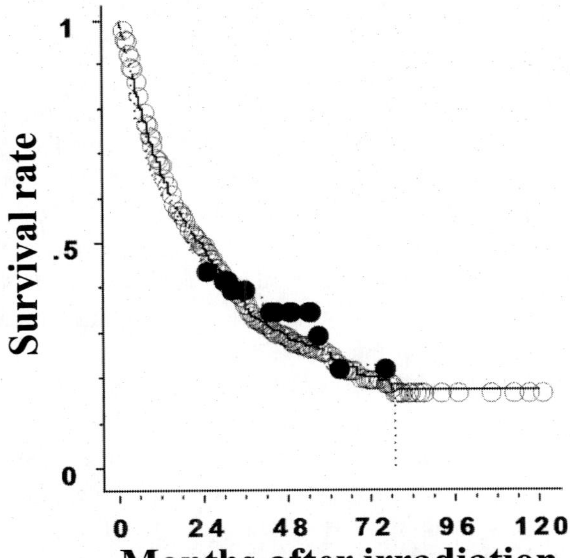

Figure 3. Survival curves for PCNSL patients receiving no spinal irradiation (○, n = 975) and those receiving spinal irradiation (●, n = 54).

Craniospinal irradiation has infrequently been used in the treatment of PCNSL. Although the JASTRO surveys of PCNSL patients seen between 1985 and 2009 indicated that the incidence of meningeal dissemination at the diagnosis of PCNSL was 13% to 19%, spinal irradiation was employed in only 1.6% to 8.3% of the patients [23, 31-33, 35]. Figure 3 shows survival curves for PCNSL patients treated with or without spinal irradiation in the above-mentioned surveys. Patients who did not receive whole spinal irradiation had a 5-year survival rate of 25.5% ($n = 975$), while those who did had a rate of 23% ($n = 54$; $P = 0.97$).

Optimal Radiation Dose and Fractionation

Conventional fractionation has been employed in the treatment of PCNSL. Since normal brain tissue is considered to have a low α / β ratio of about 2-3 Gy, it is generally not recommended to use a high dose per fraction. Except for palliative treatment, a 2-Gy daily fraction remains the standard. Accelerated fractionation or accelerated hyperfractionation may be another option for rapidly growing tumors. One small phase I study investigated accelerated hyperfractionation using 1.5 Gy twice daily to a total whole-brain dose of 45 Gy in combination with chemotherapy with high-dose MTX, idarubicin, dexamathazone, cytosine arabinoside, and cisplatin [38]. Bromodeoxyuridine infusion was delivered 2-3 days prior to whole-brain radiotherapy and then weekly during radiotherapy. With a patient number of 12, disease control was modest, but neurotoxicity was found to be unacceptable. It is not clear whether this neurotoxicity was related to the use of accelerated hyperfractionation or bromodeoxyuridine infusion. Another small pilot study with ten patients investigated 2 Gy twice daily to a whole-brain dose of 50 Gy delivered over only 13 days without weekend interruptions [39]. Nine of the ten patients died and the median survival time was only 17 months. The authors concluded that the accelerated schedule of radiation therapy was ineffective and associated with unacceptable toxicity.

Hyperfractionation using 1.0-1.2 Gy twice daily has also been evaluated in a few studies. To reduce late CNS toxicity, the use of a lower dose per fraction is considered to deserve investigation. In an Radiation Therapy Oncology Group (RTOG) study 9310 investigating pre-radiation chemotherapy including MTX, vincristine and procarbazine, the radiation dose and fractionation were changed from 45 Gy in 25 fractions to 36 Gy with 1.2 Gy twice daily over 3 weeks [40]. Although the hyperfractionation schedule represented a 25% reduction in biologically effective tumor dose as compared to the standard fractionation, progression-free survival and overall survival were not significantly affected in the RTOG study. The hyperfractionation regimen delayed leukoencephalopathy but did not eliminate severe neurotoxicity from chemoradiation. Another study with 30 patients employed hyperfractionated whole-brain radiation to 45 Gy with 1.0 Gy twice daily in combination with MTX (8 g/m^2), cytarabine and thiotepa followed by autologous stem-cell transplantation [41]. The 5-year overall survival probability was as high as 69% for all patients and 87% for 23 patients who received high-dose chemotherapy and autologous stem-cell transplantation. Five of the 30 patients (17%) developed leukoencephalopathy, and this rate was evaluated as "moderate" compared with data in the literature. From these studies, hyperfractionated radiotherapy seems to worth further investigation. The use of hyperfractionation was reported in another small study with eight patients [42]. The investigators used a whole-brain dose of as high as 64.8 Gy in 54 fractions over 5.5 weeks. Six patients deteriorated neurologically without evidence of tumor recurrence, and the marked toxicity prompted study closure.

No randomized trial has been carried out regarding the optimal total radiation dose. With 41 patients, the RTOG 8315 study investigated an escalation of the total dose to 60 Gy (40 Gy to the whole brain followed by a 20-Gy focal boost), but the results were not considered superior to those obtained by lower doses of radiation (e.g., 50 Gy) [5, 40]. Thus, the standard radiation dose in the primary treatment of PCNSL, when used alone, seems to remain as 50 Gy. With the development of MTX-containing chemotherapy, however, attempts are being made to reduce radiation doses (or even defer radiotherapy). In a phase II study with 57 patients, however, the reduction of the whole-brain dose from 45 to 30.6 Gy appeared to be associated with an increased recurrence rate [43]. On the other hand, in a phase II study enrolling 30 patients, only 23.4 Gy were given to patients who achieved a complete response after chemotherapy, and the disease control was reported to be satisfactory [44]. Figure 4 shows survival data from the above-mentioned Japanese surveys according to the total radiation dose. Patients who did not complete the planned radiotherapy were excluded. The 5-year survival rate was 24% for patients receiving 30-39.9 Gy, 31.6% for those receiving 40-49.9 Gy, 24.7% for those treated with 50-53.9 Gy and 20.6% for those receiving 54 Gy or more. Significant differences were observed between the 40-49.9 Gy group and the other three groups (all $P < 0.05$). This trend was more marked when patients undergoing MTX-containing chemotherapy were analyzed. Although these results were retrospectively obtained, they suggested a better outcome when treated with moderate radiation doses.

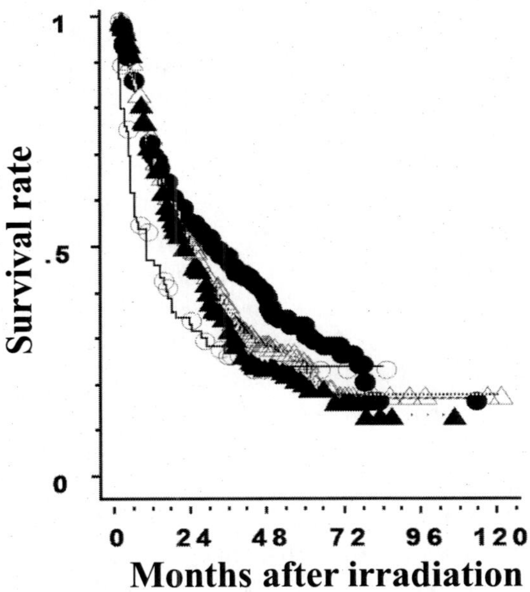

Figure 4. Survival curves for PCNSL patients treated with a total dose of 30-39.9 Gy (○, n = 82), those treated with 40-49.9 Gy (●, n = 273), those treated with 50-53.9 Gy (△, n = 361) and those treated with 54 Gy or more (▲, n = 295).

As stated above, some groups are investigating the omission of radiation therapy in elderly patients; even in younger patients, they attempt to defer radiation and reserve it until recurrence. Regarding the issue, a randomized trial was performed involving 551 patients by the German Primary CNS Lymphoma Study Group [26]. The trial compared high-dose MTX alone with high-dose MTX plus whole-brain radiotherapy to 45 Gy given as 1.5 Gy once daily. In the group treated without whole-brain radiation, high-dose cytarabine was administered when a complete response was not obtained by high-dose MTX. Also, the group of patients could receive radiation therapy at recurrence. The results clearly showed higher progression-free survival rates in the group treated with chemotherapy plus whole-brain radiation, but overall survival did not differ significantly between the two groups; it seems that radiation given as second-line treatment contributed to this result in part. Several weak points for this trial have been pointed out, including a long patient accrual period (9 years), a low rate of patients treated per protocol, and low overall survival rates in both arms. Therefore, it should be further investigated in future studies whether or not the omission or deferral of radiation therapy is really justified.

Newer Radiation Technique and Modalities

Some groups have reported the use of stereotactic radiosurgery in the treatment of PCNSL [45, 46]. Its use in recurrent cases that have already undergone conventional full-dose radiation may be partly justified, but considering the spread of tumor cells around enhancing tumor masses, the use of radiosurgery in the first-line treatment of PCNSL is not in common sense. Recurrent cases already receiving full-dose radiation and primary cases that are unable to undergo standard radiotherapy may be palliatively treated with a gammaknife, cyberknife, tomotherapy, or a linac-based radiosurgery system. Radiation doses may be determined on a case-by-case basis. The results of radiosurgical treatment for recurrent PCNSL indicate acceptable toxicity and a modest survival time [45, 46]. As expected, local control was relatively favorable, but high recurrence rates outside of the treatment volume have been reported.

As a first-line treatment, intensity-modulated radiation therapy (IMRT) deserves consideration. In the treatment of glioblastoma, the simultaneous integrated boost technique is being increasingly used [47, 48]. If this technique is used, whole-brain or margin areas for focal radiation with generous margins can be uniformly treated with a standard dose, while tumor mass areas can be simultaneously boosted. For example, the whole brain or wide-margin regions around a tumor mass can be treated with 40 Gy in 20 fractions, while tumor masses can be treated with 2.4 or 2.5 Gy per fraction to the same 20 fractions. In my opinion, this type of IMRT should be employed in as many patients with primary malignant brain tumors as possible in the near future.

The use of particle beams has not yet been reported. The advantage of proton beams that stop at the target can be utilized for focal radiotherapy or as a boost. So, with the increase in device numbers, the use of proton therapy may be investigated in the future. On the contrary, carbon-ion therapy may not be indicated for PCNSL at present in view of the relatively high CNS toxicity reported in patients treated with carbon-ion beams [49].

Conclusion and Future Direction

The role of radiation therapy seems to have somewhat decreased in the treatment of PCNSL. However, there appears a trend to reevaluate radiation therapy to cure the disease. Radiation has greater effects on local tumor control than chemotherapy, so the utilization of radiation therapy, even with lower doses than previously used, should be investigated in the near future, especially in younger patients, with the goal to cure the disease. Randomized trials are encouraged based on this issue.

Conflict of Interests

The author declares no potential conflict of interests.

References

[1] Littman P, Wang CC. Reticulum sarcoma of the brain. A review of the literature and a study of 19 cases. *Cancer* 1975;35:1412-20.

[2] Leibel SA, Sheline GE. Radiation therapy for neoplasms of the brain. *J Neurosurg* 1987;66:1-22.

[3] Shibamoto Y, Tsutsui K, Dodo Y, et al. Improved survival rate in primary intracranial lymphoma treated by high-dose radiation and systemic vincristine-doxorubicin-cyclophosphamide-prednisolone chemotherapy. *Cancer* 1990;65:1907-12.

[4] Watne K, Scott H, Hager B, et al. Primary malignant lymphoma of the brain. A report of 24 cases from the Norwegian Radium Hospital. *Acta Oncol* 1992;31:545-50.

[5] Nelson DF, Martz KL, Bonner H, et al. Non-Hodgkin's lymphoma of the brain: can high dose, large volume radiation therapy improve survival? Report on a prospective trial by the Radiation Therapy Oncology Group (RTOG): RTOG 8315. *Int J Radiat Oncol Biol Phys* 1992;23:9-17.

[6] Hayabuchi N, Shibamoto Y, Nakamura K, et al. Stage I and II aggressive B-cell lymphomas of the head and neck: radiotherapy alone as a treatment option and the usefulness of the new prognostic index B-ALPS. *Int J Radiat Oncol Biol Phys* 2003;55:44-50.

[7] Martinet S, Ozsahin M, Belkacemi Y, et al. Outcome and prognostic factors in orbital lymphoma: a Rare Cancer Network study on 90 consecutive patients treated with radiotherapy. *Int J Radiat Oncol Biol Phys* 2003;55:892-8.

[8] Schultz C, Scott C, Sherman W, et al. Preirradiation chemotherapy with cyclophosphamide doxorubicin, vincristine, and dexamethazone for primary CNS lymphomas: initial report of Radiation Therapy Oncology Group protocol 88-06. *J Clin Oncol* 1996;14:556-64.

[9] O'Neill BP, O'Fallon JR, Earle JD, et al. Primary central nervous system non-Hodgkin's lymphoma (PCNSL): survival advantages with combined initial therapy? A final report of the North Central Cancer Treatment Group (NCCTG) study 86-72-52. *Int J Radiat Oncol Biol Phys* 1999;43:559-63.

[10] Shibamoto Y, Sasai K, Oya N, et al. Systemic chemotherapy with vincristine, cyclophosphamide, doxorubicin and prednisolone following radiotherapy for primary central nervous system lymphoma: a phase II study. *J Neurooncol* 1999;42:161-7.

[11] Mead GM, Bleehen NM, Gregor A, et al. A Medical Research Council randomized trial in patients with primary cerebral non-Hodgkin lymphoma. Cerebral radiotherapy with and without cyclophosphamide, doxorubicin, vincristine, and prednisone chemotherapy. *Cancer* 2000;89:1359-70.

[12] Glass J, Gruber ML, Chef L, et al. Preirradiation MTX chemotherapy of primary central nervous system lymphoma: long-term outcome. *J Neurosurg* 1994;81:188-95.

[13] Blay JY, Conroy T, Chevreau C, et al. High-dose MTX for the treatment of primary cerebral lymphomas: analysis of survival and late neurologic toxicity in a retrospective series. *J Clin Oncol* 1998;16:864-71.

[14] Brada M, Hjiyiannakis D, Hines F, et al. Short intensive primary chemotherapy and radiotherapy in sporadic primary CNS lymphoma. *Int J Radiat Oncol Biol Phys* 1998;40:1157-62.

[15] Ferreri AJM, Reni M, Villa E. Therapeutic management of primary central nervous system lymphoma: lessons from prospective trials. *Ann Oncol* 2000;11:927-37.

[16] Abrey LE, Yahalom J, DeAngelis LM. Treatment for primary CNS lymphoma: the next step. *J Clin Oncol* 2000;18:3144-50.

[17] Reni M, Ferreri AJ, Guha-Thakurta N, et al. Clinical relevance of consolidation radiotherapy and other main therapeutic issues in primary central nervous system lymphomas treated with upfront high-dose MTX. *Int J Radiat Oncol Biol Phys* 2001;51:419-25.

[18] Calderoni A, Aebi S. Combination chemotherapy with high-dose MTX and cytarabine with or without brain irradiation for primary central nervous system lymphomas. *J Neurooncol* 2002;59:227-30.

[19] DeAngelis LM, Seiferheld W, Schold SC, et al. Combination chemotherapy and radiotherapy for primary central nervous system lymphoma: Radiation Therapy Oncology Group study 93-10. *J Clin Oncol* 2002;20:4643-8.

[20] Poortmans PMP, Kluin-Nelemans HC, Haaxma-Reiche H, et al. High-dose methotrexate-based chemotherapy followed by consolidating radiotherapy in non-AIDS-related primary central nervous system lymphoma: European Organization for Research and Treatment of Cancer Lymphoma Group Phase II trial 20962. *J Clin Oncol* 2003;21:4483-8.

[21] Bessel EM, Graus F, Lopez-Guillermo A, et al. Primary non-Hodgkin's lymphoma of the CNS treated with CHOD/BVAM or BVAM chemotherapy before radiotherapy: long-term survival and prognostic factors. *Int J Radiat Oncol Biol Phys* 2004;59:501-8.

[22] DeAngelis LM. Whither whole brain radiotherapy for primry CNS lymphoma? *Neuro Oncol* 2014;16:1032-4.

[23] Shibamoto Y, Ogino H, Suzuki G, et al. Primary central nervous system lymphoma in Japan: changes in clinical features, treatment and prognosis during 1985-2004. *Neuro Oncol* 2008;10:560-8.

[24] Rubin P, Gashu DM, Hansen JT, et al. Disruption of the blood-brain barrier as the primary effect of CNS irradiation. *Radiother Oncol* 1994;31:51-60.

[25] DeAngelis LM. Primary central nervous system lymphoma: a curable brain tumor. *J Clin Oncol* 2004;24:4471-3.

[26] Thiel E, Korfel A, Martus P, et al. High-dose methotrexate with or without whole brain radiotherapy for primary CNS lymphoma (G-PCNSL-SG-1): a phase 3, randomized, non-inferiority trial. *Lancet Oncol* 2010;11:1036-47.

[27] Shibamoto Y, Hayabuchi N, Hiratsuka J, et al. Is whole-brain irradiation necessary for primary central nervous system lymphoma? Patterns of recurrence following partial-brain irradiation. *Cancer* 2003;97:128-33.

[28] Iwabuchi M, Shibamoto Y, Sugie C, Ayakawa S, Ogino H, Baba F. Partial-brain radiotherapy for primary central nervous system lymphoma: multi-institutional experience. *J Radiat Res* 2016;57:164-8.

[29] Shibamoto Y, Sasai K, Oya N, et al. Intracranial germinoma: radiation therapy with tumor volume-based dose selection. *Radiology* 2001;218:452-6.

[30] Shibamoto Y, Ogino H, Hasegawa M, et al. Results of radiation monotherapy for primary central nervous system lymphoma in the 1990's. *Int J Radiat Oncol Biol Phys* 2005;62:809-13.

[31] Hayabuchi N, Shibamoto Y, Onizuka Y, et al. Primary central nervous system lymphoma in Japan: a nationwide survey. *Int J Radiat Oncol Biol Phys* 1999;44:265-72.

[32] Shibamoto Y, Tsuchida E, Seki K, et al. Primary central nervous system lymphoma in Japan 1995-1999: changes from the preceding 10 years. *J Cancer Res Clin Oncol* 2004;130:351-6.

[33] Kawamura T, Ishiguchi T, Shibamoto Y, et al. Results of primary central nervous system lymphoma treated by radiation and chemotherapy: retrospective analysis of twelve institutions in the Tokai district in Japan, 1995-1999. *Radiat Med* 2006;24:9-16.

[34] Ishikawa H, Hasegawa M, Tamaki Y, et al. Comparable outcomes of radiation therapy without high-dose methotrexate for patients with primary central nervous system lymphoma. Jpn. *J Clin Oncol* 2003;33:443-9.

[35] Shibamoto Y, Sumi M, Onodera S, et al. Primary CNS lymphoma treated with radiotherapy in Japan: a survey of patients treated in 2005-2009 and a comparison with those treated in 1985-2004. *Int J Clin Oncol* 2014;19:963-71.

[36] Shibamoto Y, Baba F, Oda K, et al. Incidence of brain atrophy and decline in mini-mental state examination score after whole-brain radiotherapy in patients with brain metastases: a prospective study. *Int J Radiat Oncol Biol Phys* 2008;72:1168-73.

[37] Shibamoto Y, Sumi M, Takemoto M, et al. Analysis of radiotherapy in 1054 patients with primary central nervous system lymphoma treated from 1985-2009. *Clin Oncol* 2014;26:653-60.

[38] Dabaja BS, McLaughlin P, Ha CS, et al. Primary central nervous system lymphoma: Phase I evaluation of infusional bromodeoxyuridine with whole brain accelerated fractionation radiation therapy after chemotherapy. *Cancer* 2003;98:1021-8.

[39] Laperriere NJ, Wong CS, Milosevic MF, et al. Accelerated radiation therapy for primary lymphoma of the brain. *Radiother Oncol* 1998;47:191-5.

[40] Fisher B, Seiferheld W, Schultz C, et al. Secondary analysis of Radiation Therapy Oncology Group study (RTOG) 9310: an intergroup phase II combined modality treatment of primary central nervous system lymphoma. *J Neurooncol* 2005;74:201-5.

[41] Illerhaus G, Marks R, Ihorst G, et al. High-dose chemotherapy with autologous stem-cell transplantation and hyperfractionated radiotherapy as first-line treatment of primary CNS lymphoma. *J Clin Oncol* 2006;24:3865-70.

[42] Davey P, Catton C, Ngan B, et al. Phase I study of hyperfractionated whole brain irradiation (HWBI) in the treatment of primary cerebral lymphoma. *Clin Oncol* 1993;5:159-64.

[43] Bessell EM, Lopez-Guillermo A, Villa S, et al. Importance of radiotherapy in the outcome of patients with primary CNS lymphoma : an analysis of the CHOD/BVAM regimen followed by two different radiotherapy treatments. *J Clin Oncol* 2002;20:231-6.

[44] Shah GD, Yahalom J, Correa DD, et al. Combined immunochemotherapy with reduced whole-brain radiotherapy for newly diagnosed primary CNS lymphoma. *J Clin Oncol* 2007;25:4730-5.

[45] Kenai H, Yamashita M, Nakamura T, et al. Gamma Knife surgery for primary central nervous system lymphoma: usefulness as palliative local tumor control. *J Neurosurg* 2006;105 Suppl:133-8.

[46] Sakamoto M, Oya N, Mizowaki T, et al. Initial experiences of palliative stereotactic radiosurgery for recurrent brain lymphomas. *J Neurooncol* 2006;77:53-8.

[47] Suzuki M, Nakamatsu K, Kanamori S, et al. Feasibility study of the simultaneous integrated boost (SIB) method for malignant gliomas using intensity-modulated radiotherapy (IMRT). *Jpn J Clin Oncol* 2003;33:271-7.

[48] Iuchi T, Hatano K, Narita Y, et al. Hypofractionated high-dose irradiation for the treatment of malignant astrocytomas using simultaneous integrated boost technique by IMRT. *Int J Radiat Oncol Biol Phys* 2006;64:1317-24.

[49] Miyawaki D, Murakami M, Demizu Y, et al. Brain injury after proton therapy or carbon ion therapy for head-and-neck cancer and skull base tumors. *Int J Radiat Oncol Biol Phys* 2009;75:378-84.

In: Primary Central Nervous System Lymphoma (PCNSL) ISBN: 978-1-63485-322-4
Editor: Ryuya Yamanaka

Chapter 11

CLINICAL OUTCOME OF HIGH DOSE METHOTREXATE-BASED VINCRISTINE AND PROCARBAZINE COMBINATION CHEMOTHERAPY WITHOUT RADIOTHERAPY FOR PATIENTS WITH PRIMARY CENTRAL NERVOUS SYSTEM LYMPHOMA

Ji Hwan Jang[1], Mee-Seon Kim[2] and Young Zoon Kim[1,*]
[1]Division of Neuro-Oncology and Department of Neurosurgery,
[2]Department of Pathology, Samsung Changwon Hospital,
Sungkyunkwan University School of Medicine, Changwon, South Korea

ABSTRACT

Objective. We investigated the objective response rate to high dose methotrexate (HDMTX)-based vincristine and procarbazine combination chemotherapy without radiotherapy in primary central nervous system lymphoma (PCNSL) patients as a front-line therapy, and sought to identify factors that influence response to HDMTX-based vincristine and procarbazine combination therapy.

Methods. Prospective observational analysis was performed on 109 newly diagnosed immunocompetent PCNSL patients. All patients received front-line chemotherapy of combined HDMTX (3.5 g/m2) and vincristine (1.4 mg/m2) for one day during weeks 1, 3, 5, 7, and 9, and procarbazine (100 mg/m2) for one week during weeks 1, 5, and 9 without radiotherapy.

Results. Among the 109 patients, 94 patients with PCNSL who were registered at our institute from March 2003 to August 2013 were evaluated for participation in the study. Seventy-three patients (77.7%) achieved complete or partial remission after the first combined cycle without irradiation. Higher objective response rates were observed for

* Corresponding Author address: 158 Paryong-ro, Masanhoewon-gu, Changwon, 51353, South Korea. Email: yzkim@skku.edu.

patients with: 1) age < 60 years ($p = 0.046$); 2) Eastern Cooperative Oncology Group (ECOG) performance score of <2 ($p = 0.022$); 3) low risk status as defined by the International Extranodal Lymphoma Study Group ($p = 0.004$); 4) p53 positivity ($p = 0.005$); 5) XBP-1 negativity ($p = 0.002$); 6) MUM-1 negativity ($p = 0.001$); and 7) homogenous gadolinium enhancement in MR images ($p = 0.045$). Multivariate analysis showed that ECOG performance score of < 2 ($p = 0.012$), low risk status ($p < 0.05$), positivity for p53 ($p = 0.027$), negativity for XBP-1 ($p = 0.023$), positivity for MUM-1 ($p = 0.008$), homogenous gadolinium enhancement by MRI ($p < 0.001$), and response to HDMTX-combination chemotherapy ($p < 0.001$) were associated with longer progression-free survival, and ECOG performance score of < 2 ($p = 0.009$), low risk status ($p < 0.05$), negativity for XBP-1 ($p = 0.028$), homogenous gadolinium enhancement by MRI ($p < 0.001$), and response to HDMTX-combination chemotherapy ($p < 0.001$) were associated with longer overall survival.

Conclusion. Our prospective observational study results suggest that PCNSL patients treated with HDMTX-based vincristine and procarbazine combination chemotherapy should have good clinical outcomes even without radiotherapy, which allows avoidance of radiotherapy-associated neurotoxicity.

Keywords: central nervous system, lymphoma, response, prognosis, survival, methotrexate, chemotherapy

INTRODUCTION

Primary CNS lymphoma (PCNSL) is a malignant lymphoma, most frequently diffuse large B-cell lymphoma (DLBCL), which is confined to the CNS at the time of diagnosis. PCNSL is a rare malignancy, accounting for 2.2% of CNS neoplasms in the US during the period 2005–2009 [1], with an overall incidence rate of 0.47 cases per 100,000 people per year [1]. In the past two decades, the incidence of PCNSL in the elderly, mostly in patients 50–70 years of age, has increased [1].

PCNSL is a highly aggressive tumor with a poor prognosis in untreated patients [2]; however, in contrast to most primary brain tumors, PCNSL is sensitive to corticosteroids, chemotherapy, and radiotherapy, and durable complete responses and long-term survival are possible with these treatments. However, the outcome of PCNSL is substantially poorer than that of similar stage systemic non-Hodgkin's lymphoma. The combinatorial chemotherapeutic regimen of cyclophosphamide, doxorubicin, vincristine, and prednisolone (CHOP) provides the best treatment for comparable systemic non-Hodgkin's lymphoma; however, three large, independent, multicenter trials of CHOP with cranial irradiation in PCNSL patients concluded that CHOP offered no survival advantage over radiotherapy alone [3, 4]. The apparent inability of these chemotherapeutic regimens to cross the brain-blood barrier (BBB) and eradicate microscopic disease is a major difficulty. In terms of radiotherapy, this treatment alone for PCNSL provides a median survival of only 12 to 18 months [5]; however, addition of high dose (HD) (>1 g/m2) methotrexate (MTX)-based chemotherapy to radiotherapy has been reported to result in a substantial improvement in median survival time [6-8].

Present therapeutic knowledge of PCNSL is the result of several single-group phase 2 trials, meta-analyses, and large retrospective studies. However, to date, only one randomized trial has been undertaken, and this was halted prematurely due to unsatisfactorily slow accrual [3]. The rarity of PCNSL prevents randomized trials, and the range of different opinions expressed on many of the therapeutic aspects has resulted in a lack of consensus with regard to overall strategy; therefore, the main endpoints should be investigated in a randomized setting. In addition, assessments of new front-line chemotherapy combinations in non-randomized trials, with divergent study designs and entry criteria, do not allow proper comparisons to be made between different regimens, and have resulted in only modest therapeutic progress [9, 10].

Despite limited evidence of the efficacies of specific regimens, HDMTX chemotherapy followed by whole brain radiotherapy (WBRT) is the approach most commonly used for newly diagnosed PCNSL [10, 11], and has been reported to result in a 5-year survival of 20%–35% [6, 8, 12-15]. MTX is a folate antagonist that interrupts DNA synthesis, and is the most widely studied drug in the context of PCNSL.

Following reports of a better outcome for HDMTX-based combination chemotherapy for PCNSL by the Radiation Therapy Oncology Group (RTOG) in the first multicenter trial [8], we started HD (2.5-3.5 g/m2/day) MTX-based combination chemotherapy with vincristine and procarbazine followed by WBRT to treat PCNSL patients. Although many studies have been conducted to identify prognostic factors of PCNSL, no comprehensive studies have been undertaken to identify factors that influence response to HDMTX-based combination chemotherapy.

In this chapter, we describe how we investigated objective response rates (ORR) to HDMTX-based combination chemotherapy with vincristine and procarbazine by performing a prospective observational study. Importantly, the following WBRT was routinely omitted after HDMTX-based combination chemotherapy. We calculated progression-free survival (PFS) and overall survival (OS) rates after a follow-up period of 2 years and sought to identify factors that influence ORR after HDMTX-based combination chemotherapy without following WBRT for PCNSL.

MATERIALS AND METHODS

Patients Collections

Newly diagnosed immunocompetent patients with PCNSL who were registered at our institute from March 2003 to August 2013 were evaluated for participation in the study. This study was reviewed and approved by the institutional review board of Samsung Changwon Hospital (SCMC 2003-014-00) and voluntary, informed, written consent was obtained from all patients who participated in this study. One hundred nine patients were diagnosed with CNS lymphoma, and this was confirmed by histology. Of these, eight patients refused treatment at our institute, and another seven patients did not fulfill the inclusion criteria; four had creatinine clearance below 60, two had a lymphoma in the chest, and one had severe thrombocytopenia that originated from liver cirrhosis. Therefore, clinical data for 94 patients were available, and these patients constituted the study cohort. All patients had one or more intracranial mass lesions. Histological confirmation of PCNSL by the following was required: brain biopsy or resection, CSF analysis demonstrating lymphoma cells, or vitrectomy documenting concomitant ocular lymphoma. To exclude evidence of systemic lymphoma, a negative staging evaluation by chest, abdominal, and pelvic computed tomography (CT) and by bone marrow biopsy was required. All patients underwent cranial neuroimaging at diagnosis, preferably by MRI. All patients underwent lumbar puncture and a complete ophthalmologic evaluation (including a slit-lamp examination).

Patients with newly diagnosed PCNSL were registered within 4 weeks of receiving a histological diagnosis and were considered eligible for enrollment if a pathologic diagnosis had been established and all of the following criteria were met: 1) age over 18 years; 2) Eastern Cooperative Oncology Group (ECOG) performance status grade ≤3; 3) negative HIV serology; 4) creatinine clearance ≥60; 5) no evidence of lymphoma elsewhere in the body after CT scans of the chest, abdomen, and pelvis; 6) an absolute neutrophil count of ≥ 2,000 cells/mm3 and a platelet count of ≥100,000 cells/mm3; and 7) a bilirubin of ≤2.0 mg% and a hepatic enzymes of ≤2 times the upper normal limit. The ECOG definition of performance status was used throughout [16]. Before chemotherapy, laboratory diagnosis of Epstein-Barr virus (EBV) infection was made on a single serum sample using a standard immunofluorescence test that simultaneously detects several types of antibodies to EBV-associated antigens, namely immunoglobulin M and G to the viral capsid antigen, the early antigen, and the EBV nuclear antigen.

Treatment Protocol

Our protocol was modified by the RTOG 93-10 protocol [8]. Treatment consisted of five cycles of chemotherapy administered at fortnightly intervals with a 5-day intercycle delay, as follows: methotrexate 3.5 g/m2/day for one day during weeks 1, 3, 5, 7, and 9, followed by leucovorin rescue, vincristine (1.4 mg/m2 /day with a cap at 2.0 mg/day) for one day during weeks 1, 3, 5, 7, and 9, and procarbazine (100 mg/m2/day) for one week during weeks 1, 5, and 9. Initially, all patients received intravenous methotrexate at the dose of 3.5 g/m2/day. During the chemotherapy cycle, the dose of methotrexate was altered to 3.0 g/m2/day or 2.5 g/m2/day when creatine clearance was between 50 and 60, or between 40 and 50, respectively. If creatine clearance fell below 40, we halted the schedule and delayed for as long as 2-3 weeks until recovery of creatine clearance. Methotrexate (12 mg) was injected into an Ommaya reservoir for five cycles on one day during the week following each intravenous methotrexate dose. Dexamethasone was initiated at a dose of 16 mg/day from the first cycle of HDMTX and tapered by 4 mg/day each week, providing that the patient's neurological status remained stable. If grade II or higher toxic effects as measured by the National Cancer Institute Common Toxicity Criteria version 3.0 (NCI-CTC) were observed, treatment was held up for at least 2 weeks and subsequently restarted at the same dose level in patients with grade 1 and 2 adverse effects. However, patients with grade 3 adverse effects were treated with a reduced dose regimen. Doses missed during a treatment period were not replaced. All toxicities were required to recover to normal levels before retreatment. In the case of persistent grade 2 or 3 toxicity despite discontinuation of treatment, further protocol treatment was stopped.

Follow-Up

The mean follow-up period was 41.7 months. Repeat neuroimaging was required at the completion of neoadjuvant chemotherapy; and then every 2 months for one year, every 4 months for the second year, and every 6 months thereafter. A comprehensive review of chemotherapy records was performed for assessment of adherence to the protocol, and a radiologic review was undertaken for assessment of response after neoadjuvant chemotherapy by two neuroradiologists. MRI was performed using a 1.5T clinical scanner (Signa Horizon; GE Healthcare, Milwaukee, WI, USA). Basal ganglia, the corpus callosum, brain stem, and cerebellum were defined as deep brain structures. Peritumoral edema was categorized as < 2 cm or ≥ 2 cm from the brain tumor as assessed in T2-weighted MR images. In cases of multiple brain lesions, different patterns of enhancement among lesions on MRI, regardless of the number of lesions, was considered to be heterogeneous enhancement.

Evaluation of Response to Treatment

Response to treatment was assessed by contrast-enhanced brain MRI, which was performed at most 7 days before commencement of chemotherapy, after the second and fifth HDMTX chemotherapy cycles, and 4 weeks after termination of chemotherapy. National Cancer Institute standardized response criteria regarding changes in the size of enhanced lesions on T1-weighted MR images were used to define treatment response [17]. In brief, complete remission (CR) was defined as the complete disappearance of all evidence of lymphoma; partial response (PR) as a ≥50% decrease in tumor size; progressive disease (PD) as a ≥25% increase in tumor size or the appearance of any new lesion; and stable disease (SD) as situations that did not meet any of these three previous criteria.

Risk Group as Defined by the International Extranodal Lymphoma Study Group (IELSG)

Using the prognostic scoring system devised by the IELSG, we categorized patients into three risk groups: low, intermediate, and high risk [18]. Variables found to be independently associated with survival in the present study were used to design a scoring system. These variables included age (≤ or > 60 years), ECOG performance status grade (0 to 1 versus 2 to 3), LDH serum level (normal versus elevated), protein concentration in CSF (normal versus elevated), and involvement of deep brain structures (yes versus no). Each variable was assigned a value of 0 if favorable or 1 if unfavorable. Values of these five variables were summed for calculation of final risk scores. Patients with final risk scores of 0 or 1, 2 or 3, or 4 or 5 were assigned to the low, intermediate, or high risk groups, respectively.

Immunohistochemistry and Immunofluorescence

Immunohistochemical staining was performed on formalin-fixed, paraffin-embedded tissues. In addition, MIB-1 (Ki-67) staining was performed to evaluate the proliferative activities of large neoplastic lymphocytes. Paraffin section immunohistochemistry was performed using the avidin-biotin-peroxidase technique after antigen epitope enhancement using a pressure cooker. Final detection was performed by treatment of sections with diaminobenzidine.

Anti–BCL-6 (1:100), anti-p53 (1:50), and anti-XBP-1 (1:100) antibodies were purchased from Santa-Cruz Biotechnology (Santa Cruz, CA, USA), and monoclonal anti–IL-4 (1:200) and anti-MUM-1 (1:100) antibodies were purchased from Pharmingen (San Diego, CA, USA). Anti-MUM-1 (1:100) antibody was used directly for immunofluorescence staining of tumor tissue for flow cytometric analysis (20 μl/106 cells).

Statistical Methods

Objective response was defined as complete remission or partial remission after the fifth course of HDMTX-based combination chemotherapy. OS was calculated from the date of histological diagnosis to death or the last date of follow-up, while PFS was calculated from the first day of treatment to relapse or progression, or to the last date of follow-up.

SPSS version 18.0 (SPSS Institute, Inc., Chicago, IL, USA) was used for statistical analyses. Student's t-test or a nonparametric test was used as appropriate for testing of continuous and ordinal variables. Discrete variables were analyzed using Pearson's Chi-square test. The cumulative proportions of ORR and their 95% confidence intervals (CIs), adjusted for a competing event, were calculated using the cumulative incidence method devised by Prentice et al. [19]. Survival curves were drawn using the Kaplan-Meier method with log-rank test among strata. The Cox proportional hazards method was used to identify factors associated with ORR. Variables found to be significantly associated with ORR by univariate analyses were subjected to multivariate analyses. The hazard ratios (HRs) for overall survival and progression-free survival were calculated using a Cox proportional hazards model, with ORR considered as a time-dependent covariate. Statistical significance was accepted for P values of <0.05. All tests were 2-tailed.

RESULTS

Clinical Characteristics

Total of 94 patients underwent HDMTX-based combination chemotherapy for PCNSL. All patients finished the five cycles of HDMTX chemotherapy. Mean age of patients at commencement of chemotherapy was 64.5 years (range, 37-81 years). Fifty-seven (60.6%) patients were male. Seventy-one (75.5%) patients had an ECOG performance score of <2 and 23 (24.5%) had a score of ≥2. Twenty-nine (30.9%) were categorized as high risk, 35 (37.2%) as intermediate risk, and 30 (31.9%) as low risk. Ocular involvement was found in six (6.4%) patients, and 83 patients were positive for Epstein-Barr virus antibodies which were from past infections. Surgical resection was performed in 19 (20.2%) patients and biopsy alone in 75 (79.8%) patients (Table 1).

With regard to histological features, 89 (94.5%) cases were diffuse large B-cell lymphoma, two (2.1%) cases were anaplastic large B-cell lymphoma, and three (3.2%) cases were marginal zone B-cell lymphoma. Positive staining for BCL-6 was observed in 70

(74.5%) patients, positive staining for XBP-1 in 25 (26.6%), and positive staining for MUM-1 in 45 (47.9%) (Figure 1). In terms of MRI findings, involvement of deep structures was found in 46 (48.9%) patients, homogeneous gadolinium enhancement was observed for 56 (59.6%) tumors, and heterogeneous enhancement for 38 (40.4%) (Table 2).

Table 1. Clinical characteristics of patients who underwent the high dose methotrexate based-combination chemotherapy for primary central nervous system lymphoma (N = 94)

Factors		Number	Percentage
Age	Mean	64.5	(-)
	Range	37 - 81	(-)
	<60 years	32	34.0
	≥60 years	62	66.0
Gender	Male	57	60.6
	Female	37	29.4
ECOG performance score	<2	71	75.5
	≥2	23	24.5
CSF metastasis	Yes	12	12.8
	No	82	87.2
Elevated CSF protein	Yes	59	62.8
	No	35	37.2
Elevated serum LDH	Yes	31	33.0
	No	63	67.0
Risk of international extranodal lymphoma study group	High	29	30.9
	Intermediate	35	37.2
	Low	30	31.9
Ocular involvement	Yes	6	6.4
	No	88	93.6
Epstein-Barr virus infection	Yes	83	88.3
	No	11	11.7
Surgical intervention	Resection	19	20.2
	Biopsy	75	79.8

Abbreviations: ECOG, Eastern Cooperation Oncology Group; CSF, cerebrospinal fluid; LDH, lactate dehydrogenase.

Five cycles of HDMTX-based combination chemotherapy were administered to all patients. No dose reduction was performed during the first cycle. However, during the second and third cycles, two patients received MTX at 3.0 g/m2/day, while during the fourth cycle, two patients received MTX at 2.5 g/m2/day, and three patients received MTX at 3.0 g/m2/day. During the fifth cycle, four patients received MTX at 2.5 g/m2/day and five at 3.0 g/m2/day.

Table 2. Pathological and radiological characteristics of primary central nervous system lymphoma in patients who underwent the high dose methotrexate based-combination chemotherapy (N = 94)

Factors		Number	Percentage
Histopathological feature	Diffuse large B cell lymphoma	89	94.5
	Anaplastic large B cell lymphoma	2	2.1
	Marginal zone B cell lymphoma	3	3.2
BCL-6	Positive	70	74.5
	Negative	24	25.5
p53	Positive	63	67.0
	Negative	31	33.0
IL-4	Positive	30	31.9
	Negative	64	68.1
XBP-1	Positive	25	26.6
	Negative	69	73.4
MUM-1	Positive	45	47.9
	Negative	49	52.1
Necrosis	Positive	74	78.7
	Negative	20	21.3
Ki-67	< 50%	29	30.9
	≥ 50%	65	69.1
Involvement of deep location	Yes	46	48.9
	No	48	51.1
Distance of peritumoral edema from tumor	< 2 cm	29	30.9
	≥ 2 cm	65	69.1
Gadolinium enhancement in MRI	Homogeneous	56	59.6
	Heterogeneous	38	40.4

Abbreviations: MRI, magnetic resonance image.

Response to High Dose Methotrexate-Based Combination Chemotherapy

The overall crude incidence of objective response to HDMTX chemotherapy was 77.7% (CR of 60.6% and PR of 17.1%), and the overall incidence after adjusting for competing events was 81.8% (95% CI 76.2%-87.4%). The ORR was 93.6% for patients aged < 60 years and 69.4% for those aged ≥ 60 years; these values were significantly different ($p = 0.046$). In patients with an ECOG performance score of < 2, the ORR was 87.3%, and in those with an ECOG performance score of ≥ 2, the ORR was 47.8% ($p = 0.022$). ORRs of patients in the high, intermediate, and low risk groups were 44.8%, 88.6%, and 96.7%, respectively ($p < 0.001$). However, no significant ORR differences were found for the other clinical variables studied (Table 3).

Table 3. Response to the high dose methotrexate based combination chemotherapy in patients with primary central nervous lymphoma according to clinical factors of the patients

Factors		Number	CR + PR (n = 73)	SD + PD (n = 21)	p-value
Age	<60 years	32	30 (93.6%)	2 (6.4%)	*0.046
	≥60 years	62	43 (69.4%)	19 (30.6%)	
Gender	Male	57	43 (75.4%)	14 (24.6%)	0.751
	Female	37	30 (81.1%)	7 (18.9%)	
ECOG performance score	<2	71	62 (87.3%)	9 (12.7%)	0.022
	≥2	23	11 (47.8%)	12 (52.2%)	
CSF metastasis	Yes	12	9 (75.0%)	3 (25.0%)	*0.905
	No	82	64 (74.6%)	19 (25.4%)	
Elevated CSF protein	Yes	59	44 (74.6%)	15 (25.4%)	0.854
	No	35	29 (82.9%)	6 (17.1%)	
Elevated serum LDH	Yes	31	23 (74.2%)	8 (25.8%)	0.881
	No	63	50 (79.4%)	13 (20.6%)	
Risk of international extranodal lymphoma study group	High	29	13 (44.8%)	16 (55.2%)	*0.004
	Intermediate	35	31 (88.6%)	4 (11.4%)	
	Low	30	29 (96.7%)	1 (3.3%)	
Ocular involvement	Yes	6	4 (66.7%)	2 (33.3%)	*0.463
	No	88	69 (78.4%)	19 (21.6%)	
Epstein-Barr virus infection	Yes	83	65 (78.3%)	18 (21.7%)	*0.911
	No	11	8 (72.7%)	3 (27.3%)	
Surgical intervention	Resection	19	14 (73.7%)	5 (26.3%)	0.782
	Biopsy	75	59 (78.7%)	16 (21.3%)	

Abbreviations: CR, complete remission; CSF, cerebrospinal fluid; ECOG, Eastern Cooperation Oncology Group; LDH, lactate dehydrogenase; PD, progressive disease; PR, partial remission; SD, stable disease.

*Fisher's exact test, and others are student t-test.

In terms of the molecular features of the brain tumors, the ORR was 87.3% for patients positive for p53 expression, and 58.1% for those negative for p53 (p = 0.005). Those positive for XBP-1 had an ORR of 52.0%, and those negative for XBP-1 an ORR of 87.0% (p = 0.002), while those positive for MUM-1 had an ORR of 62.2%, and those negative for MUM-1 an ORR of 91.8% (p = 0.001). Patients with heterogeneous gadolinium enhancement on MR images had an ORR of 65.8%; however, those with homogeneous enhancement had an objective response of 85.7% (p = 0.045). We found no other histopathological and radiological variables with significant effects on ORR (Table 4). The crude ORRs of tumors that were heterogeneously or homogeneously enhanced were 60.7% and 91.0%, respectively, and ORRs after adjusting for competing events were 64.2% (95% CI 56.7%-70.3%) and 89.8% (95% CI 81.6%-95.8%), respectively. This finding confirms that an enhancing pattern independently predicts objective response to HDMTX-based chemotherapy.

Table 4. Response to the high dose methotrexate based combination chemotherapy in patients with primary central nervous lymphoma according to pathological and radiological characteristics

Factors		Number	CR + PR (n = 73)	SD + PD (n = 21)	p-value
Histopathological feature	DLBCL	89	70 (78.7%)	19 (22.3%)	*0.237
	Others	5	3 (60.0%)	2 (40.0%)	
BCL-6	Positive	70	55 (78.6%)	15 (21.4%)	0.887
	Negative	24	18 (75.0%)	6 (25.0%)	
p53	Positive	63	55 (87.3%)	8 (12.7%)	0.005
	Negative	31	18 (58.1%)	13 (41.9%)	
IL-4	Positive	30	21 (70.0%)	9 (30.0%)	0.286
	Negative	64	52 (81.3%)	12 (18.7%)	
XBP-1	Positive	25	13 (52.0%)	12 (48.0%)	0.002
	Negative	69	60 (87.0%)	9 (13.0%)	
MUM-1	Positive	45	28 (62.2%)	17 (37.8%)	0.001
	Negative	49	45 (91.8%)	7 (8.2%)	
Necrosis	Positive	74	55 (74.3%)	19 (25.7%)	0.124
	Negative	20	18 (90.0%)	2 (10.0%)	
Ki-67	<50%	29	20 (69.0%)	9 (31.0%)	0.081
	≥50%	65	53 (81.5%)	12 (19.5%)	
Involvement of deep location	Yes	46	36 (78.3%)	10 (21.7%)	0.858
	No	48	37 (77.1%)	11 (22.9%)	
Distance of peritumoral edema from tumor	<2 cm	29	21 (72.4%)	8 (27.6%)	0.741
	≥2 cm	65	52 (80.0%)	13 (20.0%)	
Gadolinium enhancement in MRI	Homogeneous	56	48 (85.7%)	8 (14.3%)	0.045
	Heterogeneous	38	25 (65.8%)	13 (34.2%)	

Abbreviations: CR, complete remission; DLBCL, diffuse large B cell lymphoma; MRI, magnetic resonance image; PD, progressive disease; PR, partial remission; SD, stable disease. *Fisher's exact test, and others are student t-test.

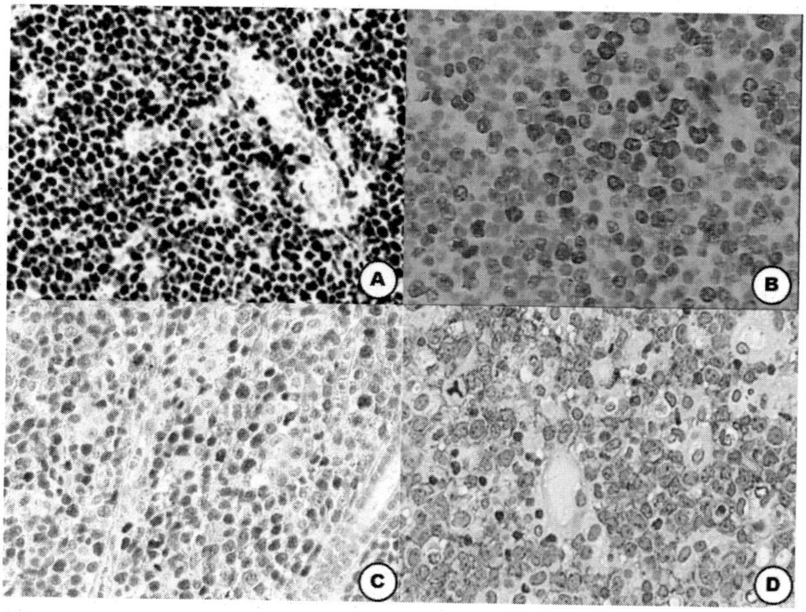

Figure 1. A representative example of primary central nervous system diffuse large B-cell lymphoma showing immunohistochemical positive expression of A) BCL-6, B) MUM-1, C) TP53, and D) XBP-1. (Original magnification x 400).

Table 5. Factors predisposing progression-free survivals (PFS)

Variables		Median PFS (month)	Univariate analysis		Multivariate analysis	
			HR (95% CI)	p-value	HR (95% CI)	p-value
Age (years)	< 60	22.2	2.24 (1.35-3.13)	0.023	1.86 (1.09-2.63)	0.224
	≥ 60	18.0				
Gender	Female	19.9	1.28 (0.42-2.14)	0.715	N A.	
	Male	21.0				
ECOG status	< 2	23.5	4.05 (2.61-5.49)	<0.001	2.76 (1.52-3.90)	0.012
	≥ 2	13.8				
CSF metastasis	No	20.9	1.43 (0.56-2.30)	0.524	N A.	
	Yes	19.1				
Risk of IELSG	Low	30.2	5.27 (3.86-6.68)	<0.001	3.42 (1.76-5.08)	<0.001
	Intermediate	18.9	1.95 (0.92-2.93)	0.227	1.94 (0.91-2.97)	0.138
	High	15.3				
Ocular involvement	Yes	20.9	1.39 (0.71-2.07)	0.695	N.A.	
	No	19.1				
Surgical intervention	Resection	20.3	1.04 (0.28-1.81)	0.904	N.A.	
	Biopsy	19.9				
Response to treatment	CR + PR	21.2	4.21 (2.18-6.24)	0.001	9.28 (4.87-13.69)	<0.001
	SD + PD	12.5				
Histopathology	DLBC	20.7	1.01 (0.31-1.69)	0.927	N.A.	
	Others	20.0				
BCL-6	Positive	21.5	1.82 (0.88-2.76)	0.261	N.A.	
	Negative	19.1				
p53	Positive	22.3	3.08 (1.63-4.53)	0.018	2.63 (1.16-4.10)	0.027
	Negative	18.0				
IL-4	Negative	20.8	1.61 (0.52-2.71)	0.448	N.A.	
	Positive	19.2				
XBP-1	Negative	25.6	4.47 (3.06-5.88)	<0.001	2.70 (1.64-3.76)	0.023
	Positive	13.7				
MUM-1	Negative	23.3	3.49 (1.87-5.11)	0.010	3.03 (1.87-4.19)	0.008
	Positive	18.3				
Necrosis	Negative	20.4	1.32 (0.75-1.89)	0.737	N.A.	
	Positive	19.5				
Ki-67	≥ 50%	20.9	2.03 (0.94-3.12)	0.086	1.96 (0.82-3.10)	0.127
	< 50%	18.4				
Enhancement in MRI	Homo-geneous	26.8	2.55 (1.57-3.53)	0.028	3.38 (1.94-4.82)	<0.001
	Hetero-geneous	15.9				

Abbreviations: CI, Confidence Interval; CR, complete remission; CSF, cerebrospinal fluid; ECOG, Eastern Cooperation Oncology Group; HR, Hazard Ratio; IELSG, International Extranodal Lymphoma Study Group; MRI, magnetic resonance image; LDH, lactate dehydrogenase; NA, not assessed; PD, progressive disease; PR, partial remission; SD, stable disease.

Progression-Free Survival

Median PFS was 20.2 months (95% CI 16.2-24.8 months). In univariate analysis for clinical features predisposing to PFS, median PFS was 22.2 months for those <60 years and

18.0 months for those ≥60 years (HR of 2.24; $p = 0.023$). Patients with an ECOG performance score of <2 had a median PFS of 23.5 months, and those with an ECOG performance score of ≥2 had a median PFS of 13.8 months (HR of 4.05; $p < 0.018$). Median PFSs in the high, intermediate, and low risk groups were 15.3, 18.9, and 30.2 months, respectively ($p < 0.001$). Patients with an objective response had a median PFS of 21.2 months, and those without an objective response had a median PFS of 3.1 months (HR of 4.21; $p = 0.001$). Those factors such as patient's age, ECOG performance score, responsiveness to HDMTX-base chemotherapy, and risk group that had an association with PFS in univariate analysis were subjected to multivariate analysis. However, among clinical features, gender, CSF metastasis, the level of CSF protein, serum LDH level, ocular involvement, and the method of surgical intervention were not associated with PFS even in univariate analysis (Table 5).

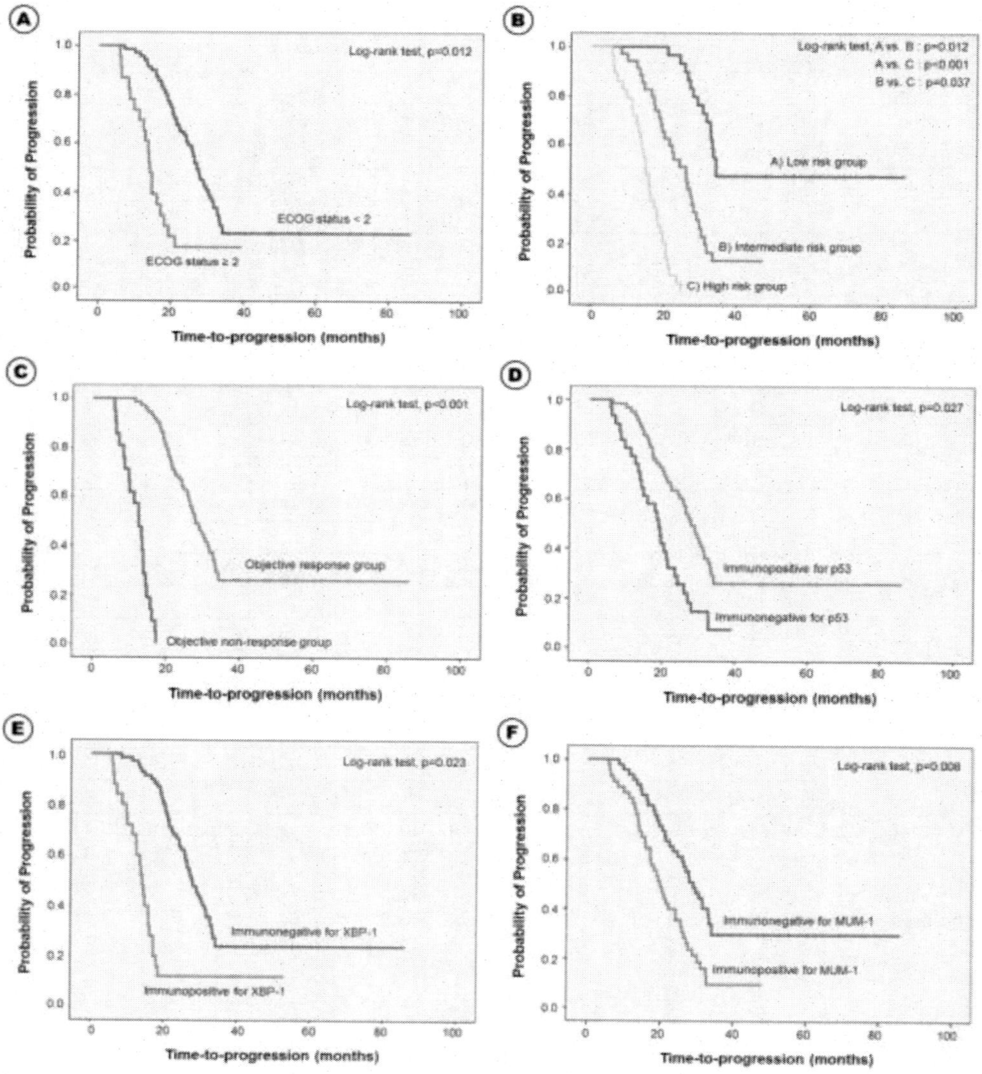

Figure 2. (Continued)

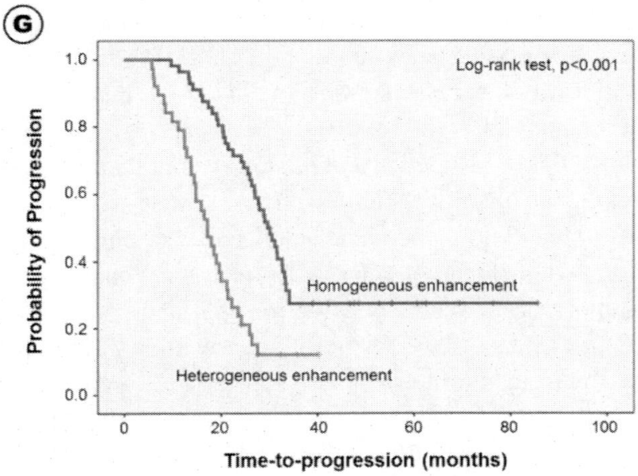

Figure 2. Kaplan-Meier survival curves analysis of factors predicting longer progression-free survival: A) ECOG status, B) risk group of International Extranodal Lymphoma Study Group, C) response to HDMTX-based chemotherapy, D) immunoreactivity for p53, E) immunoreactivity for XBP-1, F) immunoreactivity for MUM-1, and G) enhancement with gadolinium in MR images.

In terms of histopathological and radiological characteristics of PCNSLs, median PFS was 22.3 months for patients positive for p53 expression, and 18.0 months for patients negative for p53 (HR of 3.08; $p = 0.018$). Patients negative for XBP-1 had a greater median PFS than those positive for XBP-1 (27.3 months versus 13.7 months, respectively; HR of 4.47, $p < 0.001$). Patients positive for MUM-1 had a median PFS of 18.3 months, and those negative for MUM-1 had a median PFS of 23.3 months (HR of 3.49; p = 0.0[illegible]0). Of particular interest, median PFS was 17.3 months for patients with a heterogeneously gadolinium-enhanced PCNSL, and 31.2 months for those with a homogeneously-enhanced PCNSL (HR of 2.55; $p = 0.028$). However, histopathological type, BCL-6 immunoreactivity, IL-4 immunoreactivity, necrosis, Ki-67 index, involvement of deep structures, and peritumoral edema were not associated with PFS in univariate analysis (Table 5).

In multivariate analysis, ECOG performance status (HR of 2.76; $p = 0.012$), risk of IELSG (low risk versus high risk; HR of 3.42, $p < 0.001$), response group to treatment (HR of 9.28; $p < 0.001$), positive IHC staining of p53 (HR of 2.63; $p = 0.027$), negative IHC staining of XBP-1 (HR of 2.70; $p = 0.023$), negative IHC staining of MUM-1 (HR of 3.03; $p = 0.008$), and homogeneous enhancement in MRI (HR of 3.38; $p < 0.001$) were independently associated with longer PFS in PCNSL patients who were treated with HDMTX-based combination chemotherapy (Table 5). The factors that had a strong association with longer PFS were analyzed by Kaplan-Meier survival methods and the log-rank test (Figure 2). Age and Ki-67 status, which were associated with PFS in univariate analysis, did not have an independent association with PFS after multi-factor adjustment.

Overall Survival

Median OS and the 2-year survival rate were 35.3 months (95% CI 2[illegible].2-39.5 months) and 73.8%, respectively. Furthermore, in univariate analysis for clinical factors predisposing to PFS, median OS was 37.8 months in patients with an ECOG performance score of <2 and 21.1 months in those with a performance score of ≥2 (HR of 4.85; $p < 0.001$). Patients in the high, intermediate, and low risk groups had OSs of 24.2, 34.7, and 47.9 months, respectively, and these were significantly different ($p < 0.05$). As expected, patients who achieved an objective response to HDMTX-based combination chemotherapy survived longer. The median OS of patients who experienced an objective response was 40.8 months, whereas the median OS of patients who did not experience an objective response was 17.5 months (HR of 5.22; $p < 0.001$). In terms of histopathological and radiological characteristics of PCNSLs, the median OS was 41.7 months in patients positive for p53, and 25.3 months in those negative for p53 (HR of 4.92; $p < 0.001$). IHC positivity and negativity for XBP-1 expression were found to be associated with median OS rates of 22.5 and 39.8 months, respectively (HR of 4.68; $p < 0.001$). Of particular interest, homogeneous gadolinium enhancement was found to be associated with a longer median OS (43.2 months versus 29.8 months; HR of 4.09, $p = 0.017$). However, age, gender, CSF metastasis, the level of CSF protein, serum LDH level, ocular involvement, the method of surgical intervention, histopathological type, BCL-6 immunoreactivity, IL-4 immunoreactivity, MUM-1 immunoreactivity, necrosis, Ki-67 index, involvement of deep structures, and peritumoral edema were not associated with OS in univariate analysis (Table 6).

In multivariate analysis, the HR of an ECOG performance score of <2 over a score of ≥2 or longer OS was 2.81 (95% CI, 1.57-4.05; $p = 0.009$), and the HRs of a high risk over intermediate risk, and a high risk over a low risk were 2.42 (95% CI, 1.48-3.36; $p = 0.041$) and 4.44 (95% CI, 2.86-6.02; $p < 0.001$), respectively. The HR of the presence over the absence of an objective response to HDMTX chemotherapy for longer OS was 7.28 (95% CI, 3.45-11.11; $p < 0.001$). The HR of negativity versus positivity for XBP-1 expression for longer OS was 3.00 (95% CI, 1.68-4.32; $p = 0.028$), and the HR of homogenous versus heterogeneous enhanced PCNSL for longer OS was 4.02 (95% CI, 2.08-5.96; $p < 0.001$). Similarly, these factors had a good association with longer OS as determined by Kaplan-Meier survival analysis and the log-rank test (Figure 3). Although p53 expression was found to be associated with longer OS by univariate analysis, multivariate analysis revealed no significant association (Table 6).

Follow-Up and Clinical Course

All patients were followed-up for 2 years or longer, and the mean follow-up time from the date of histopathological diagnosis was 41.7 months (range, 25. 2 – 73.8 months). During the follow-up period, 65 (69.1%) patients died. Of these, eight patients (8.5%) died during treatment: four patients (4.3%) succumbed to rapid progression of PCNSLs, two (2.1%) to acute renal failure, and two (2.1%) to sepsis. In patients with disease progression, acute cerebral edema and hydrocephalic crisis were the cause of death. Acute renal failure and sepsis were attributed to toxicity of HDMTX-based combination chemotherapy. Six of the patients who died were older than 60 years. There were no deaths from other systemic diseases e.g., acute myocardiac infarction, pulmonary embolism, or complications of diabetes.

Seventy-three patients (77.7%) experienced disease recurrence. Median time to recurrence was 20.2 months (95% CI 16.2-24.8 months). After recurrence, all patients were treated with HDMTX-based combination chemotherapy again at first and second recurrence.

Seven patients had recurrent disease three times or more; four patients were treated with cytarabine arabinoside chemotherapy and three patients were treated with WBRT for palliative purposes.

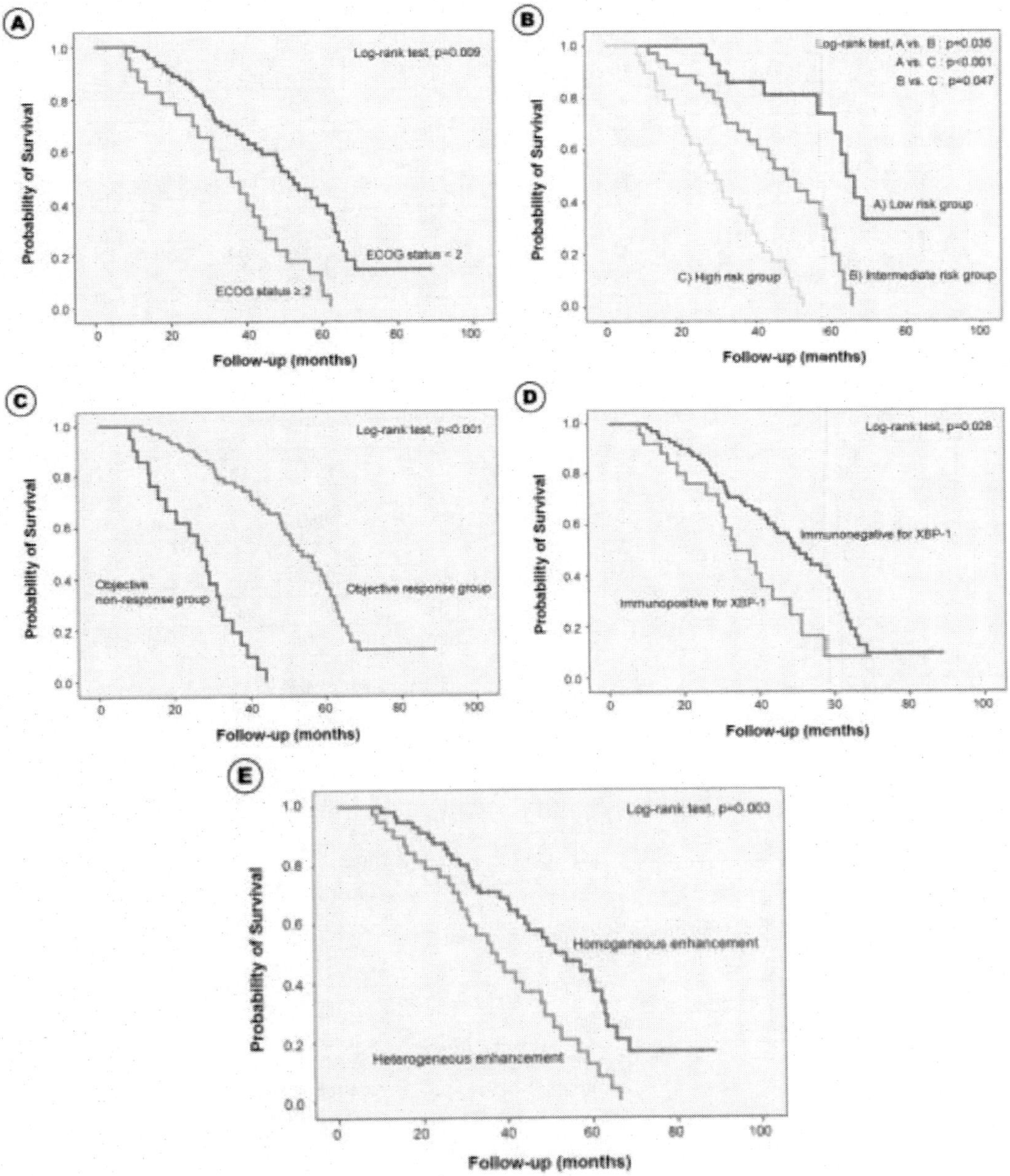

Figure 3. Kaplan-Meier survival curves analysis for factors predicting longer overall survival: A) ECOG status, B) risk group of International Extranodal Lymphoma Study Group, C) response to HDMTX-based chemotherapy, D) immunoreactivity for XBP-1, and F) enhancement with gadolinium in MR images.

Table 6. Factors predisposing overall survivals (OS)

Variables		Median OS (month)	Univariate analysis		Multivariate analysis	
			HR (95% CI)	p-value	HR (95% CI)	p-value
Age (years)	<60	47.1	2.41 (0.92-3.90)	0.112	1.75 (0.94-2.56)	0.401
	≥60	42.8				
Gender	Female	46.3	1.34 (0.46-2.22)	0.631	N.A.	
	Male	42.0				
ECOG status	<2	51.2	4.85 (3.04-6.67)	<0.001	2.81 (1.57-4.05)	0.009
	≥2	36.2				
CSF metastasis	No	47.1	1.26 (0.45-2.07)	0.763	N.A.	
	Yes	43.2				
Risk of IELSG	Low	57.9	6.31 (4.27-8.35)	<0.001	4.44 (2.86-6.02)	<0.001
	Intermediate	44.7	3.86 (2.05-5.67)	0.026	2.42 (1.48-3.36)	0.041
	High	34.2				
Ocular involvement	Yes	46.5	1.12 (0.28-1.96)	0.812	N.A.	
	No	45.1				
Surgical intervention	Resection	47.8	1.32 (0.64-2.01)	0.529	N.A.	
	Biopsy	45.1				
Response to treatment	CR + PR	50.8	5.22 (3.48-6.96)	<0.001	7.28 (3.45-11.11)	<0.001
	SD + PD	27.5				
Histopathology	Others	46.7	1.20 (0.34-2.06)	0.826	N.A.	
	DLBC	45.1				
BCL-6	Positive	46.1	1.88 (0.86-2.89)	0.305	N.A.	
	Negative	42.4				
p53	Positive	51.7	4.92 (2.85-6.98)	<0.001	1.38 (0.84-1.92)	0.652
	Negative	40.3				
IL-4	Negative	49.0	1.93 (0.91-2.95)	0.276	N.A.	
	Positive	42.8				
XBP-1	Negative	49.8	4.68 (2.91-6.45)	<0.001	3.00 (1.68-4.32)	0.028
	Positive	32.5				
MUM-1	Negative	46.1	2.54 (0.93-4.15)	0.105	2.15 (0.95-3.30)	0.054
	Positive	43.1				
Necrosis	Negative	46.3	1.37 (0.61-2.13)	0.116	1.94 (0.88-3.00)	0.083
	Positive	42.8				
Ki-67	≥ 50%	46.6	3.04 (0.98-5.09)	0.059	1.36 (0.66-2.06)	0.582
	< 50%	2.4				
Enhancement in MRI	Homogeneous	53.2	4.09 (1.84-6.34)	0.017	4.02 (2.08-5.96)	<0.001
	Heterogeneous	39.8				

Abbreviations: CI, Confidence Interval; CR, complete remission; CSF, cerebrospinal fluid; ECOG, Eastern Cooperation Oncology Group; HR, Hazard Ratio; IELSG, International Extranodal Lymphoma Study Group; MRI, magnetic resonance image; LDH, lactate dehydrogenase; NA, not assessed; PD, progressive disease; PR, partial remission; SD, stable disease.

A total of 41 patients (43.6%) suffered from several adverse effects: 33 patients (35.1%) from grade 1 adverse effects, 24 patients (25.5%) from grade 2 adverse effects, nine patients (9.6%) from grade 3 adverse effects, and four patients (4.2%) from grade 4-5 adverse effects (Table 7). Nine patients who had experienced the grade 3 adverse effects had a break time to wait for full recovery from toxicity, and all of them recovered. However, four of them could not tolerate the toxicity after retreatment with HDMTX-based combination chemotherapy, even at a reduced dose.

Table 7. Adverse effects measured by the National Cancer Institute Common Toxicity Criteria version 3.0 (NCI-CTC)

	Grade 1	Grade 2	Grade 3	Grade 4-5
Myelosuppression	9	5	2	0
Mucositis	3	2	0	0
Diarrhea	2	1	0	0
Nausea/Vomiting	2	2	0	0
Renal toxicity	3	3	1	0
Skin reaction	2	1	0	0
Pulmonary toxicity	1	1	0	0
Neurotoxicity	8	8	5	2
Hepatobiliary toxicity	3	1	0	0
Infective disorder	0	0	1	2
Total	33 (35.1%)	24 (25.5%)	9 (9.6%)	4 (4.2%)

DISCUSSION

Until the early 1990s, WBRT alone was considered standard primary treatment for PCNSL. However, long-term disease control with WBRT alone is poor, with a median overall survival of 12–16 months and a 2-year overall survival of 28–40% [30, 31]. HDMTX–based chemotherapy followed by WBRT was therefore initiated in many institutes and became the standard therapy for PCNSL. CR rates of 69–87%, median PFS of >20 months, and 2-year OS of 62–85% were reported in several phase II studies of combined chemotherapy and radiotherapy [6, 8, 13, 14, 20, 21]. However, the combination of HDMTX and WBRT is potentially neurotoxic. Severe cognitive dysfunction occurred in all patients over 60 years of age treated with HDMTX and intraventricular MTX followed by WBRT and systemic HD cytarabine. In extreme cases, this dysfunction led to dementia with incontinence and ataxia, leaving affected patients dependent on assistants [22]. Consequently, the role of WBRT in the primary therapy of PCNSL has increasingly been questioned.

Recently, one randomized trial (the G-PCNSL-SG1 study) investigated immediate consolidation of WBRT (30 doses of 1.5 Gy) in the primary treatment of PCNSL after complete response to HDMTX-based chemotherapy versus deferred WBRT at relapse. Patients treated with WBRT experienced some benefit in terms of PFS: 18.3 versus 11.9 months (95% CI 7.3–16.5, $p = 0.13$), but without significant effect on OS: median 32.4 months with WBRT versus 37.1 months without WBRT (95% CI 0.8–1.4, $p = 0.70$) [23]. In these prospective studies, median OS reached 35.3 months with omitting WBRT, which was similar to the results of the G-PCNSL-SG1 study. PFS in our study was much longer than that in the G-PCNSL-SG1 study (20.2 versus 11.9 months).

Although many reports have shown that several factors influence the prognosis of PCNSL, no study to date has assessed the factors that influence objective response to

HDMTX-based combination chemotherapy for PCNSL. Ferri et al. [18] suggested that age, performance status, LDH serum level, HDMTX, and the use of HD cytarabine are significantly associated with overall response rate. Their therapeutic modalities included radiotherapy alone, radiotherapy followed by chemotherapy, chemotherapy alone, and chemotherapy followed by radiotherapy. However, their chemotherapeutic regimen was highly heterogeneous, that is, it involved MTX followed by alkylating agents, HD cytarabine, and anthracycline. Other regimens included alkylating agent alone, the CHOP regimen, an HD cytarabine-based regimen, HDMTX alone, HDMTX plus alkylating agents, HDMTX plus CHOP-like regimens, and others. Furthermore, no previous studies have investigated how the molecular features of PCNSL can influence objective response to HDMTX-based combination chemotherapy.

We found that age, performance status, and low risk status as defined by the IELSG, expression of p53, XBP-1, and MUM-1, and patterns of gadolinium enhancement in MR images significantly affected objective response. Ferri et al. [24] also studied predictors of treatment outcome in PCNSL patients, and consistent with our study, found that age, performance status, and a lower prognostic score (as defined by the IELSG) influenced the overall response rate to HDMTX-based combination chemotherapy. However, in our study, unlike the previous study, multivariate analysis showed no relationship between age and longer PFS or OS; the cause of this discrepancy is not known.

Rubenstein et al. [25] suggested that PCNSL has several distinct clinical features: 1) a short response duration to combined modality therapy; 2) a unique proclivity to grow in the CNS; and 3) a heightened responsiveness to MTX. In terms of the prognostic significance of biologic phenotypes, diffuse large B-cell lymphoma (DLBCL) cases with germinal center B-cell patterns expressing BCL-6 have been demonstrated to have a better prognosis than DLBCL cases with activated B-cell expressing MUM-1 [25, 26]. However, other groups observed no difference in survival between DLBCL patients based on BCL-6 expression [27, 28]. One report in fact showed that BCL-6 expression was associated with a poor prognosis [29]. In our study, BCL-6 expression was not associated with PFS or OS, while absence of expression of MUM-1 was associated with longer PFS in multivariate analysis. Multivariate analysis showed that absence of XBP-1 expression was associated with longer PFS and OS. Rubenstein et al. also suggested that XBP-1 was among the genes that showed the most significant differential expression in PCNSL, and that strong XBP-1 protein expression in dense tumor cell populations was associated with the vasculature [25]. Further studies are needed to determine the role(s) of these biomarkers.

Of particular interest, we found that patterns of gadolinium enhancement were predictive of response to HDMTX. According to a report by Algazi et al. contrast enhancement was uniform in 55 to 60% of PCNSL cases [30]. They suggested that the apparent diffusion coefficient (ADC) is correlated with cellular density in PCNSL, and that pre-therapeutic ADC (a possible surrogate marker of cellular density) is predictive of clinical outcome. Low cellularity, which reduces the ADC within contrast-enhancing regions, may permit a high influx of contrast into the tumor; therefore, PCNSLs showing homogeneous gadolinium enhancement have lower cellularity and a higher objective response due to the smaller tumor cell burden. Unfortunately, because ADC mapping was not performed on many of the MR images, we were unable to investigate the association between ADC and response to HDMTX-based combination chemotherapy.

Although we showed that several factors, including age < 60 years, good performance status, low risk status of IELSG, expression of p53, XBP-1, and MUM-1, and homogeneous MRI enhancement patterns are associated with objective response to HDMTX-based combination chemotherapy for PCNSL, several study shortcomings limit our conclusions. First, HDMTX is known to be the primary treatment for PCNSL and has been successfully incorporated into multi-drug chemotherapy regimens, which has in turn been associated with notable improvements in response and survival. We commenced this decade-long study in 2003; thus, it is somewhat dated in terms of current practice. In fact, results of combination chemotherapies with other drugs, such as high-dose cytarabine [24], temozolomide [31], and cyclophosphamide [32] have also been reported. In addition, the recently introduced extremely high dose MTX mono-chemotherapy (>8 g/m2/day) [33], and development of targeted drugs, such as rituximab [15], have improved the prognosis for PCNSL. To establish the advantage of HDMTX-based procarbazine and vincristine combination chemotherapy for PCNSL over other guaranteed treatments, a prospective randomized clinical trial is essential. Second, samples were examined as paraffin-embedded tissues and we did not investigate alterations in proteins that have previously been found to be associated with response to treatment. Therefore, the present research did not shed light on pathophysiologic mechanisms. Third, we did not perform ADC mapping using MR images during the early period of this study in most patients, which could have confirmed the positive association between homogeneous gadolinium enhancement and high signal intensity on the ADC map. Therefore, we could not examine the association between homogeneous enhancement and low tumor cellularity. Accordingly, we could not evaluate the strength of the association between responsiveness to HDMTX-based chemotherapy and low cellularity PCNCL. Fourth, the number of patients in this study was relatively small. Randomized and prospective studies of more patients are required to verify our hypotheses.

CONCLUSION

In this chapter, based on prospective analysis, we found that front-line HDMTX-based combination chemotherapy achieved good clinical outcomes even without radiotherapy compared to a previous study that performed HDMTX chemotherapy followed by radiotherapy. We found that an age of <60 years, an ECOG performance score of <2, low or intermediate risk of IELSG, immunohistochemical positivity for p53, immunohistochemical negativity for XBP-1 or MUM-1, and homogenous gadolinium enhancement in MRI were associated with a good PCNSL patient response to front-line HDMTX-based combination chemotherapy without radiotherapy. In particular, most patients who underwent these treatments tolerated the treatment well. Therefore, we suggest that HDMTX-based combination chemotherapy alone is an effective therapeutic option for patients who are at risk of neurotoxicity from radiotherapy.

ACKNOWLEDGMENTS

The authors would like to thank Young Min Kim, MD, and Mi-Ok Sunwoo, MD, (Department of Radiology, Samsung Changwon Hospital) for their review of the neuroradiological images, Young Wook Kim, MD (Department of Biostatistics, Samsung Changwon Hospital) for assistance with statistical analysis, and Eun Hee Lee, MD (Department of Pathology, Samsung Changwon Hospital) for performing the immunohistochemical staining.

DISCLOSURE

This study was supported financially by Samsung Biomedical Research Institute (SBRI) grants. The authors disclose there are no conflicts of interest in the materials, methods, or findings of this manuscript.

REFERENCES

[1] Dolecek, T., Propp, J. M., Stroup, N. E. and Kruchko, C. CBTRUS statistical report: primary brain and central nervous system tumors diagnosed in the United States in 2005–2009. *Neuro Oncol* 2012; 14 (suppl. 5): v1–v49).

[2] Maher EA, Fine HA. Primary CNS lymphoma. *Semin Oncol* 1999; 26: 346-356.

[3] Mead GM, Bleehen NM, Gregor A, Bullimore J, Shirley D, Rampling RP, Trevor J, Glaser MG, Lantos P, Ironside JW, Moss TH, Brada M, Whaley JB, Stenning SP. A medical research council randomized trial in patients with primary cerebral non-Hodgkin lymphoma: cerebral radiotherapy with and without cyclophosphamide, doxorubicin, vincristine, and prednisone chemotherapy. *Cancer* 2000; 89: 1359–1370.

[4] Schultz C, Scott C, Sherman W, Donahue B, Fields J, Murray K, Fisher B, Abrams R, Meis-Kindblom J. Preirradiation chemotherapy with cyclophosphamide, doxorubicin, vincristine, and dexamethasone for primary CNS lymphomas: Initial report of Radiation Therapy Oncology Group protocol 88-06. *J Clin Oncol* 1996; 14: 556-554.

[5] Nelson DF. Radiotherapy in the treatment of primary central nervous system lymphoma (PCNSL). J Neurooncol 1999; 43: 241-247.

[6] Abrey LE, Yahalom J, DeAngelis LM. Treatment for primary CNS lymphoma: The next step. *J Clin Oncol* 2000; 18: 3144-3150.

[7] Ferreri AJ, Reni M, Dell'Oro S, Ciceri F, Bernardi M, Camba L, Ponzoni M, Terreni MR, Tomirotti M, Spina M, Villa E. Combined treatment with high-dose methotrexate, vincristine and procarbazine, without intrathecal chemotherapy, followed by consolidation radiotherapy for primary central nervous system lymphoma in immunocompetent patients. *Oncology* 2001; 60: 134-140.

[8] DeAngelis LM, Seiferheld W, Schold SC, Fisher B, Schultz CJ; Radiation Therapy Oncology Group Study 93-10. Combination chemotherapy and radiotherapy for primary central nervous system lymphoma: Radiation Therapy Oncology Group Study 93-10. *J Clin Oncol* 2002; 20: 4643–4648.

[9] Ferreri AJ, Reni M, Villa E. Therapeutic management of primary central nervous system lymphoma: lessons from prospective trials. *Ann Oncol* 2000; 11: 927–937.

[10] Ferreri AJ, Abrey LE, Blay JY, Borisch B, Hochman J, Neuwelt EA, Yahalom J, Zucca E, Cavalli F, Armitage J, Batchelor T. Summary statement on primary central nervous system lymphomas from the Eighth International Conference on Malignant Lymphoma, Lugano, Switzerland, June 12 to 15, 2002. *J Clin Oncol 2003*; 21: 2407–2414.

[11] Ferreri AJ, Reni M, Pasini F, Calderoni A, Tirelli U, Pivnik A, Aondio GM, Ferrarese F, Gomez H, Ponzoni M, Borisch B, Berger F, Chassagne C, Iuzzolino P, Carbone A, Weis J, Pedrinis E, Motta T, Jouvet A, Barbui T, Cavalli F, Blay JY. A multicenter study of treatment of primary CNS lymphoma. *Neurology* 2002; 58: 1513–1520.

[12] Herrlinger U, Küker W, Uhl M, Blaicher HP, Karnath HO, Kanz L, Bamberg M, Weller M. NOA-03 trial of high-dose methotrexate in primary central nervous system lymphoma: final report. *Ann Neurol* 2005; 57: 843–847.

[13] O'Brien PC, Roos DE, Pratt G, Liew KH, Barton MB, Poulsen MG, Olver IN, Trotter GE; Trans-Tasman Radiation Oncology Group. Combined modality therapy for primary central nervous system lymphoma: long-term data from a phase II multicenter study (Trans-Tasman Radiation Oncology Group). *Int J Radiat Oncol Biol Phys* 2006; 64: 408–413.

[14] Ferreri AJ, Dell'Oro S, Foppoli M, Bernardi M, Brandes AA, Tosoni A, Montanari M, Balzarotti M, Spina M, Ilariucci F, Zaja F, Stelitano C, Bobbio F, Corazzelli G, Baldini L, Ponzoni M, Picozzi P, Caligaris Cappio F, Reni M. MATILDE regimen followed by radiotherapy is an active strategy against primary CNS lymphomas. *Neurology* 2006; 66: 1435–1438.

[15] Shah GD, Yahalom J, Correa DD, Lai RK, Raizer JJ, Schiff D, LaRocca R, Grant B, DeAngelis LM, Abrey LE. Combined immunochemotherapy with reduced whole-brain radiotherapy for newly diagnosed primary CNS lymphoma. *J Clin Oncol* 2007; 25: 4730–4735.

[16] Oken MM, Creech RH, Tormey DC, Horton J, Davis TE, McFadden ET, Carbone PP. Toxicity and response criteria of the Eastern Cooperative Oncology Group. *Am J Clin Oncol* 1982; 5: 649-655.

[17] Cheson BD, Horning SJ, Coiffier B, Shipp MA, Fisher RI, Connors JM, Lister TA, Vose J, Grillo-López A, Hagenbeek A, Cabanillas F, Klippensten D, Hiddemann W, Castellino R, Harris NL, Armitage JO, Carter W, Hoppe R, Canellos GP. Report of an international workshop to standardize response criteria for non-Hodgkin's lymphomas. NCI Sponsored International Working Group. *J Clin Oncol* 1999; 17: 1244.

[18] Ferreri AJ, Blay JY, Reni M, Pasini F, Spina M, Ambrosetti A, Calderoni A, Rossi A, Vavassori V, Conconi A, Devizzi L, Berger F, Ponzoni M, Borisch B, Tinguely M, Cerati M, Milani M, Orvieto E, Sanchez J, Chevreau C, Dell'Oro S, Zucca E, Cavalli F. Prognostic scoring system for primary CNS lymphomas: The International Exranodal Lymphoma Study Group Experience. *J Clin Oncol* 2003; 21: 266-272.

[19] Chen BE, Kramer JL, Greene MH, Rosenberg PS. Competing risks analysis of correlated failure time data. *Biomechanics* 2008; 64: 172-179.

[20] Poortmans PM, Kluin-Nelemans HC, Haaxma-Reiche H, Van't Veer M, Hansen M, Soubeyran P, Taphoorn M, Thomas J, Van den Bent M, Fickers M, Van Imhoff G, Rozewicz C, Teodorovic I, van Glabbeke M; European Organization for Research and Treatment of Cancer Lymphoma Group. High-dose methotrexate-based chemotherapy

followed by consolidating radiotherapy in non-AIDS-related primary central nervous system lymphoma: European Organization for Research and Treatment of Cancer Lymphoma Group phase II trial 20962. *J Clin Oncol* 2003; 21: 4483–4488.

[21] Korfel A, Martus P, Nowrousian MR, Hossfeld DK, Kirchen H, Brücher J, Stelljes M, Birkmann J, Peschel C, Pasold R, Fischer L, Jahnke K, Thiel E; German primary central nervous system lymphoma Study Group (G-PCNSL-SG). German Primary Central Nervous System Lymphoma Study Group (G-PCNSL-SG). Response to chemotherapy and treating institution predict survival in primary central nervous system lymphoma. *Br J Haematol* 2005; 128: 177–183.

[22] Abrey LE, DeAngelis LM, Yahalom J. Long-term survival in primary CNS lymphoma. *J Clin Oncol* 1998; 16: 859–863.

[23] Thiel E, Korfel A, Martus P, Kanz L, Griesinger F, Rauch M, Röth A, Hertenstein B, von Toll T, Hundsberger T, Mergenthaler HG, Leithäuser M, Birnbaum T, Fischer L, Jahnke K, Herrlinger U, Plasswilm L, Nägele T, Pietsch T, Bamberg M, Weller M. High-dose methotrexate with or without whole brain radiotherapy for primary CNS lymphoma (G-PCNSL-SG-1): a phase 3, randomized, non-inferiority trial. *Lancet* Oncol 2010; 11: 1036–1047.

[24] Ferreri AJ, Reni M, Foppoli M, Martelli M, Pangalis GA, Frezzato M, Cabras MG, Fabbri A, Corazzelli G, Ilariucci F, Rossi G, Soffietti R, Stelitano C, Vallisa D, Zaja F, Zoppegno L, Aondio GM, Avvisati G, Balzarotti M, Brandes AA, Fajardo J, Gomez H, Guarini A, Pinotti G, Rigacci L, Uhlmann C, Picozzi P, Vezzulli P, Ponzoni M, Zucca E, Caligaris-Cappio F, Cavalli F; Andres JMF, Michele R, Marco F. High-dose cytarabine plus high-dose methotrexate versus high-dose methotrexate alone in patients with primary CNS lymphoma: a randomized phase 2 trial. *Lancet* 2009; 374: 1512–1520.

[25] Rubenstein JL, Fridlyand J, Shen A, Aldape K, Ginzinger D, Batchelor T, Treseler P, Berger M, McDermott M, Prados M, Karch J, Okada C, Hyun W, Parikh S, Haqq C, Shuman M. Gene expression and angiotropism in primary CNS lymphoma. *Blood* 2006; 107: 3716-3723.

[26] Chang CC, McClintock S, Cleveland RP Trzpuc T, Vesole DH, Logan B, Kajdacsy-Balla A, Perkins SL. Immunohistochemical expression patterns of germinal center and activation B-cell markers correlate with prognosis in diffuse large B-cell lymphoma. *Am J Surg Pathol* 2004; 28: 464–470.

[27] Lin CH, Kuo KT, Chuang SS. Kuo SH, Chang JH, Chang KC, Hsu HC, Tien HF, Cheng AL. Comparison of the expression and prognostic significance of differentiation markers between diffuse large B-cell lymphoma of central nervous system origin and peripheral nodal origin. *Clin Cancer Res* 2006; 12: 1152–1156.

[28] Sugita Y, Tokunaga O, Nakashima A. Shigemori M. SHP-1 expression in primary central nervous system B-cell lymphomas in immunocompetent patients reflects maturation stage of normal B cell counterparts. *Pathol Int* 2004; 54: 659–666.

[29] Momota H, Narita Y, Maeshima AM, Miyakita Y, Shinomiya A, Maruyama T, Muragaki Y, Shibui S. Prognostic value of immunohistochemical profile and response to high-dose methotrexate therapy in primary CNS lymphoma. *J Neurooncol* 2010; 98: 341-348.

[30] Algazi AP, Kadoch C, Rubenstein JL. Biology and treatment of primary central nervous system lymphoma. *Neurotherapeutics* 2009; 6: 587-597.

[31] Antonio MPO, Luc T, Oliver C, Charlotte C, Maryline B, Khe HX. Temozolomide and methotrexate for primary central nervous system lymphoma in the elderly. *J Neurooncol* 2007; 85: 207-211.

[32] Silvani A, Salmaggi A, Eoli M Lamperti E, Broggi G, Marras CE, Fariselli L, Milanesi I, Fiumani A, Gaviani P, Erbetta A, Giovagnoli AR, Pollo B, Botturi A, Boiardi A. Methotrexate based chemotherapy and deferred radiotherapy for primary central nervous system lymphoma (PCNSL): single institution experience. *J Neurooncol* 2007; 82: 273–279.

[33] Ferreri AJ, Crocchiolo R, Assaanelli A, Govi S, Reni M. High-dose chemotherapy supported by autologous stem cell transplantation in patients with primary central nervous system lymphoma: facts and opinions. *Leuk Lymphoma* 2008; 49: 2042-2047.

In: Primary Central Nervous System Lymphoma (PCNSL) ISBN: 978-1-63485-322-4
Editor: Ryuya Yamanaka

Chapter 12

FAREWELL TO WHOLE-BRAIN RADIOTHERAPY IN THE TREATMENT OF PRIMARY CENTRAL NERVOUS SYSTEM LYMPHOMA

Yasuo Iwadate, MD, PhD*
Departments of Neurological Surgery, Chiba University,
Graduate School of Medicine, Chuo-ku, Chiba, Japan

ABSTRACT

High-dose methotrexate (HD-MTX) has dramatically improved median overall survival (OS) for primary central nervous system lymphoma (PCNSL) to 34-46 months from the 12-18 months obtained with whole-brain radiotherapy (WBRT) alone. However, HD-MTX alone is not curative for most patients with PCNSL. HD-MTX frequently causes neurotoxicity when combined with WBRT and hematological toxicity when combined with other chemotherapeutic agents. For further improvement of OS without such adverse events, application of recently-advanced modalities such as highly-localized radiotherapy appears an important option for residual tumors after HD-MTX. We should pursue cure of this disease with minimal damage to the normal brain, which enables full return to the previous social activities of the patient.

Keywords: PCNSL, MTX, methotrexate, high dose, radiotherapy

INTRODUCTION

Primary central nervous system lymphoma (PCNSL) is an aggressive disease that is typically fatal within months when not treated with cytotoxic therapies [1]. Although whole-brain radiotherapy (WBRT) results in impressive initial response on imaging studies and improved progression-free survival (PFS) and overall survival (OS), tumor recurrences

* Corresponding Author address: Yasuo Iwadate, M.D., Ph.D. 1-8-1, Inohana, Chuo-ku, Chiba, 260-8670, Japan, Telephone: +81-43-226-2158, FAX number: +81-43-226-2159, Email: iwadatey@faculty.chiba-u.jp.

inevitably occur and limit OS to no longer than around 18 months [1]. The discrepancy between the good initial response and limited survival benefit suggests that PCNSL is essentially not radiosensitive. To enhance the moderate effectiveness of WBRT, combined use of chemotherapy has been trialed, initially with the CHOP regimen that is widely used for systemic lymphoma [2]. Many of these trials failed to show any prolongation of survival, and only high-dose methotrexate (HD-MTX) has proven effective, with a median OS approximately three times longer than that with WBRT alone [3-5]. Despite such dramatic improvement in survival, this encouraging therapeutic combination was soon found to be accompanied by a major risk of neurotoxicity resulting in dementia, changes in personality, and gait disturbance [6, 7]. Neurotoxicity results in the patient dependence in activities of daily living (ADL) and deprives them of their previous social activities [8]. Cure of this disease, while minimizing damage to the normal brain, is worth pursuing to achieve the full return of the patient to previous social activity. In other words, we should provide a minimum requirement for therapies to the individual patients. In Japan, neurosurgeons are central to the diagnosis, treatments, rehabilitation, and outpatient-based follow-up of patients with PCNSL and thus have a role to play in defining the balance between therapeutic efficacy and neurotoxicity for any treatment modalities [8].

HD-MTX

MTX is an antimetabolite for folic acid, and was first used with moderate efficacy to treat brain infiltration of lymphoma or leukemia by intrathecal (IT) injection [9]. In the 1970s, intravenous (IV) injection of MTX in high doses was demonstrated to yield cytotoxic concentrations in the cerebrospinal fluid (CSF) that are more uniform and stable than those achieved with the IT route [10]. Although MTX does not penetrate the blood-brain barrier (BBB), the high serum concentrations obtained with high-dose administration can enable penetration of the BBB. IV administration of 1 g/m^2 yields an intracerebral concentration within the therapeutic window, and 3 g/m^2 achieves effective concentrations both in brain parenchyma and CSF [10, 11]. The optimal dose for HD-MTX has not yet been examined in a prospective study. Retrospective studies have shown no difference in therapeutic efficacy with doses of 3-8 g/m^2 (Tables 1-3). Carrabba et al. found the dose of 3.5 g/m^2 offered the optimal balance of efficacy and adverse effects [12]. Systemic adverse events could be avoided by the forced drug excretion obtained with hydration and administration of leucovorin as an antidote [4]. HD-MTX was first combined with WBRT which was considered as an effective therapy for PCNSL at that time [3-5]. This combination therapy remarkably prolonged patient survival in terms of both PFS and OS, but at a high cost of neurotoxicity. After establishment of the significance and limitations of HD-MTX combined with WBRT in the treatment of PCNSL, therapeutic trials were directed at two different purposes. To pursue disease cure or longer survival, multidrug regimens including HD-MTX were combined with standard WBRT [12-14]. To avoid neurotoxicity, radiotherapy was omitted or reduced in dose or field [15-18]. Currently, many authors describe HD-MTX as the sole standard of care for patients with PCNSL, with or without WBRT [19].

RADIOTHRAPY

Complete disappearances of enhancing tumor masses on magnetic resonance imaging (MRI) are frequently observed following conventional radiotherapy [2]. This excellent initial response has made WBRT a widely used therapeutic option for PCNSL. Since MST improved to 12-18 months from 3.3 months with supportive care and 4.6 months with surgery alone, WBRT was considered the sole effective therapeutic modality until the 1970s [3-5]. The recently published guideline from the International Lymphoma Radiation Oncology Group recommends 30-36 Gy of consolidation WBRT after HD-MTX for PCNSL [20]. However, it must be emphasized that WBRT is never curative for PCNSL, unlike the situation for germinoma [2, 21]. When treated with WBRT alone without effective systemic chemotherapy, PCNSL usually results in local recurrences in the irradiated field [21]. Concerning the optimal dose of radiotherapy, no prospective randomized studies have yet been reported. Based on retrospective data, a dose of 50 Gy or more may be necessary to control tumor growth [21, 22]. A total dose of 60 Gy to the tumor bed (WBRT of 40 Gy + local boost of 20 Gy) was trialed by the Radiation Therapy Oncology Group (RTOG) 8315 study, resulting in OS of only 11.6 months [23]. These accumulated data showed that PCNSL is difficult to eradicate by using radiotherapy alone. PCNSL is recognized as less sensitive to radiotherapy than other systemic lymphomas [24]. Consolidation WBRT after HD-MTX remains controversial, but the latest recommendation offers radiotherapy may be a therapeutic option only for patients with residual or progressive disease after chemotherapy [19].

The role of radiotherapy in the treatment of other systemic extra-nodal lymphomas had been established not only for localized disease (stage I), but also for more diffuse types following chemotherapy [20]. Some researchers have insisted that treatment with chemotherapy alone at increasing intensity would submit the patient to an increasing risk of hematologic toxicities, which may be avoided with the use of radiotherapy [25]. However, although systemic lymphoma is more radiosensitive than PCNSL, many medical oncologists have started to reconsider reducing the optimal radiation field from the whole-organ, on the balance of therapeutic benefits and late adverse events [26]. For PCNSL, the whole-brain field has traditionally been used, because this tumor is highly invasive to the surrounding brain. Recent advances in MRI have achieved much greater resolutions than available with computed tomography (CT), although we still cannot trace theoretically all microscopic lesions with imaging techniques. The relatively low resolution of imaging studies in the pre-MRI era was one of the reasons whole-brain radiation fields were needed. The greater precision of imaging studies and the current state of radiation techniques should enable highly localized radiotherapy sparing the majority of normal organs without compromising patient survival [27].

CURRENT TREATMENT STRATEGIES FOR PCNSL

HD-MTX Combined with WBRT

HD-MTX was first combined with WBRT, and markedly improved median OS to 34-46 months from the 12-18 months obtained with WBRT alone [3-5]. Median PFS was also improved to 24-35 months. Although no randomized studies have compared HD-MTX + WBRT with WBRT alone, combined therapy is definitely superior to WBRT alone. Indeed, researchers typically considered such a randomized study as unnecessary or even unethical [3-5, 8]. However, combined therapy was soon shown to cause severe neurotoxicity that impairs ADL and deprives the patient of social activity [6-8]. The G-PCNSL-SG-1 prospective randomized study clearly showed that neurotoxicity was more common with WBRT + HD-MTX than with HD-MTX-based chemotherapy alone [28].

Table 1. Multidrug regimen including HD-MTX combined with WBRT

Study	N	Drug	MTX dose	RR (%)	M-PFS (m)	M-OS (m)
DeAngelis LM	98	VCR, PAZ	2.5 g/m^2	94	24	36.9
Pootmans PM	52	Teniposide, BCNU	3 g/m^2	81	27	46
Ferreri AJ	79	Ara-C	3.5 g/m^2	40	22	33

WBRT: whole-brain radiotherapy, HD-MTX: high-dose methotrexate.
Ara-C: Cytarabine, BCNU: Carmustine, PAZ: Procarbazine, VCR: Vincristine.

Multidrug Regimen Including HD-MTX Combined with WBRT

To obtain more favorable survival rates, the first approach is to further increase the therapeutic intensity, by adding other chemotherapeutic agents to the established HD-MTX plus WBRT. Three major reports have examined this type of strategy (Table 1), achieving median OS of 37, 46, and 33 months, not so much better than simple HD-MTX + WBRT [12-14]. Although increased initial responses and better PFS can be obtained with drug combination therapies, whether such benefits translate into long-term tumor control and prolonged survival is doubtful. A further problematic issue is that treatment-related death was reported to occur in approximately 10% of patients in all three trials. DeAngelis et al. stated that the multidrug regimen with WBRT was associated with higher rates of neurotoxicity and all treatment-related death (8 of 98 patients treated: 8%) occurred in the patients with neurotoxicity [12]. Since some retrospective studies have demonstrated the efficacy of HD-cytarabine (AraC) combined with HD-MTX + WBRT, Ferreri et al. conducted a randomized phase II trial using the multidrug regimen. The result showed the superiority of the HD-MTX plus HD-AraC group, with a 3-year PFS rate of 38% compared to 21% for the HD-MTX group, whereas OS was not prolonged [14]. In contrast, hematologic toxicity of grade III or more was observed in 92% of the combined group, in contrast to 15% of the HD-MTX group. As a result, treatment-related death was more frequent in the combined group (8%) than in the HD-MTX-alone group [14].

HD-MTX Alone Omitting WBRT

Omission of WBRT was expected to be less toxic to the normal brain, preserving cognitive functions without compromising OS, based on the hypothesis that the survival prolongation of HD-MTX + WBRT may be largely attributable to the effects of HD-MTX. No randomized studies have simply compared HD-MTX alone with HD-MTX + WBRT. However, Thiel et al. reported results from a randomized phase III trial comparing regimens with and without WBRT based on HD-MTX + ifosfamide multidrug chemotherapy, and concluded that no difference was observed in OS between regimens with and without WBRT [28]. Several retrospective studies employed HD-MTX alone omitting WBRT for PCNSL (Table 3). Most of these studies used an intensified HD-MTX (8 g/m^2) [18, 29-33]. Gerstner et al. reported excellent results with a median PFS of 13 months and a median OS of 55 months [31]. Iwadate et al. reported similar results of a median PFS of 15 months and a median OS of 52 months using a standard HD-MTX of 3.5 g/m^2 (Figure 1A) [18]. Radiological complete response was observed in 45% of patients and salvage therapy with HD-MTX alone appeared effective for almost all recurrent patients (Figure 1B). Importantly, 11 of 42 patients (26%) survived without any tumor recurrence after 3 courses of HD-MTX alone [18]. Although median PFS in these studies was shorter than in WBRT-employing regimens, median OS was comparable to that with WBRT + HD-MTX. In contrast, Herrlinger et al. reported a median OS of 25 months and neurotoxicity in long-term survivors using a HD-MTX of 8 g/m^2 alone without WBRT and expressed doubts about omitting WBRT from first-line treatments [32].

Table 2. High-dose methotrexate alone without whole-brain radiotherapy

Study	N	MTX dose	RR (%)	M-PFS (m)	M-OS (m)
Guha-Thakurta	31	8 g/m^2	100	10	30
Batchelor	25	8 g/m^2	74	12.8	55.4
Herrlinger	37	8 g/m^2	35	—	25
Cobert	121	8 g/m^2	85	37	84
Iwadate	42	3.5 g/m^2	78	15	52

Table 3. Multidrug regimen including HD-MTX without radiotherapy

Study	N	Drug	MTXdose	RR (%)	M-PFS (m)	M-OS (m)
Hoang-Xuan	50	CCNU, PAZ	1 g/m^2	48	6.8	14.3
Pels	65	Ara-C, VCR, Ifos, CPM	5 g/m^2	71	21	50
Abrey	22	PAZ, VCR, Ara-C	3.5 g/m^2	90	—	33
Omuro	23	TMZ	3 g/m^2	55	8	35
Fritsch	28	RIT, PAZ, CCNU	3 g/m^2	82	3y-PFS: 31%	3y-OS: 31%
Gerard	23	PAZ,VCR	3.5 g/m^2	65	4.6	41.1

Ara-C: Cytarabine, CCNU: Lomustine, CPM: Cyclophosphamide, Ifos: Ifosphamide.
PAZ: Procarbazine, RIT: Rituximab, TMZ: Temozolomide, VCR: Vincristine.

The literature for HD-MTX alone provided three lessons. First, despite the inferiority of initial response and PFS in the chemotherapy-alone group, OS does not differ between HD-MTX + WBRT and HD-MTX alone. Second, the frequency and severity of neurotoxicity are higher with HD-MTX + WBRT than with HD-MTX alone. Third, HD-MTX alone is effective enough to achieve long-term remission for 20-30% of patients. For these responsive patients who achieve CR, additional consolidation therapies such as WBRT or HD-AraC did not prolong OS compared with HD-MTX alone and would only cause toxic effects [34]. Another important issue is a comparison between a decline in ADL caused by the short PFS and that by neurotoxicity. The ADL decline from short PFS is usually recovered with salvage chemotherapy, whereas that from neurotoxicity would gradually progressive day by day and is never recovered.

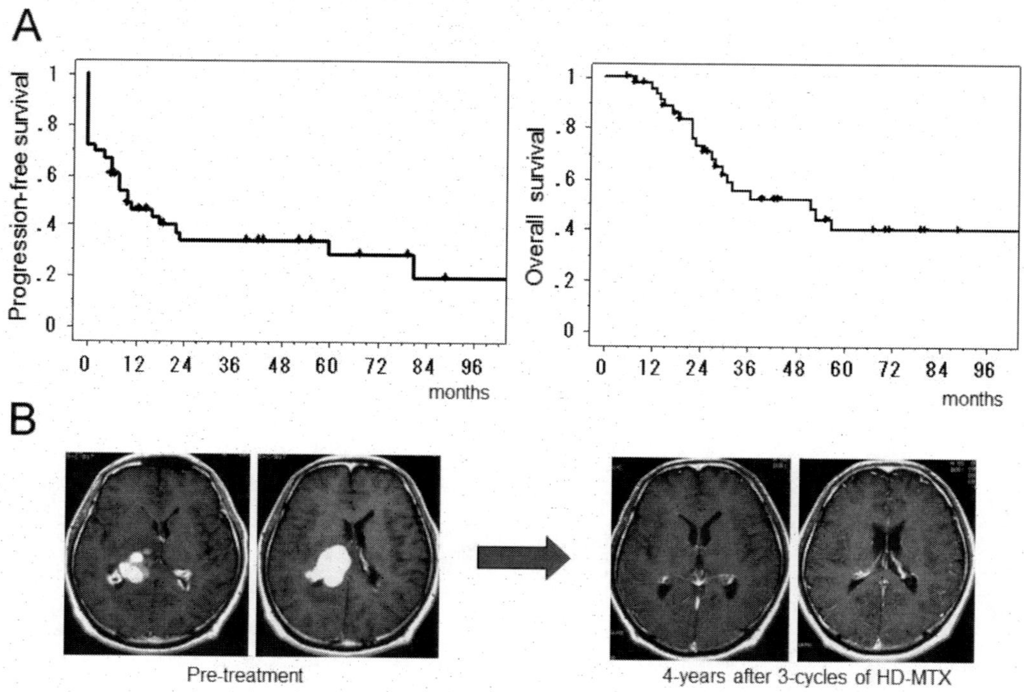

Figure 1. A: Kaplan-Meier survival curves for progression-free survival (left panel) and for overall survival (right panel). B: A typical case who showed a complete response after 3 courses of high-dose methotrexate. This patient returned to the previous social activity and is stable without recurrence for more than 4 years.

Multidrug Regimen Including HD-MTX Omitting WBRT

This approach replaced WBRT with additional chemotherapeutic agents to avoid neurotoxicity. Table 2 summarizes the therapeutic results of such treatments [16, 17, 28, 35-38]. All these trials included moderate doses of HD-MTX (3-5 g/m^2) and cytotoxic drugs such as ifosfamide, nitrosoureas, or procarbazine. First, Hoang-Xuan et al. used a moderate dose of HD-MTX (1 g/m^2) combined with lomustine and procarbazine for elderly patients over 60 years old, achieving a median PFS of 7 months and a median OS of 14 months [35]. They described chemotherapy alone as an appropriate regimen for elderly patients to avoid WBRT. Pels et al. achieved a median PFS of 21 months and a median OS of 50 months, whereas treatment-related death occurred in 9% of patients [36]. More recently, the randomized phase III trial reported by Thiel et al. compared multidrug chemotherapy regimens with and without WBRT [28]. Patients enrolled in the chemotherapy-alone arm who did not accomplish CR were administered HD-AraC. Median PFS was 18 months and median OS was 32 months with WBRT, compared with 12 months and 37 months for treatment without WBRT. Although PFS was significantly prolonged by WBRT, OS did not differ significantly between treatment arms. The results led the authors to describe that omission of WBRT from first-line treatment as justified [28].

HD-MTX Combined with Localized Radiotherapy

Since PCNSL is highly infiltrative into any part of the brain, partial radiotherapy was considered insufficient for this disease. This notion may be correct when treatment is restricted to radiation therapy alone, but we now have a powerful chemotherapy regimen in the form of HD-MTX, and the role of radiotherapy is consolidation after HD-MTX. In this situation, most infiltrative areas may be eradicated, and the tumor core, which may be supported by the host microenvironment similar to the neural stem-cell niche, may be resistant to various cytotoxic therapies [39]. To eradicate such tumors remaining in a niche biologically suited to their survival, not only the tumor cells but also host non-tumor cells in the niche should be targeted [39]. For this purpose, radiotherapy rather than chemotherapy would be appropriate, especially highly localized radiotherapies such as stereotactic radiosurgery (SRS).

The efficacy of partial brain radiotherapy for PCNSL has recently been reported by some researchers. Shibamoto et al. reported that reducing radiation field to partial brain with a 4 cm margin or more is as effective as WBRT [40]. However, the 4-cm margin of targets would include almost all important structures of the brain, such as the limbic system. Hirono et al. recently published the first systematic report for a novel strategy of first-line SRS instead of WBRT for patients who did not achieve a complete response (CR) after three cycles of HD-MTX [41]. Twenty patients were treated with HD-MTX plus SRS, achieving a local control rate of 86% at 2 years and median PFS after SRS of 17 months. Median OS was 52 months, which is rather excellent giving that these patients did not include the most promising group for long-term survival, that is, those who accomplished CR following HD-MTX. Interestingly, 8 of 20 patients (40%) demonstrated a PFS of more than 24 months, suggesting that residual tumors after HD-MTX are really restricted to the specific niche and most infiltrative tumor cells might have been eradicated by HD-MTX. The high local control rate obtained with SRS suggests that residual PCNSL cells after HD-MTX are mostly located within the tumor mass showing gadolinium-enhancement on MRI and can be eradicated with single-fraction irradiation of 15 Gy using a gamma knife unit [41].

FUTURE DIRECTION OF PCNSL TREATMENT

WBRT Disrupts the Protective Function of the Brain against Tumor Invasion

PCNSL infiltrates into surrounding normal brain tissues to breakdown established complex neural networks. However, many inhibitory or repulsive guidance molecules involved in axonal growth during development also restrict axonal regeneration and cellular infiltration in cases of CNS injury in adults. These mechanisms also restrict tumor cell infiltration into the brain parenchyma once the neuron-glia network is established [42]. The main players are inhibitory molecules in CNS myelin including Nogo, myelin-associated glycoproteins, semaphorins, ephrins, netrin, and slit, as well as proteoglycans associated with astrocytes [42]. Neural stem cells (NSCs) and neurons themselves possess inhibitory functions against neighboring tumor cells. In particular, endogenous NSCs have been shown to be recruited to an experimental brain tumor sites to exhibit anti-tumor activities [43, 44]. Loss of NSCs is thus directly associated not only with cognitive dysfunctions, but also declines in defense mechanisms [42, 45]. These mechanisms have evolved to protect the established neuron-glia network necessary for the maintenance of higher brain function in individuals. Innate inhibitory mechanisms may be injured by WBRT, which could favor tumor infiltration and lead to long-term cognitive impairment (Figure 2). DeAngelis et al. actually showed a direct association between treatment-related neurotoxicity and treatment-related deaths in the report for Radiation Therapy Oncology Group Study 93-10, although deaths were not proven to result from tumor progression [13]. The final report of a phase III randomized study concerning WBRT clearly showed that OS is not prolonged by WBRT, despite prolongation of PFS [46]. The breakdown of innate inhibitory mechanisms is one of the reasons the PFS benefit resulting from the addition of WBRT to first-line treatment does not translate to an OS benefit, although the absence of OS benefits for early radiotherapy have usually been attributed to the effectiveness of salvage radiotherapy at recurrence. Survival after progression was considered to be longer in radiation-free patients in whom the innate protective mechanisms of the brain are preserved, compared to patients in the first-line radiation group [42].

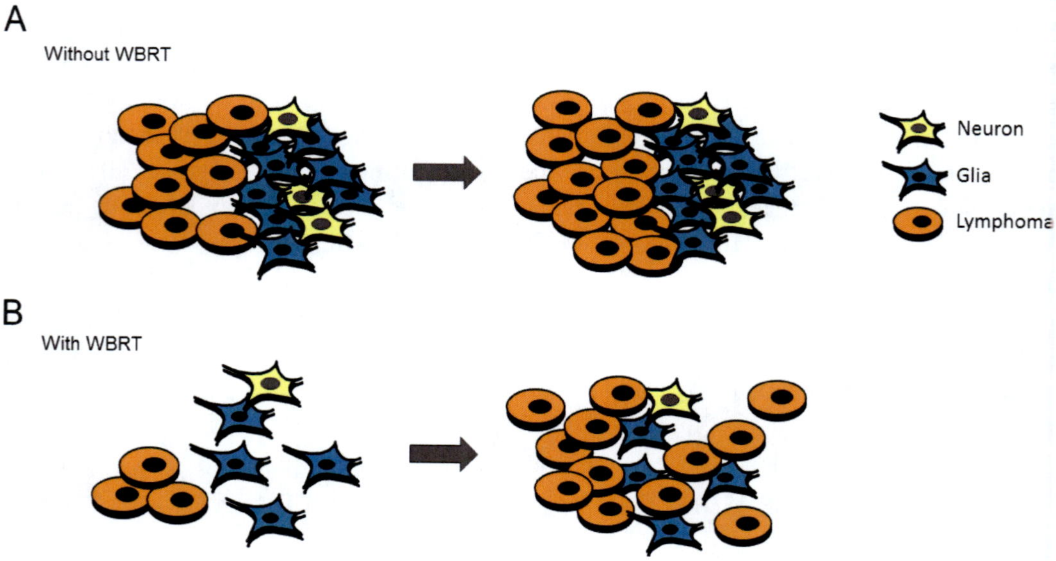

Figure 2. A schema for the loss of neuron-glia network caused by whole-brain radiotherapy (WBRT) in relation to tumor cell infiltration. A: When not receiving WBRT. The neuron-glia network are maintained to restrict tumor infiltration. B: When receiving WBRT. The reduced neuron-glia network permits tumor cell infiltration.

Inclusion of WBRT Should Not Come First

As described above, most retrospective analyses have failed to demonstrate a role for WBRT in prolonging OS compared with HD-MTX omitting WBRT as a first-line treatment. Furthermore, many studies have confirmed that addition of WBRT is associated with higher risk of neurotoxicity. These data suggest that the recent issue of "whether omitting WBRT from first-line treatment can be justified" seems curious. The issue should be "whether addition of WBRT into the first-line treatment of PCNSL can be justified." Inclusion of WBRT aimlessly into routine clinical practice would not be ethically justifiable outside of clinical trials. If we pursue cure in younger patients, the risk of inducing cognitive impairment for their remaining lifetime should be avoided. In cases of elderly patients, WBRT should not be used because of the increased sensitivity of this population to treatment-associated neurotoxicity directly associated with treatment-related death. Since HD-MTX has a highly PCNSL-specific killing effect that can eradicate infiltrating tumor cells unprotected by a firm scaffold, combining treatment modalities should target the remaining PCNSL cells that may be supported by microenvironments within the "tumor niche." Such remaining cells can be radio- and chemo-resistant, and thus would not be fully eradicated by systemically administered chemotherapeutic agents even at high doses, instead needing more intense radiotherapy localized to the niche. WBRT is a relic from the pre-MRI era before modern technological advances in precision radiotherapy. The inclusion of WBRT into PCNSL treatment should not come first, as the conclusion of a story should not come first.

Other Drugs for Combination with HD-MTX

As described previously, addition of CHOP, nitrosourea, procarbazine, or vincristine to HD-MTX has proven unsuccessful, primarily due to severe hematological toxicities. The frequency of treatment-related death increased significantly. A prospective randomized study showed addition of HD-AraC to HD-MTX was not superior to HD-MTX alone in terms of OS [46]. Since these chemotherapeutic agents were ineffective as single drug regimens, addition of the drugs rather decreases the possible dose of MTX, which would not be beneficial for prolongation of survival of patients with PCNSL.

Temozolomide (TMZ) is an alkylating agents mainly used for malignant gliomas, and has also shown some degree of efficacy against PCNSL [47]. For recurrent cases, the CR rate has been reported as 31% and 1-year survival rate as 31%. Kurzwelly et al. reported that first-line treatment with TMZ alone without WBRT achieved a CR rate of 47% and median OS of 21 months in elderly patients [48]. When combined with HD-MTX, median OS in elderly patients was 35 months also in the elderly patients. However, Omuro et al. recently reported results from a randomized phase II study in which HD-MTX + temozolomide without WBRT was less toxic, but not beneficial for OS prolongation [48].

Rituximab has also been shown to be effective for recurrent cases both as monotherapy and in combined multidrug therapy [50]. Two randomized control studies are now under examination. When sensitivity to HD-MTX is not expected to be high or for recurrent cases after HD-MTX, combination therapy including TMZ or rituximab would represent an option for treatment.

Conclusion

HD-MTX is highly active against PCNSL including infiltrated tumor cells, and some patients can be cured using HD-MTX alone. We should not over-treat these patients, to allow the preservation of the higher brain functions necessary to maintain social activities. On the other hand, many patients cannot be cured using HD-MTX alone. Recurrences after HD-MTX may contain the highly chemo- and radio-resistant cells, warranting locally-intensified therapies such as highly localized radiotherapy, rather than multidrug chemotherapies at high doses. We should pursue cure of this disease with a view to minimize damage to the normal brain, taking advantage of recent advances in techniques for the precision localization for radiotherapy.

References

[1] Hochberg FH, Baehring JM, Hochberg EP. Primary CNS lymphoma. *Nat Clin Prac Neurol* 3: 24-35, 2007.

[2] Nelson DF. Radiotherapy in the treatment of primary central nervous system lymphoma (PCNSL). *J Neurooncol* 43: 241-247, 1999.

[3] Glass J, Gruber ML, Cher L, Hochberg FH. Preirradiation methotrexate chemotherapy of primary central nervous system lymphoma: long-term outcome. *J Neurosurg* 81: 188-195, 1994.

[4] Hiraga S, Arita N, Ohnishi T, et al. Rapid infusion of high-dose methotrexate resulting in enhanced penetration into cerebrospinal fluid and intensified tumor response in primary central nervous system lymphomas. *J Neurosurg* 91: 221-230, 1999.

[5] O'Brien PC, Roos DE, Pratt G, et al. Combined modality therapy for primary central nervous system lymphoma: long-term data from phase II multicentrer study (Trans-Taman Radiation Oncology Group). *Int J Radiat Oncol Biol Phys* 64: 408-413, 2006.

[6] Abrey LE, DeAngelis, Yahalom J. Long-term survival in primary CNS lymphoma. *J Clin Oncol* 16: 859-863, 1998.

[7] Correa DD, Shi W, Abrey LE, et al. Cognitive functions in primary CNS lymphoma after single or combined modality regimens. *Neuro Oncol* 14: 101-108, 2012.

[8] Iwadate Y. [II. Primary treatment of CNS lymphoma with high-dose MTX]. *Gan To Kagaku Ryoho* 39: 892-897, 2012.

[9] Herbst KD, Corder MP, Justice GR. Successful treatment with methotrexate of a multicentric lymphoma of the central nervous system. *Cancer* 38: 1476-1478, 1976.

[10] Shapiro WR, Young DF, Mehta BM. Methotrexate: Distribution in cerebrospinal fluid after intravenous, ventricular and lumbar injections. *N Engl J Med* 293: 161-166, 1975.

[11] Lippens RJ, Winograd B. Methotrxate concentration levels in the cerebrospinal fluid during high-dose methotrexate infusions: an unreliable prediction. *Pediatr Hematol Oncol* 5: 115-124, 1988.

[12] Carrabba MG, Reni M, Foppoli M, et al. Treatment approach for primary CNS lymphomas. *Expert Opin Pharmacother* 11: 1263-1276, 2010.

[13] DeAngelis LM, Seiferheld W, Schold SC, et al. Combination chemotherapy and radiotherapy for primary central nervous system lymphoma: Radiation Therapy Oncology Group Study 93-10. *J Clin Oncol* 20: 4643-4648, 2002.

[14] Pootmans PMP, Kluin-Nelemans HC, Haaxma-Reiche H, et al. High-dose methotrexate-based chemotherapy followed by consolidating radiotherapy in Non-AIDS-related primary central nervous system lymphoma: European Organization for Research and Treatment of Cancer Lymphoma Group Phase II Trial 20962. *J Clin Oncol* 21: 4483-4488, 2003.

[15] Ferreri AJ, Reni M, Foppoli M, et al. High-dose cytrabine plus high-dose methotrexate versus high-dose methotrexate alone in patients with primary CNS lymphoma: a randomized phase 2 trial. *Lancet* 374: 1512-1520, 2009.

[16] Cher L, Glass J, Harsh GR, et al. Therapy of primary CNS lymphoma with methotrexate-based chemotherapy and deferred radiotherapy: Preliminary results. *Neurology* 46: 1757-1759, 1996.

[17] Freilich RJ, Delattre JY, Monjour A, DeAngelis LM. Chemotherapy without radiation therapy as initial treatment for primary CNS lymphoma in older patients. *Neurology* 46: 435-439, 1996.

[18] Iwadate Y, Suganami A, Yamanaka R, et al. Non-deep-seated primary CNS lymphoma: therapeutic responses and a molecular signature. *J Neurooncol* 117: 261-268, 2014.

[19] Hoang-Xuan K, Bessell E, Bromberg J, et al. Diagnosis andtretament of primary CNS lymphoma in immunocompetent patients: guidelines from the European Association for Neuro-Oncology. *Lancet Oncol* 16; e322-e332, 2015.

[20] Yahalom J, Illidge T, Specht L, et al. Modern radiation therapy for extranodal lymphoma: Field and dose guidelines from the International Lymphoma Radiation Oncology Group. *Int J Radiat Oncol Biol Phy* 92; 11-31, 2015.

[21] Shibamoto Y. Radiation therapy for primary central nervous system lymphoma. *Oncol Review* 7: 27-33, 2013.

[22] Murray K, Kun L, Cox J. Primary malignant lymphoma of the central nervous system. Results of treatment of 11 cases and review of the literature. *J Neurosurg* 65: 600-607, 1986.

[23] Nelson DF, Martz KL, Bonner H, et al. Non-Hodgkin's lymphomas of the brain: can high dose, large volume radiation therapy improve survival? Report on a prospective trial by the Radiation Therapy Oncology Group (RTOG): RTOG 8315. *Int J Radiat Oncol Biol Phys* 23: 9-17, 1992.

[24] Weller M. The vanishing role of whole-brain radiotherapy for primary central nervous system lymphoma. *Neuro-Oncol* 16: 1035-1036, 2014.

[25] Mendes F, Domingues C, Teixo R, et al. The importance of radiotherapy on diffuse large B cell lymphoma tretamnet: a current review. *Cancer Meta Rev* 34: 511-525, 2015.

[26] Hu C, Deng C, Zou W, Zhang G, Wang J. The role of consolidative radiotherapy after a complete response to chemotherapy in the treatment of diffuse large B-cell lymphoma in the Rituximab era: Results from a systematic review with a meta analysis. *Acta Hematol* 134: 111-118, 2015.

[27] Eng T, Ha CS. Image-guided radiation therapy in lymphoma management. *Radiat Oncol J* 33: 161-171, 2015.

[28] Thiel E, Korfel A, Martus P, et al. High-dose methotrexate with or without whole brain radiotherapy for primary CNS lymphoma (G-PCNSL-SG-1): a phase 3, randomized, non-inferiority trial. *Lancet Oncol* 11: 1036-1047, 2010.

[29] Guha-Thakurta N, Damek D, Pollack C, Hochberg FH. Intravenous methotrexate as initial treatment for primary central nervous system lymphoma: Response to therapy and quality of life of patients. *J Neurooncol* 43: 259-268, 1999.

[30] Batchelor T, Carson K, O'Neill A, et al. Treatment of primary CNS lymphoma with methotrexate and deferred radiotherapy: a report of NABTT 96-07. *J Clin Oncol* 21: 1044-1049, 2003.

[31] Gerstner ER, Carson KA, Grossman SA, Batchelor TT. Long-term outcome in PCNSL patients treated with high-dose methotrexate and deferred radiation. *Neurology* 70: 401-402, 2008.

[32] Herrlinger U, Kuker W, Uhl M, et al. NOA-03 trial of high-dose methotrexate in primary central nervous system lymphoma: final report. *Ann Neurol* 57: 843-847, 2005.

[33] Cobert J, Hochberg E, Woldenberg N, Hochberg F. Monotherapy with methotrexate for primary central nervous system lymphoma has single agent activity in the absence of radiotherapy: a single institution cohort. *J Neurooncol* 98: 385-393, 2010.

[34] Ekenel M, Iwamoto FM, Ben-Porat LS, et al. Primary central nervous system lymphoma: the role of consolidation treatment after a complete response to high-dose methotrexate-based chemotherapy. *Cancer* 113; 1025-1033, 2008.

[35] Hoang-Xuan K, Taillandier L, Chinot O, et al. Chemotherapy alone as initial treatment for primary CNS lymphoma in patients older than 60 years: a multicenter phase II study (26952) of the European Organization for Research and Treatment of Cancer Brain Tumor Group. *J Clin Oncol* 21: 2726-2731, 2003.

[36] Pels H, Schmidt-Wolf IG, Glamacher A, et al. Primary central nervous system lymphoma: results of a pilot and phase II study of systemic and intraventricular chemotherapy with deferred radiotherapy. *J Clin Oncol* 21: 4489-4495, 2003.

[37] Abrey LE, Yahalom J, DeAngelis LM. Treatment for primary CNS lymphoma: the next step. *J Clin Oncol* 18: 3144-3150, 2000.

[38] Gerard LM, Imarie KR, Mangel J, et al. High-dose methotrexate based chemotherapy with deferred radiation for treatment of newly diagnosed primary central nervous system lymphoma. *Leuk Lymphoma* 52: 1882-1890, 2011.

[39] Ye J, Wu D, Wu P, et al. The cancer stem cell niche: cross talk between cancer stem cells and their microenvironment. *Tumour Biol* 35: 3945-3951, 2014.

[40] Shibamoto Y, Hayabuchi N, Hiratsuka J, et al. Is whole-brain irradiation necessary for primary central nervous system lymphoma/ Pattern of recurrence following partial-brain irradiation. *Cancer* 97: 128-133, 2003.

[41] Hirono S, Iwadate Y, Higuchi Y, et al. Stereotactic radiosurgery in combination with up-front high-dose methotrexate as a first-line treatment for newly diagnosed primary central nervous system lymphoma. *J Neurooncol* 123: 237-244, 2015.

[42] Iwadate Y, Fukuda K, Matsutani T, Saeki N. Intrinsic protective mechanisms of neuron-glia network against glioma invasion. *J Clin Neurosci.* 2016.

[43] Walzlein JH, Synowitz M, Engel B, et al. The antitumorigenic response of neural precursors depends on subventricular proliferation and age. *Stem Cells* 26: 2945-2954, 2008.

[44] Glass R, Synowitz M, Kronrnberg G, et al. Glioblastoma-induced attraction of endogenous neural precursor cells is associated with improved survival. *J Neurosci* 25: 2637-46, 2005.

[45] Liedo PM, Alonso M, Grubb MS, et al. Adult neurogenesis and functional plasticity in neuronal circuits. *Nat Rev Neurosci* 7: 179-193, 2006.

[46] Korfel A, Thiel E, Martus P, et al. Randomized phase III study of whole-brain radiotherapy for primary CNS lymphoma. *Neurology* 84: 1242-1248, 2015.

[47] Reni M, Zaja F, Mason W, et al. Temozolomide as salvage treatment in primary brain lymphomas. *Br J Cancer* 96: 864-867, 2007.

[48] Kurzwelly D, Glas M, Roth P, et al. Primary CNS lymphoma in the elderly: Temozolomide therapy and MGMT status. *J Neurooncol* 97: 389-392, 2010.

[49] Omuro AM, Taillandier L, Chinot O, et al. Temozolomide and methotrexate for primary central nervous system lymphoma in the elderly. *J Neurooncol* 85: 207-211, 2007.

[50] Shah GD, Yahalom J, Correa DD, et al. Combined immunochemotherapy with reduced whole-brain radiotherapy foe newly diagnosed primary CNS lymphoma. *J Clin Oncol* 25: 4730-4735, 2007.

In: Primary Central Nervous System Lymphoma (PCNSL) ISBN: 978-1-63485-322-4
Editor: Ryuya Yamanaka

Chapter 13

TEMOZOLOMIDE CHEMOTHERAPY FOR PRIMARY CENTRAL NERVOUS SYSTEM LYMPHOMA

Keishi Makino* and Junichi Kuratsu
Department of Neurosurgery, Kumamoto University, Kumamoto, Japan

ABSTRACT

High-dose methotrexate is effective in the initial treatment of primary central nervous system lymphoma (PCNSL). Since treatment options in patients with progressive or recurrent PCNSL are limited, the prognosis remains poor. Temozolomide, a well-tolerated oral alkylating agent that permeates the blood brain barrier, is effective against malignant glioma and recurrent PCNSL cases. Recently, temozolomide has been demonstrated to have modest efficacy in a number of retrospective and prospective studies, with and without rituximab, with an objective response rate of 14–53% and one-year overall survival rate of 31–71%. However, progression-free survival was 2–2.8 months. Although some patients were elderly and had been heavily pre-treated, temozolomide produced a complete response and was well tolerated without any major toxicity.

Keywords: primary central nervous system lymphoma, salvage chemotherapy, temozolomide, MGMT

INTRODUCTION

The principal drug in the management of primary central nervous system lymphoma (PCNSL) is high-dose methotrexate (HD-MTX), which yields a complete response rate of 30–65%. [1-3] However, 10–35% of tumors were refractory to the HD-MTX regimen, and up to 60% of complete responders manifest tumor recurrence during follow-up. [4, 5] Thus,

* Correspondence to: Keishi Makino, Department of Neurosurgery, Kumamoto University. E-mail: kmakino@fc.kuh.kumamoto-u.ac.jp.

PCNSL remains an incurable disease, and attempts to improve survival with HD-MTX-based combination therapies have been undertaken.

There are few agents with demonstrable activities against PCNSL. Most active agents used for extra-cerebral non-Hodgkin's lymphomas do not penetrate the blood-brain barrier (BBB) at sufficient concentrations to be effective against PCNSL, and agents that penetrate the BBB do not tend to be effective or have unacceptable toxicities [6, 7].

Temozolomide is an oral alkylating agent that spontaneously undergoes chemical conversion to the cytotoxic metabolite 5-(3 methyl-1-triazeno) imidazole-4-carboxamide at physiological pH without metabolic conversion. This metabolite depletes the deoxyribonucleic acid (DNA)-repair enzyme O^6 methylguanine-DNA methyltransferase (MGMT) in various cell types. Alkylating agents are generally effective against non-Hodgkin's lymphoma, and temozolomide has good CNS penetration and a favorable toxicity profile [8, 9]. The use of single-agent temozolomide as salvage therapy for PCNSL has been described in case reports [10-12]. In this chapter, we review reports regarding temozolomide chemotherapy against PCNSL.

Results and Discussion

Use of Temozolomide for PCNSL in the Elderly

Although HD-MTX-based chemotherapy is the standard therapy for patients with PCNSL, PCNSL that develops in the elderly is associated with lower response rates, earlier relapses, and higher incidence of acute and late-delayed toxicities as compared to younger patients. [13] Thus, temozolomide has been used as a first-line treatment for PCNSL in the elderly. For instance, Kurzwelly et al. reported the use of temozolomide as the first-line monotherapy (100–200 mg/m^2 on days 1-5 of a 28-day cycle) in 17 patients with PCNSL (median age, 75 years [range 62–90]). [14] The complete response rate was 47%, median progression-free survival was 5 months, and median overall survival was 21 months. Regarding toxicity, two patients (12%) developed grade 3 and 4 hematoxicity.

In addition, Omuro et al. reported outcomes of a consecutive series of 23 PCNSL elderly patients (median age, 68 years [range 60–79]). [15] They gave induction chemotherapy with methotrexate (3 g/m^2 on days 1, 10, and 20) and temozolomide (100 mg/m^2 on days 1–5); for patients achieving a partial or complete response, they gave monthly maintenance therapy with methotrexate (3 g/m^2 on day 1) and temozolomide (100 mg/m^2 on days 1–5). The complete response rate was 55%, median event-free survival was 8 months, and median overall survival was 35 months. Regarding severe toxicities (grade 3 or 4), three patients developed nephrotoxicity, and five patients developed hematoxicity.

Use of Temozolomide for Salvage Therapy

Temozolomide has been evaluated in a number of retrospective [16-18] and prospective [19, 20] studies as salvage therapy, with and without rituximab (Table 1). Reni et al. reported the results of a phase II trial assessing temozolomide effectiveness in 36 patients (median age,

60 years [range 34–81]) with recurrent PCNSL and who had previously been treated with HD-MTX-containing chemotherapy with or without radiotherapy; [19] 23 patients (78%) were experiencing a first recurrence, and eight had multiple recurrent diseases after having failed other salvage regimens. Temozolomide (150 mg/m^2 on days 1–5 of a 28-day cycle) was administered to all patients and yielded a 31% response rate, with nine complete and two partial responses. Median progression-free survival was 2.8 months, median overall survival was 3.9 months, and one-year overall survival was 31%. Regarding toxicity, two patients developed grade 4 neutropenia, one developed grade 4 thrombocytopenia, and one developed grade 3 vomiting.

In addition, one retrospective study reported results from 17 patients (median age, 68 years) with refractory or relapsed PCNSL, [16] all of whom were treated with temozolomide (150–200 mg/m^2 for 5 days in the course of 28 days). The response rate was 47% (complete response, 29%; partial response, 18%). Median progression-free survival was 1.9 months, median overall survival was 6.7 months, and one-year overall survival rate was 35%. Regarding toxicity, one patient developed grade 3 thrombocytopenia, and one patient developed neutropenia.

Table 1.

Treatment	Study	No.	mAge	CR + PR (%)	mPFS	mOS	1-year OS (%)	N (%)	PLT (%)	Other tox (%)
Temozolomide [Reni et al.]	Prospective	36	60	25 + 6	2.8	4	31	6	3	3
Temozolomide [Makino et al.]	Retrospective	17	68	29 + 18	1.9	6.7	35	6	6	0
Temozolomide [Wong]	Retrospective	7	60	0 +14	2	4	n.d.	14	14	14
Temozolomide + Rituximab [Enting et al]	Retrospective	15	69	40 + 13	2.2	14	n.d.	7	27	7
Temozolomide + Rituximab [Nayak et al.]	Prospective	14	63	14 + 0	7 weeks	n.r.	71	0	0	0

mAge: median age; CR: complete response; PR: partial response; mPFS: median progression-free survival (months); mOS: median overall survival (months); N: grade 3–4 neutropenia; PLT: grade3-4 thrombocytopenia; Other tox: other grade 3–4 toxicity; n.d.: not done; n.r.: not reached.

Another retrospective study reported results from seven patients (median age, 60 years), [17] all of whom were treated with temozolomide (150–200 mg/m^2 for 5 days in a 28-day cycle). The objective response rate was 14%. Median progression-free survival was 2 months, and median overall survival was 4 months. Regarding toxicity, one patient developed grade 2 thrombocytopenia, and one patient developed grade 3 neutropenia.

In addition, Enting et al. evaluated the efficacy of a combination of rituximab (750 mg/m^2; days 1, 8, 15, 22 in a 28-day cycle) and temozolomide (100–200 mg/m^2 for days 1–7 and 15–21 in a 28-day cycle) for recurrent or refractory PCNSL [18] in 15 patients (median age, 69 years). The objective response rate was 53%, with a complete response in six patients and a partial response in two patients. Median progression-free survival was 2.2 months, and median overall survival was 14 months. Regarding toxicity, four patients developed grade 3 thrombocytopenia, one patient developed grade 3 anemia, and one patient developed grade 3 leukopenia.

Furthermore, Nayak et al. reported the results of a prospective multicenter phase II trial using rituximab and temozolomide in 16 immunocompetent patients (median age, 63 years) with progressive or recurrent PCNSL. [20] Fourteen of sixteen patients were evaluable for response. The 28-day cycle treatment schedule included an induction phase with rituximab (750 mg/m^2) on days 1, 8, 15, and 22 and temozolomide (150 mg/m^2) days 1–7 and 15–21, followed by six cycles of consolidation temozolomide (150–200 mg/m^2 for 5 days in the course of 28 days), followed by maintenance with methylprednisolone (1 g every 28 days). The objective response rate was 14%. Median progression-free survival was 7 weeks, median overall survival was not reached. No patients experienced any serious adverse events or grade 3–5 toxicities.

O6-Methylguanine-DNA methyltransferase (MGMT) gene promoter methylation (mMGMT) should be highly predictive of survival in temozolomide-treated glioblastoma patients. [21] Accordingly, several reports investigated mMGMT status in PCNSL patients treated with temozolomide. Among these, Makino et al. evaluated mMGMT in 11 of 17 patients using a methylation-specific polymerase chain reaction assay. [16] Of the 11 patients, mMGMT was found in four (36.4%) of them. However, there was no statistical difference in median overall survival between patients with mMGMT (11.1 months) and those without mMGMT (6.7months). In addition, Jiang et al. analyzed MGMT expression using immunohistochemistry [22] in 15 of 20 patients treated with temozolomide. Of the 15 patients, five with low MGMT level exhibited a response; of these, four exhibited a complete response, and one exhibited a partial response; in contrast, only one of 10 patients with high MGMT level exhibited a response (complete response).

Conclusion

Temozolomide is well tolerated and of moderate toxicity, thus it may be a good candidate agent for induction, consolidation, and maintenance therapy for patients with PCNSL and for salvage treatment.

References

[1] Herrlinger U, Schabet M, Brugger W, Kortmann RD, Kuker W, Deckert M, Engel C, Schmeck-Lindenau HJ, Mergenthaler HG, Krauseneck P, Benohr C, Meisner C, Wiestler OD, Dichgans J, Kanz L, Bamberg M, Weller M: German Cancer Society Neuro-Oncology Working Group NOA-03 multicenter trial of single-agent high-dose methotrexate for primary central nervous system lymphoma. *Ann Neurol* 51: 247-252, 2002.

[2] Guha-Thakurta N, Damek D, Pollack C, Hochberg FH: Intravenous methotrexate as initial treatment for primary central nervous system lymphoma: response to therapy and quality of life of patients. *J Neurooncol* 43: 259-268, 1999.

[3] Batchelor T, Carson K, O'Neill A, Grossman SA, Alavi J, New P, Hochberg F, Priet R: Treatment of primary CNS lymphoma with methotrexate and deferred radiotherapy: a report of NABTT 96-07. *J Clin Oncol* 21: 1044-1049, 2003.

[4] Reni M, Ferreri AJ: Therapeutic management of refractory or relapsed primary central nervous system lymphomas. *Ann Hematol* 80 Suppl 3: B113-117, 2001.

[5] Reni M, Ferreri AJ, Villa E: Second-line treatment for primary central nervous system lymphoma. *Br J Cancer* 79: 530-534, 1999.

[6] Reni M, Ferreri AJ: Is withdrawal of consolidation radiotherapy an evidence-based strategy in primary central nervous system lymphomas? *J Clin Oncol* 22: 1165-1167, 2004.

[7] Ferreri AJ, Abrey LE, Blay JY, Borisch B, Hochman J, Neuwelt EA, Yahalom J, Zucca E, Cavalli F, Armitage J, Batchelor T: Summary statement on primary central nervous system lymphomas from the Eighth International Conference on Malignant Lymphoma, Lugano, Switzerland, June 12 to 15, 2002. *J Clin Oncol* 21: 2407-2414, 2003.

[8] Herrlinger U, Kuker W, Platten M, Dichgans J, Weller M: First-line therapy with temozolomide induces regression of primary CNS lymphoma. *Neurology* 58: 1573-1574, 2002.

[9] Reni M, Mason W, Zaja F, Perry J, Franceschi E, Bernardi D, Dell'Oro S, Stelitano C, Candela M, Abbadessa A, Pace A, Bordonaro R, Latte G, Villa E, Ferreri AJ: Salvage chemotherapy with temozolomide in primary CNS lymphomas: preliminary results of a phase II trial. *Eur J Cancer* 40: 1682-1688, 2004.

[10] Makino K, Nakamura H, Kudo M, Takeshima H, Kuratsu J: Complete response to temozolomide treatment in an elderly patient with recurrent primary central nervous system lymphoma--case report. *Neurol Med Chir (Tokyo)* 47: 229-232, 2007. doi:JST.JSTAGE/nmc/47.229 [pii].

[11] Reni M, Ferreri AJ, Landoni C, Villa E: Salvage therapy with temozolomide in an immunocompetent patient with primary brain lymphoma. *J Natl Cancer Inst* 92: 575-576, 2000.

[12] Strik HM, Spreer A, Nagel H, Jacob S, Jung W, Kitze B, Bahr M: Clinical response following adjuvant Temozolomide in a patient with primary cerebral lymphoma. *Anticancer Res* 24: 4121-4125, 2004.

[13] Hoang-Xuan K, Chinot OL, Taillandier L: Treatment of primary central nervous system lymphoma in the elderly. *Seminars in oncology* 30: 53-57, 2003.

[14] Kurzwelly D, Glas M, Roth P, Weimann E, Lohner H, Waha A, Schabet M, Reifenberger G, Weller M, Herrlinger U: Primary CNS lymphoma in the elderly: temozolomide therapy and MGMT status. *J Neurooncol* 97: 389-392, 2010.

[15] Omuro AM, Taillandier L, Chinot O, Carnin C, Barrie M, Hoang-Xuan K: Temozolomide and methotrexate for primary central nervous system lymphoma in the elderly. *J Neurooncol* 85: 207-211, 2007.

[16] Makino K, Nakamura H, Hide T, Kuratsu J: Salvage treatment with temozolomide in refractory or relapsed primary central nervous system lymphoma and assessment of the MGMT status. *J Neurooncol* 106: 155-160, 2012. doi:10.1007/s11060-011-0652-z.

[17] Wong SF, Gan HK, Cher L: A single centre study of the treatment of relapsed primary central nervous system lymphoma (PCNSL) with single agent temozolomide. *J Clin Neurosci* 19: 1501-1505, 2012. doi:10.1016/j.jocn.2012.04.001.

[18] Enting RH, Demopoulos A, DeAngelis LM, Abrey LE: Salvage therapy for primary CNS lymphoma with a combination of rituximab and temozolomide. *Neurology* 63: 901-903, 2004. doi:63/5/901 [pii].

[19] Reni M, Zaja F, Mason W, Perry J, Mazza E, Spina M, Bordonaro R, Ilariucci F, Faedi M, Corazzelli G, Manno P, Franceschi E, Pace A, Candela M, Abbadessa A, Stelitano C, Latte G, Ferreri AJ: Temozolomide as salvage treatment in primary brain lymphomas. *Br J Cancer* 96: 864-867, 2007. doi:10.1038/sj.bjc.6603660.

[20] Nayak L, Abrey LE, Drappatz J, Gilbert MR, Reardon DA, Wen PY, Prados M, Deangelis LM, Omuro A: Multicenter phase II study of rituximab and temozolomide in recurrent primary central nervous system lymphoma. *Leuk Lymphoma* 54: 58-61, 2013. doi:10.3109/10428194. 2012.698736.

[21] Hegi ME, Diserens AC, Gorlia T, Hamou MF, de Tribolet N, Weller M, Kros JM, Hainfellner JA, Mason W, Mariani L, Bromberg JE, Hau P, Mirimanoff RO, Cairncross JG, Janzer RC, Stupp R: MGMT gene silencing and benefit from temozolomide in glioblastoma. *N Engl J Med* 352: 997-1003, 2005. doi:10.1056/NEJMoa043331.

[22] Jiang X, Reardon DA, Desjardins A, Vredenburgh JJ, Quinn JA, Austin AD, Herndon JE, 2nd, McLendon RE, Friedman HS: O6-methylguanine-DNA methyltransferase (MGMT) immunohistochemistry as a predictor of resistance to temozolomide in primary CNS lymphoma. *J Neurooncol* 114: 135-140, 2013. doi:10. 1007/s11060-013-1162-y.

In: Primary Central Nervous System Lymphoma (PCNSL) ISBN: 978-1-63485-322-4
Editor: Ryuya Yamanaka

Chapter 14

SALVAGE THERAPY WITH HIGH-DOSE CYTARABINE FOR PRIMARY CENTRAL NERVOUS SYSTEM LYMPHOMA

Hiroshi Kanno*
Department of Neurosurgery, International University of Health and Welfare Atami Hospital, Japan

ABSTRACT

Primary central nervous system lymphoma (PCNSL) is an aggressive intrinsic malignant tumor in found in the CNS. This tumor mostly develops in elderly patients over 50 years and very frequently recurs following remission. Although combination with high-dose methotrexate (HD-MTX) and high-dose cytarabine (HD-Ara C) was proposed as a candidate for the gold standard therapy several years ago, HD-MTX followed by whole-brain radiotherapy (WBRT) is still commonly used as the initial standard therapy because of its fewer side effects except for renal impairment. However, PCNLS treated with HD-MTX mostly always recurs. In spite of the high rate of recurrence of PCNSL following HD-MTX, salvage therapy or second-line therapy for PCNSL has not yet been established. Relapsed/refractory PCNSL has been often treated with HD-AraC-based chemotherapy. Here, we describe ESHAP (etoposide, solumedrol, HD-AraC, platinum agent) therapy, which is one of the HD-AraC-based chemotherapies. Fourteen PCNSL patients treated with ESHAP therapy showed a high complete-response (CR) rate and long progression-free and survival overall. Although hematopoietic toxicities above Grade 2 level developed in most of the cases, the side effects were controllable. In conclusion, ESHAP therapy contributed to long survival of PCNSL patients and was useful as a salvage therapy for PCNSL.

Keywords: primary CNS lymphoma, salvage therapy, high-dose cytarabine, ESHAP therapy

* Corresponding Author address: Hiroshi Kanno, Department of Neurosurgery, International University of Health and Welfare Atami Hospital, 13-1 Higashikaigan-cho, Atami, Shizuoka, 413-0012 Japan. Email: hiroshikannomd@nifty.com.

INTRODUCTION

At present the first-line therapy for primary central nervous system lymphoma (PCNSL) is high-dose methotrexate (HD-MTX) followed by whole-brain radiotherapy (WBRT) with 24-36 Gy. The high rate of complete remission achieved with the first-line therapy for PCNSL and complete response (CR) to this first-line therapy ranges from 42% to 61%, with overall survival between 14 and 55 months (Nobors, 2015). Unfortunately, however, most PCNSL patients who initially achieved CR eventually suffer a relapse and die within a year. Re-challenge with HD-MTX may be useful in patients with prior exposure (Plotkin et al., 2004). Several other regimens, including temozolomide (Reni, 2004), rituximab(Shulz, 2004), rituximab plus temozolomide (Enting, 2004), topotecan (Voloschin, 2008), premetrexated (Raizer, 2012), high-dose cytarabine (Chamberlain, 2015), etoposide plus ifomide and cytarabine (Arellano-Rodrigo, 2003), methylpredonisolone plus high-dose cytarabine, epoposide, and cisplatin/caroboplatin (del Rio, 2011; Ungur, 2015), dexamethasone plus high-dose cytarabine and cisplatin/carboplatin (del Rio, 2011) and additional whole-brain radiotherapy (Zacher, 2014) or stereotactic radiotherapy (Hirono, 2015) have shown activity against the recurrence or progression of the disease. Although salvage therapies mostly produce a second complete remission with consequent symptomatic and survival improvement, the optimal schedule for salvage therapy has not yet been identified, and none has been established as a standard therapy. Among salvage therapies for PCNSL, high-dose cytarabine (HD-AraC)-based chemotherapy shows a high CR rate and produces long survival in spite of its hematopoietic toxicity (Chamberlain, 2015; Arellano-Rodrigo, 2003; del Rio, 2011; Ungur, 2015). Herein, I describe a salvage therapy with HD-AraC, in particular ESHAP (etoposide, solumedrol, HD-Ara C, platinum agent) therapy (del Rio, 2011; Ungur, 2015).

METHODS

Chemotherapy Regimen

The ESHAP therapy regimen (Velasquez et al., 1994) was as follows: continuous drip intravenous infusion of cisplatin (25 mg/m^2/day) or carboplatin (80 mg/m^2 /24 h) for 4 days, drip intravenous infusion of etoposide (40 mg/m^2/2 h) for 4 days, drip intravenous infusion of methylprednisolone (solumedrol, 500 mg/body for 5 days), and drip intravenous infusion of cytarabine (2 g/m^2) on the 5 th day. Lactated ringer solution (2000 ml/day) was continuously infused for 5 days. Granisetron hydrochloride (3 mg) was used for 5 days. From the 7 th day, the granulocyte colony-stimulating factor (G-CSF) analog filgrastim (75 mg or 150 mg) was used daily until the white blood cell count exceeded 10,000/mm^3. Exclusion criteria (contraindication) were as follow: platelet count below 100,000/mm^3, Eastern Cooperative Oncology Group (ECOG) performance status (PS) score with the use of the ESHAP regimen above 2, creatinine clearance (CCr) below 40 ml/min, age below 18 years, white blood cell count below 2000/mm^2, hemoglobin below 9 g/dl or C-reactive protein above 5 mg/dl. The ESHAP regimen was applied ever 4 weeks for at least 2 and up to 6 cycles. The ESHAP regimen was approved by the institutional review board (IRB) for chemotherapy.

Patients with PCNSL

Patients included 11 males and 3 females, and the age of the patients ranged from 43 to 76 years. The follow-up period ranged from 12 to 75 months. All 14 patients' tumors were histologically verified as non-Hodgkin diffuse large B cell lymphoma. Other types of PCNSL were excluded. All 14 patients underwent high-dose MTX therapy followed by folinate calcium rescue as the first-line chemotherapy except for CCr below 70 ml/min. PCNSL patients that had only the first-line chemotherapy (HD-MTX) followed by WBRT and no relapse were excluded. All 14 patients underwent at least 2 courses of ESHAP regimen. Three patients underwent ESHAP therapy because of being refractory to treatment, whereas the remaining 11 patients underwent EHAP therapy because of a relapse.

Chemotherapy Assessment

Chemotherapy results were assessed by Gd-enhanced MRI as follow: complete response (CR, enhanced area not shown), partial response (PR, enhanced area reduction above 50%), stable disease (SD, enhanced area not changed), and progressive disease (PD, enhanced area increased). The rate of CR plus PR was assessed as effective. In addition, progression-free survival and overall survival since ESHAP therapy and overall survival since the onset were examined, as shown in Table 1.

RESULTS

Effectiveness and Survival

All 14 patients underwent at least 2 courses of ESHAP regimen, with a mean of 3.1 courses. The period of progression-free survival ranged from 3 to 48 months, with a median of 16 months. The period of overall survival since the onset ranged from 11 to 122 months, with a median of 39.5 months. The period of overall survival since the end of ESHAP therapy ranged from 7 to 75 months, with a median of 20 months. The time to progression since the initial therapy ranged from 2 to 47 months, with a median of 16 months. The CR rate was 78.6%; and the PR rate, 14.3%. Effectiveness rate (CR plus PR) was 92.9%; whereas the SD rate was 7.1% and the PD, zero. Among 14 patients, 7 died and 7 remain alive (Table 1).

Illustrative Case

The MRI of a PCNSL patient (Case 9, 58 years, male) treated with ESHAP therapy is shown in Figure 1. The patient developed motor dysfunction, and the MRI showed an enhanced mass in bilateral thalamus. He was initially treated with 3 courses of HD-MTX, but the tumor was not fully reduced. Therefore, he was treated with 2 courses of the ESHAP therapy regimen, and CR was recognized.

Table 1. PCNSL patients treated with ESHAP therapy

Case No	Age	Sex	ECOG PS	Op	Reason of ESHAP use	Initial therapy	Additional radiation	No. of courses of ESHAP	PFS (month)	OS since ESHAP (month)	OS since onset (month)	TTP after initial therapy (month)	D/A	Response
1	68	M	1	T	Relapsed	HD-MTX+WBR30	—	4	20	23	38	15	D	CR
2	72	M	2	P	Relapsed	HD-MTX+WBR40	—	3	10	12	14	2	D	PR
3	74	F	2	B	Refractory	HD-MTX	SRT	3	7	9	11	2	D	PR
4	58	M	1	P	Relapsed	HD-MTX+WBR40	—	3	8	11	13	3	D	CR
5	68	M	1	B	Relapsed	HD-MTX	—	4	75+	75+	122+	47	A	CR
6	64	M	1	B	Relapsed	HD-MTX	—	3	16	20	22	6	D	CR
7	55	F	1	P	Relapsed	HD-MTX+WBR30	SRT	2	16	20	36	20	D	CR
8	71	F	1	T	Relapsed	HD-MTX+WBR30	—	3	27+	27+	43+	16	A	CR
9	58	M	0	B	Refractory	HD-MTX+WBR30	—	6	14	47	52	32	D	CR
10	43	M	0	P	Relapsed	HD-MTX+WBR30	WBR24	4	31+	31+	56+	25	A	CR
11	47	M	1	B	Relapsed	HD-MTX+WBR30	—	2	18+	18+	46+	29	A	SD
12	67	M	1	P	Relapsed	HD-MTX+WBR30	—	3	16+	16+	27+	11	A	CR
13	46	M	1	P	Relapsed	HD-MTX+WBR30	—	2	25+	25+	53+	28	A	CR
14	76	M	1	T	Refractory	HD-MTX	SRT	2	23+	23+	41+	17	A	CR

Op, operation; ECOG PS, performance status; D, died; A, alive; M, male; F, female; T, total removal; P, partial removal; B, biopsy; WBR40, whole-brain radiotherapy (40Gy); WBR30, whole-brain radiotherapy (30Gy); WBR24, whole-brain radiotherapy (24Gy); SRT, stereotactic radiotherapy; OS, overall survival; TTP, time to progression; PFS, progression free survival.

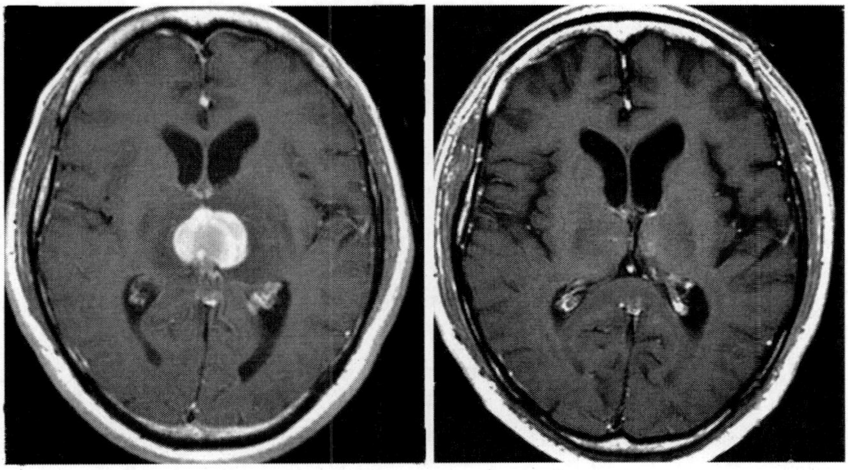

Figure 1. Left, Gd-enhanced T1-weighted MRI of a PCNLS patient before ESHAP therapy. PCNSL was found in bilateral thalamus. Right, Gd-enhanced T1-weighted MRI of a PCNLS patient after ESHAP therapy. PCNSL disappeared.

Side Effects

Side effects of ESHAP therapy developed in all patients. The major side effect was myelosuppression. Toxicity was graded according to the National Cancer Institute Common Toxicity Criteria for Adverse Events (NCI-CTCAE) version 4.0. Grade 2 hematopoietic toxicity was found in 4 patients; and Grade 3, in 10 patients. Grade 3 hematopoietic toxicity included leucopenia and/or thrombocytopenia. Eight patients needed platelet transfusion due to thrombocytopenia, and 2 required infusion with irradiated red cell concentrates due to anemia. However, death due to side effect was not found. Grade 2 alopecia was found in 3 patients; and Grade 1 alopecia, in 5 patients.

Discussion

Until combination therapy with HD-MTX plus HD-AraC was proposed as a candidate for the gold standard therapy for PCNSL (Ferreri, 2009), PCNSL patients had been treated with 3 or 4 courses of HD-MTX followed by WBRT. In the future, this new combination therapy may be established as the standard therapy for PCNSL. Up to now, however, HD-MTX therapy has been commonly used as the first-line chemotherapy due to its fewer side effects. Most PCNSL patients suffer a recurrence after the first-line therapy, and are scarcely completely cured. Therefore, the second-line or salvage therapy at relapse remains an unsolved problem. HD-MTX therapy is effective for most PCSNL patients, but some of them show resistance. In addition, as an initial therapy, HD-MTX is effective for PCNSL; but at relapse HD-MTX often is ineffective. As for systemic diffuse large B-cell lymphoma, the first-line therapy is R-CHOP (rituximab, cyclophophamide, hydoxydaunorubin, vincristine, predonisolone; Hebermann, 2006) with/without irradiation. The second-line chemotherapy is usually based on HD-AraC, particularly ESHAP (etoposide, methylpredonisolone, high-dose cytarabine, cisplatin; Velasques, 1994)/DHAP (dexamethasone, high-dose cytarabine, cisplatin) therapy (Velasques, 1988), which is adequate for gathering hemotopoietic stem cells. Thereafter, strong chemotherapy is performed; and autologous hematopoietic stem cell transplantation is applied to recover the impaired bone marrow. However, not only ESHAP/DHAP therapy but also autologous hematopoietic cell transplantation for PCNSL is scarcely reported (Schmitz, 2015; Madle, 2015). Although elderly patients occasionally show a delayed recovery from reversible myelosuppression, G-CFS or blood transfusion can improve the status of hematopoietic toxicity. A high concentration of cytarabine fascinates to pass through the blood-brain-barrier. Therefore, chemotherapy including cytarabine is potentially effective for brain tumors sensitive to cytarabine. Therefore, as the second-line therapy for PCNSL, a chemotherapy regimen including cytarabine is considered to be useful.

In conclusion, the present study showed HD-AraC-based ESHAP therapy to have great effectiveness as a salvage chemotherapy for PCNLS and to contribute to the long survival of PCNSL patients. However, the goal of overall survival and progression-free survival of patients given ESHAP therapy is not fully satisfied, because some PCNSL patients may be possibly refractory to a positive response to the chemotherapy.

References

Arellano-Rodrigo, E., López-Guillermo, A., Bessell, E. M., Nomdedeu, B., Montserrat, E., Graus, F. (2003) Salvage treatment with etoposide (VP-16), ifosfamide and cytarabine (Ara-C) for patients with recurrent primary central nervous system lymphoma. *Eur J Haematol.* 70, 219-224.

Chamberlain, M. C. (2016) High-dose cytarabine salvage therapy for recurrent primary CNS lymphoma. *J Neurooncol* 126, 545-550.

del Rio MS, Choquet, S., Hoang-Xuan, K., Glaisner, S., Fourme, E., Janvier, M., Soussain, C. (2011) Platine and cytarabine-based salvage treatment for primary central nervous system lymphoma. *J Neurooncol.* 105, 409-414.

Enting, R. H., Demopoulos, A., DeAngelis, L. M., Abrey, L. E. (2004) Salvage therapy for primary CNS lymphoma with a combination of rituximab and temozolomide. Neurology. 63, 901-903.

Ferreri, A. J., Reni, M., Foppoli, M., Martelli, M., Pangalis, G. A., Frezzato, M., Cabras, M. G., Fabbri, A., Corazzelli, G., Ilariucci, F., Rossi, G., Soffietti, R., Stelitano, C., Vallisa, D., Zaja, F., Zoppegno, L., Aondio, G. M., Avvisati, G., Balzarotti, M., Brandes, A. A., Fajardo, J., Gomez, H., Guarini, A., Pinotti, G., Rigacci, L., Uhlmann, C., Picozzi, P., Vezzulli, P., Ponzoni, M., Zucca, E., Caligaris-Cappio, F., Cavalli, F., International Extranodal Lymphoma Study Group (IELSG).(2009) High-dose cytarabine plus high-dose methotrexate versus high-dose methotrexate alone in patients with primary CNS lymphoma: a randomised phase 2 trial. Lancet. 374, 1512-1520.

Habermann, T. M., Weller, E. A., Morrison, V. A., Gascoyne, R. D., Cassileth, P. A., Cohn, J. B., Dakhil, S. R., Woda, B., Fisher, R. I., Peterson, B. A., Horning, S. J. (2006) Rituximab-CHOP versus CHOP alone or with maintenance rituximab in older patients with diffuse large B-cell lymphoma. J Clin Oncol. 24, 3121-3127.

Hirono, S., Iwadate, Y., Higuchi, Y., Serizawa, T., Nagano, O., Matsutani, T., Saeki, N. Stereotactic radiosurgery in combination with up-front high-dose methotrexate as a first-line treatment for newly diagnosed primary central nervous system lymphoma. (2015) *J Neurooncol.* 123, 237-244.

Madle, M., Krämer, I., Lehners, N., Schwarzbich, M., Wuchter, P., Herfarth, K., Egerer, G., Ho, A. D., Witzens-Harig, M. (2015) The influence of rituximab, high-dose therapy followed by autologous stem cell transplantation, and age in patients with primary CNS lymphoma. Ann Hematol. 94:1853-1857.

Nabors, L. B., Portnow, J., Ammirati, M., Baehring, J., Brem, H., Brown, P., Butowski, N., Chamberlain, M. C., Fenstermaker, R. A., Friedman, A., Gilbert, M. R., Hattangadi-Gluth, J., Holdhoff, M., Junck, L., Kaley, T., Lawson, R., Loeffler, J. S., Lovely, M. P., Moots, P. L., Mrugala, M. M., Newton, H. B., Parney, I., Raizer, J. J., Recht, L., Shonka, N., Shrieve, D. C., Sills, A. K. Jr, Swinnen, L. J., Tran, D., Tran, N., Vrionis, F. D., Weiss, S., Wen, P. Y., McMillian, N., Engh, A. M. (2015) Central Nervous System Cancers, Version 1.2015. J Natl Compr Canc Netw. 13:1191-1202.

Plotkin, S. R., Betensky, R. A., Hochberg, F. H., Grossman, S. A., Lesser, G. J., Nabors, L. B., Chon, B., Batchelor, T. T. (2004) Treatment of relapsed central nervous system lymphoma with high-dose methotrexate. Clin Cancer Res. 10:5643-5646.

Reni, M., Mason, W., Zaja, F., Perry, J., Franceschi, E., Bernardi, D., Dell'Oro, S., Stelitano, C., Candela, M., Abbadessa, A., Pace, A., Bordonaro, R., Latte, G., Villa, E., Ferreri, A. J. (2004) Salvage chemotherapy with temozolomide in primary CNS lymphomas: preliminary results of a phase II trial. Eur J Cancer. 40:1682-1688.

Schulz, H., Pels, H., Schmidt-Wolf, I., Zeelen, U., Germing, U., Engert, A. (2004). Intraventricular treatment of relapsed central nervous system lymphoma with the anti-CD20 antibody rituximab. Haematologica. 89(6):753-754.

Raizer, J. J., Rademaker, A., Evens, A. M., Rice, L., Schwartz, M., Chandler, J. P., Getch, C. C., Tellez, C., Grimm, S. A. (2012) Pemetrexed in the treatment of relapsed/refractory primary central nervous system lymphoma. Cancer. 118:3743-3748.

Ungur, R., Tempescul, A., Berthou, C., Bagacean, C., Radeanu, D., Muresan, A., Zdrenghea, M. ESHAP chemotherapy is efficient in refractory/relapsed primary central nervous system lymphoma: report of four cases. (2015) *Onco Targets Ther.* 8:2771-2773.

Velasquez, W. S., Cabanillas, F., Salvador, P., McLaughlin, P., Fridrik, M., Tucker, S., Jagannath, S., Hagemeister, F. B., Redman, J. R., Swan, F. (1988) Effective salvage therapy for lymphoma with cisplatin in combination with high-dose Ara-C and dexamethasone (DHAP). *Blood.* 71, 117-122.

Velasquez, W. S., McLaughlin, P., Tucker, S., Hagemeister, F. B., Swan, F., Rodriguez, M. A., Romaguera, J., Rubenstein, E., Cabanillas, F. (1994) ESHAP--an effective chemotherapy regimen in refractory and relapsing lymphoma: a 4-year follow-up study. *J Clin Oncol.* 12, 1169-1176.

Voloschin, A. D., Betensky, R., Wen, P. Y., Hochberg, F., Batchelor, T. (2008) Topotecan as salvage therapy for relapsed or refractory primary central nervous system lymphoma. J Neurooncol. 86:211-215.

Zacher, J., Kasenda, B., Engert, A., Skoetz, N. (2014) The role of additional radiotherapy for primary central nervous system lymphoma. Cochrane Database Syst Rev. 6, CD009211.

In: Primary Central Nervous System Lymphoma (PCNSL)
Editor: Ryuya Yamanaka
ISBN: 978-1-63485-322-4

Chapter 15

SALVAGE THERAPY FOR PRIMARY CENTRAL NERVOUS SYSTEM LYMPHOMA

Ryuya Yamanaka*
Laboratory of Molecular Target Therapy for Cancer, Graduate School for Medical Science, Kyoto Prefectural University of Medicine,
Kyoto, Japan

ABSTRACT

Methotrexate-based chemotherapy with or without radiation therapy is the most accepted treatment for primary central nervous system lymphoma (PCNSL), and patients with PCNSL have a median overall survival of 10 to 79 months. Failure after first-line treatment has been reported in most patients with PCNSL. Salvage therapy improves outcomes although many different treatments have been used. As such, conclusions cannot be made regarding an optimal treatment schedule. This review analyzes the efficacy of salvage therapy, excluding temozolomide and cytarabine, by focusing on data from papers that report salvage therapy use. Well-designed, randomized trials will resolve issues, such as the best second-line chemotherapy regimen.

Keywords: Chemotherapy, primary central nervous system lymphoma, recurrence, refractory, salvage therapy

INTRODUCTION

Several phase II studies combining chemotherapy with radiotherapy were performed in the last decade. The systemic use of high-dose methotrexate (HD-MTX)-based chemotherapy

* Corresponding Author address: Ryuya Yamanaka, M.D., Ph.D., Laboratory of Molecular Target Therapy for Cancer, Graduate School for Medical Science, Kyoto Prefectural University of Medicine, 465 Kajii-cho, Kamigyoku, Kyoto 602-8566, Japan, TEL: 81-75-212-5429, FAX: 81-75-212-5423, Email: ryaman @koto.kpu-m.ac.jp.

with or without radiation therapy for newly diagnosed PCNSL has improved the median overall survival (OS) from 10 to 79 months [1–14]. However, salvage treatment is necessary for 10–35% of patients with refractory disease and for another 30–60% or more who have a relapse [15]. Moreover, the prognoses for patients who are refractory or who relapse after initial therapy are poor [15]. Treatment options for patients with recurrent PCNSL are limited; there is no standard second-line treatment. Salvage treatment may improve outcomes and quality of life even if the optimal salvage regimen is not known. Reni et al. reported median OS rates of 14 months for patients who underwent salvage therapy and 2 months for patients who received no treatment [15]. Use of novel therapeutic agents with clear activity are warranted for recurrent PCNSL. Since the use of temozolomide and cytarabine as salvage therapy is described in chapters 13 and 14 respectively, the present chapter analyzes the impact of second-line treatment with other agents on survival of PCNSL patients by reviewing recent articles and provides some therapeutic recommendations for management of patients with refractory or relapsed PCNSL.

SALVAGE TREATMENT AFTER FAILURE WITH HD-MTX (TABLE 1)

Table 1. Salvage therapy for relapsed or refractory PCNSL

Treatment Regimen	Clinical Trial Design	Patient Population (refractory, recurrent)	Median Age	Response Rate (%)	mPFS[e] (month)	mOS[d] (month)	Reference
HD-MTX[b]	Retrospective	22	58	92	61.9	91.9	[16]
HD-MTX	Retrospective	39 (0,39)	66	85	16	41	[17]
ProMACE-MOPP Hybrid	Retrospective	9 (2,7)	62.6	90	10	30	[18]
Rituximab	Phase II	12 (0,12)	64	36	2	20.9	[23]
Pemetrexed	Phase II	11	69.8	55	5.7	10.1	[26]
Pemetrexed+ Rituximab	Retrospective	27 (9,18)	53.5	62.9	6.9	11.2	[28]
Topotecan	Phase II	27 (14,13)	51	33	2	8.4	[31]
Topotecan	Phase II	15	56	40	2	33	[32]
Bendamustine	Retrospective	12	59	50	3.5	5.5	[34]
Lenalidomide	Retrospective	6 (0,6)	73.5	50	n.d.[f]	4	[36]
Zevalin	Phase II	10 (0,10)	53.5	40	n.d.	n.d.	[37]
PCV[g]	Retrospective	7 (2,5)	57	86	2	12	[38]
Carboplatin+CPA[a]+VP-16[h]	Retrospective	37	57.5	35	3	6.8	[43]
HDC-ASCT[c]	Phase II	43 (21,22)	52	50	11.6	18.3	[48]
Radiotherapy	Retrospective	27 (17,10)	67	74	9.7	10.9	[53]
Radiotherapy	Retrospective	48 (24,24)	59.5	79	10	16	[54]

[a] CPA, cyclophosphamide;
[b] HD-MTX, high-dose methotrexate;
[c] HDC-ASCT, high-dose chemotherapy supported by autologous peripheral blood stem cell transplant,
[d] mOS, median overall survival;
[e] mPFS, median progression-free survival;
[f] n.d., not determined;
[g] PCV, lomustine + procarbazine + vincristine;
[h] VP-16, etoposide.

HD-MTX

Plotkin et al. [16] reported on 22 relapsed patients who had initially achieved a complete response (CR) with HD-MTX as a retrospective study. The median time to first relapse was 24.4 months (range, 2–100 months), reinduction with same HD-MTX schedule resulted in response rates of 91% to the first salvage attempt (20 of 22 patients) and 100% to the second salvage attempt (4 of 4 patients).

A median progression-free survival (PFS) of 61.9 months and an OS of 91.9 months were noted. Hematologic grade 3/4 toxicities were observed in 1.7% of patients. Pentsova et al. [17] also reported on 39 patients who received MTX rechallenge. The median time from initial diagnosis was 26 months. The objective response rate was 85%, the median PFS was 16 months, and the median OS was 41 months. Grade 3/4 toxicities included pulmonary toxicity in 2 patients, reversible nephrotoxicity in 4 patients, leucoencephalopathy in 2 patients, and neutropenia in 7 patients. Rechallenge with HD-MTX remained effective for relapsed patients who initially responded to HD-MTX, suggesting retained chemosensitivity to MTX. However, HD-MTX should be avoided for patients who received prior whole brain radiation therapy (WBRT) and patients with significant renal insufficiency.

We previously reported the efficacy of salvage therapy using repetition for a modified ProMACE-MOPP hybrid of MTX containing a polychemotherapeutic regimen in patients with PCNSL [18]. Nine relapsed patients were retreated with a 90% objective response rate. The median CR duration was 13.2 months, and the median OS after initial relapse was 30 months. The major acute toxicity was grade 3/4 leucopenia, which was noted in 24.3% of patients. Additional treatment with a ProMACE-MOPP hybrid regimen was still effective for relapsed disease.

Rituximab

Rituximab, a humanized anti-CD20 monoclonal antibody, achieves a cerebrospinal fluid (CSF) concentration that is only 0.1% of matched plasma levels after systemic administration, suggesting poor blood brain barrier (BBB) penetration [19]. However, most PCNSLs have marked contrast enhancement on neuroimaging, indicative of a disrupted BBB, and Rituximab may enter PCNSLs with associated BBB disruption. Rituximab improves survival when combined with CHOP therapy in patients with systemic diffuse large B-cell lymphoma (DLBCL) [20]. Approximately 70–90% of PCNSLs are DLBCLs or its variant [21, 22], and rituximab is now part of combination therapy in some PCNSL regimens Twelve CD20+ PCNSL patients with relapsed or refractory disease who received prior methotrexate-based therapy were enrolled in a phase II trial of rituximab monotherapy [23]. Rituximab was intravenously administered at a dose 375 mg/m^2 weekly for a maximum of 8 cycles. The objective response rate was 36%, with a median PFS of 57 days (95% confidence interval (CI) 29–175 days) and a median OS of 20.9 months (95% CI 2.9–47 months). Four patients experienced grade 3/4 toxicities, consisting of allergic reaction, fatigue, anxiety, and pain. Rituximab monotherapy combined with other chemotherapeutic agents in patients with relapsed or refractory PCNSL warrants further study.

Pemetrexed

Pemetrexed targets purine synthesis by inhibiting thymidylate synthase and dihydrofolate reductase. It targets pyrimidine synthesis by inhibiting glycinamide ribonucleotide formyltransferase and aminoimidazole carboxamide formyltransferase. This gives pemetrexed a broader spectrum of activity than methotrexate [24]. Although the CSF penetration of pemetrexed is less than 2% [25], it can be potentially active in patients with PCNSL that have disrupted BBBs. Raizer et al. [26] reported a phase II trial in 11 relapsed or refractory patients who were given 900 mg/m^2 pemetrexed every 3 weeks. The response rate was 55%, and the disease control rate was 91%. The 6-month PFS (PFS-6) was 45%, with a median PFS of 5.7 months (95% CI, 1.6–21.4 months) and a median OS of 10.1 months (95% CI, 2.4–33.3 months). The most common adverse events were hematologic, and the most severe adverse event was pneumonia combined with neutropenia in 1 patient.

Zhang et al. [27] also reported on 18 patients who received pemetrexed as salvage therapy. The overall response rate was 64.7%, with a median PFS of 5.8 months. Zhao et al. [28] reported on 27 patients who received combination rituximab and pemetrexed as second-line treatment. Rituximab (375 mg/m^2) was administered on day 0, and pemetrexed (500 mg/m^2) was administered on day 1, every 3 weeks. The response rate was 62.9%, with a median PFS of 6.9 months (95% CI, 5.6–8.3 months) and a median OS of 11.2 months (95% CI, 9.1–13.4 months). None of the patients experienced grade 4 toxicity. Pemetrexed may not exhibit cross-resistance with HD-MTX since the majority of these patients had received prior HD-MTX. Pemetrexed treatment resulted in relatively minimal toxicity. However, neurotoxicity should be further investigated since this drug is a dihydrofolate reductase, similar to methotrexate.

Topotecan

Topotecan, a semi-synthetic camptothecin derivative and a specific inhibitor of topoisomerase I in the S-phase of the cell cycle, has documented efficacy in patients with relapsed systemic non-Hodgkin's lymphoma [29]. It penetrates the BBB, reaching concentrations in CSF of more than 30% of those in plasma [30]. Fischer et al. [31] report the results of a prospective study on topotecan chemotherapy in 27 relapsed or refractory patients. Fourteen patients were refractory, and 13 relapsed after a median of 6.0 months. A 30-min daily topotecan infusion of 1.5 mg/m^2 for 5 days was administered every 3 weeks. The response rate was 33%, with a median event-free survival (EFS) of 2.0 months (9.1 months in responders), a PFS-6 of 52%, a median OS of 8.4 months (9–28 months in responders), and a 1-year survival rate of 39%. The average survival time of refractory patients was 9.5 months, and that of recurrent patients was 3.4 months. The refractory patients had additional radiation therapy after topotecan treatment, which is the reason for longer survival time in this subgroup. However, five patients achieved long-term remissions, lasting for 7.5, 10.5, 15.8, >24.1, and 28.6 months, with topotecan alone. Grade 3/4 leucopenia occurred in 26% of patients, and thrombocytopenia occurred in 11% of the patients. Voloschin et al. [32] reported a phase II study of 15 refractory or relapsed patients treated with intravenous topotecan (1.5 mg/m^2) for five days during each 21-day cycle. The response rate was 40%, with a median PFS of 2 months and a median OS of 33 months. Most patients were treated with WBRT.

Eleven out of 15 patients had grade 3/4 neutropenia, and three patients had grade 3 thrombocytopenia. Topotecan as monotherapy has activity in relapsed and refractory PCNSL with tolerable toxicity.

Bendamustine

Bendamustine, an alkylating agent, is a mechlorethamine derivative that contains a purine-like benzimidazole ring and appears to lack cross-resistance to other alkylator agents with established activity in B cell systemic lymphomas [33]. Bendamustine penetrates the BBB, as shown by tissue distribution studies [33]. Chamberlain et al. [34] reported on 12 HD-MTX refractory patients treated with bendamustine at the time of their second recurrences. A cycle of bendamustine was 2 days of treatment (100 $mg/m^2/day$) administered every 4 weeks. The radiographic response rate was 50%, with a median PFS of 3.5 months (range, 1–14 months) and a PFS-6 of 33%. Grade 3 toxicities, such as anemia, fatigue, hyperglycemia, nausea, neutropenia, and lymphopenia, were observed in 5 patients. Bendamustine had modest single-agent activity with manageable toxicity.

Lenalidomide

Lenalidomide is an immunomodulatory agent, derived from thalidomide, with antitumor activities. Lenalidomide functions by modifying cytotoxic T cell and natural killer cell activity [35]. Its efficacy is well known in multiple myeloma and non-Hodgkin's lymphoma. Houillier et al. [36] reported on 6 recurrent patients treated with lenalidomide as third- to fifth-line therapy, using a standard dose of 25 mg/day on days 1–21 of a 28-day cycle by oral administration. Two patients, including 1 patient with long-lasting remission (> 24 months), achieved CR. No patients experienced any grade 3/4 toxicity. Lenalidomide showed moderate activity in heavily pretreated patients and was well tolerated in elderly patients.

^{90}Y-Iibritumomab Tiuxetan (Zevalin)

^{90}Y-Ibritumomab tiuxetan (Zevalin) is a murine anti-CD20 antibody covalently linked to the high-energy beta emitter Yttrium-90 by the chelator tiuxetan [37]. Although monoclonal antibodies are large molecules that get excluded by an intact BBB, they could leak across tumor vasculature into PCNSL and induce radiolysis in both the targeted and adjacent lymphoma cells. Maza et al. [37] reported a phase II trial that evaluated the efficacy, toxicity, and biodistribution of Zevalin in 10 relapsed patients. Four patients responded. One patient had a CR lasting > 30 months, and three patients had short-term responses of less than 4 weeks. All patients experienced grade 3/4 hematotoxicity without acute neurotoxicity. Penetration of a therapeutic antibody into PCNSL and significant clinical activity was shown by single-photon emission computed tomography imaging with ^{111}In ibritumomab tiuxetan. Due to limited response duration and considerable hematotoxicity, future investigations should focus on a multimodal approach with additional chemotherapy.

Lomustine + Procarbazine + Vincristine (PCV)

Procarbazine and lomustine (CCNU) penetrate the BBB, and the mechanism of action as an alkylating agent differs from the antimetabolite methotrexate. Herrlinger et al. [38] reported on 7 patients with recurrent or refractory disease as a retrospective study. The regimen consist of procarbazine 60 mg/m^2 (days 8–21), CCNU 110 mg/m^2 (day 1), and vincristine 2 mg (days 8 and 29). The response rate was 86%, with a median PFS of 2 months, a median OS of 12 months (range, 1–39 months) and a 1-year survival rate of 58%. Toxic hepatitis or allergic dermatitis due to procarbazine was seen in one patient. Severe leucoencephalopathy and neuropsychological deficits were noted in 2 of the patients after PCV treatment.

Carboplatin (IA) + Cyclophosphamide + Etoposide

Carboplatin, a second-generation platinum analog, has efficacy in multiple cancers and has been used in combination with several agents for relapsed systemic lymphoma [39]. The safety and efficacy of intra-arterial (IA) chemotherapy with osmotic BBB disruption has been documented [40–42]. Opening tight junctions with mannitol allows increased drug levels to reach the CNS [40–42]. Tyson et al. [43] reported a retrospective study of 37 relapsed patients who were treated with IA carboplatin-based chemotherapy with BBB disruption. Mannitol was infused (5–10 mL/s for 30 s) into an internal carotid or vertebral artery. Cyclophosphamide was administered intravenously (IV) at a dose of 330–660 mg/m^2 20 min before the mannitol infusion, and carboplatin was administered IA at a dose of 200–400 mg/m^2 over 10 min, starting within 5 min after the mannitol infusion. Etoposide was administered IA or IV at a dose of 200–400 mg/m^2. This protocol was repeated every 4 weeks for up to 1 year. The overall response rate was 35%, with a median PFS for patients with CR and PR of 9.1 months, a median OS of 6.8 months (range, 11–91.0 months). Seven out of 37 patients survived longer than 27 months. However, grade 3/4 hematological adverse events were observed in 41% of the patients, and grade 3/4 non-hematological adverse events, such as 3% ototoxicity, 11% vascular toxicity, 21% infection, 3% pulmonary toxicity, and 11% neurotoxicity, were observed.

Rituximab + Ifosfamide + Etoposide (R-IE)

Ifosfamide and etoposide are active agents against systemic lymphoma and cross the BBB [44, 45]. The combination of targeted agent, alkylating agent, and topoisomerase inhibitor may be an active therapeutic approach with different anticancer mechanisms from HD-MTX. Mappa et al. [46] reported the R-IE regimen (rituximab 375 mg/m^2, day 0: ifosfamide 2g/m^2/day, days 1–3; etoposide 250 mg/m^2, day 1; four cycles) administration for 22 patients as second- to third-line therapy. The overall response rate was 41%, and the 2-year survival rate after relapse was 25%. Four patients received high-dose chemotherapy supported by autologous peripheral blood stem cell transplant (HDC-ASCT). The most common grade 4 hematological toxicities were neutropenia in 50% of patients, thrombocytopenia in 23% of patients, and anemia in 14% of patients. There was only one instance of grade 4 non-hematologic toxicity, which was transient hepatotoxicity. Two previously irradiated patients developed neurologic deterioration. R-IE was exhibited some activity on its own and was successful in combination with HDC-ASCT.

HDC-ASCT

Sussain et al. [47] reported the results of HDC-ASCT in patients after failure of HD-MTX-based treatment. Salvage treatment consisted of two cycles of high-dose cytarabine and etoposide (CYVE). Intensive chemotherapy combined thiotepa, busulfan, and cyclophosphamide. Seventy-nine patients were included. Just before HDC-ASCT, 32 patients achieved CRs, and 26 patients achieved PRs. The 5-year OS rate was 51% for the entire population and 62% for patients chemosensitive to salvage treatment. The 5-year EFS rate was 37.8% in the entire population and 43.7% in chemosensitive populations. However, toxicity was not moderate. Three patients died after HDC, as a result of septic shock (n = 2) or mesenteric necrosis (n = 1), and five patients had late neurologic toxicity after HDC-ASCT [48]. HDC-ASCT should be used in clinical centers that have sufficiently trained staff [49]. The rationale for using the thiotepa-busulfan-cyclophosphamide combination was that thiotepa and busulfan are able to penetrate the BBB well [50, 51]. The CYVE regimen was used because of the lack of cross-resistance between cytarabine, etoposide, and methotrexate and for its efficacy in newly diagnosed PCNSL [52]. HDC-ASCT is an effective treatment for refractory and recurrent PCNSL and should be evaluated in further studies.

Radiation Therapy

For patients who received chemotherapy alone or low-dose radiation therapy for newly diagnosed PCNSL, radiation therapy (RT) may be selected for relapsed or refractory patients. Nguyen et al. [53] reported the efficacy of WBRT as salvage therapy in a retrospective study. This study included 17 refractory and 10 recurrent patients who failed initial HD-MTX treatment and then received salvage WBRT with a median dose of 36 Gy. The overall response rate was 74%, with a median OS from WBRT initiation of 10.9 months (range, 0.3–63.7 months) and a median PFS of 9.7 months. By univariate analysis, age < 60 years was a predictor of longer survival. Late neurotoxicity was diagnosed in 4 patients (15%) and was significantly associated with total radiation doses greater than 36 Gy. Hottinger et al. [54] also evaluated the efficacy of salvage WBRT for 24 refractory and 24 recurrent patients in a retrospective study. After WBRT, the overall response rate was 79%, with a median OS of 16 months and a median PFS of 10 months. Age < 60 years and complete response to WBRT were associated with better outcomes. Treatment-related neurotoxicity was observed in 22% of patients. Patients > 60 years old and those treated less than 6 months after HD-MTX therapy had an increased risk of neurotoxicity.

The median OS after salvage WBRT compares favorably with the 11.6 months reported for patients whose initial treatment was WBRT alone [55], suggesting that post-WBRT survival is maintained in MTX-resistant disease. However, in relapsed patients, the risk of neurotoxicity after salvage radiotherapy could be greater than in patients who received radiotherapy as an initial treatment, especially in older patients.

Discussion

There is no standard salvage therapy for relapsed or refractory PCNSL patients, but numerous regimens have been used with variable results. Treatment options for such patients include WBRT, reinduction with methotrexate in patients who previously responded to methotrexate, and alternative chemotherapy agents, such as temozolomide, topotecan, pemetrexed, bendamustine, PCV regimens, ifosfamide-etoposide-based regimens, or cisplatin-cytarabine based regimens used alone or in combination with rituximab [49]. A salvage treatment schedule should include drugs that can cross the BBB and agents with some efficacy as an initial treatment [56–58]. Radiotherapy is an option for patients not previously treated using radiation. Additional treatment with HD-MTX may be an option for patients who relapsed after prolonged remission after treatment with this agent and had not received prior radiotherapy. If the patient did not receive any consolidation treatment after HD-MTX-based induction chemotherapy, therapy with WBRT or HDC-ASCT should be considered [49]. If the patient is not suitable for WBRT or HDC-ASCT, conventional chemotherapy can be proposed as second-line treatment [49].

Apart from disease rarity, there are several difficulties associated with treatment because of the aggressive course of relapsing PCNSL that produces an impaired performance status and neurological deterioration, usually in elderly patients. Because most reported case series were undersized and retrospective studies in which patients received heterogeneous initial regimens with varied drug doses and schedules and were not adequately restaged at recurrence, no conclusions could be drawn about the optimal regimen. The development of novel agents for PCNSL is extremely warranted. Emerging novel agents for systemic diffuse large B cell lymphoma are presented in chapter 16. The inclusion of patients with relapsed or refractory PCNSL in prospective trials addressing new therapeutic agents or combination therapies should be further recommended.

References

[1] Abrey LE, Yahalom J, DeAngelis LM. Treatment for primary CNS lymphoma: The next step. *J. Clin. Oncol.* 2000; 18:3144-3150.

[2] Bessell EM, López-Guillermo A, Villá S, Verger E, Nomdedeu B, Petit J, Byrne P, Montserrat E, Graus F. Importance of radiotherapy in the outcome of patients with primary CNS lymphoma: An analysis of the CHOD/BVAM regimen followed by two different radiotherapy treatments. *J. Clin. Oncol.* 2002; 20:231-236.

[3] DeAngelis LM, Seiferheld W, Schold SC, Fisher B, Schultz CJ; Radiation Therapy Oncology Group Study 93-10. Combination chemotherapy and radiotherapy for primary central nervous system lymphoma: Radiation Therapy Oncology Group Study 93-10. *J. Clin. Oncol.* 2002; 20:4643-4648.

[4] Herrlinger U, Schabet M, Brugger W, Kortmann RD, Küker W, Deckert M, Engel C, Schmeck-Lindenau HJ, Mergenthaler HG, Krauseneck P, Benöhr C, Meisner C, Wiestler OD, Dichgans J, Kanz L, Bamberg M, Weller M. German Cancer Society Neuro-Oncology Working Group NOA-03 multicenter trial of single-agent high-dose methotrexate for primary central nervous system lymphoma. *Ann. Neurol.* 2002; 51:247-252.

[5] Batchelor T, Carson K, O'Neill A, Grossman SA, Alavi J, New P, Hochberg F, Priet R. Treatment of primary CNS lymphoma with methotrexate and deferred radiotherapy: A report of NABTT 96-07. *J. Clin. Oncol.* 2003; 21:1044-1049.

[6] Poortmans PM, Kluin-Nelemans HC, Haaxma-Reiche H, Van't Veer M, Hansen M, Soubeyran P, Taphoorn M, Thomas J, Van den Bent M, Fickers M, Van Imhoff G, Rozewicz C, Teodorovic I, van Glabbeke M; European Organization for Research and Treatment of Cancer Lymphoma Group. High-dose methotrexate-based chemotherapy followed by consolidating radiotherapy in non-AIDS-related primary central nervous system lymphoma: European Organization for Research and Treatment of Cancer Lymphoma Group Phase II Trial 20962. *J. Clin. Oncol.* 2003; 21:4483-4488.

[7] Korfel A, Martus P, Nowrousian MR, Hossfeld DK, Kirchen H, Brücher J, Stelljes M, Birkmann J, Peschel C, Pasold R, Fischer L, Jahnke K, Thiel E; German primary central nervous system lymphoma Study Group (G-PCNSL-SG). German primary central nervous system lymphoma Study Group (G-PCNSL-SG). Response to chemotherapy and treating institution predict survival in primary central nervous system lymphoma. *Br. J. Haematol.* 2005; 128:177-183.

[8] Omuro AM, DeAngelis LM, Yahalom J, Abrey LE. Chemoradiotherapy for primary CNS lymphoma: An intent-to-treat analysis with complete follow-up. *Neurology.* 2005; 64:69-74.

[9] Ferreri AJ, Dell'Oro S, Foppoli M, Bernardi M, Brandes AA, Tosoni A, Montanari M, Balzarotti M, Spina M, Ilariucci F, Zaja F, Stelitano C, Bobbio F, Corazzelli G, Baldini L, Ponzoni M, Picozzi P, Caligaris Cappio F, Reni M. MATILDE regimen followed by radiotherapy is an active strategy against primary CNS lymphomas. *Neurology.* 2006;66(9):1435-1438.

[10] Ferreri AJ, Reni M, Foppoli M, Martelli M, Pangalis GA, Frezzato M, Cabras MG, Fabbri A, Corazzelli G, Ilariucci F, Rossi G, Soffietti R, Stelitano C, Vallisa D, Zaja F, Zoppegno L, Aondio GM, Avvisati G, Balzarotti M, Brandes AA, Fajardo J, Gomez H, Guarini A, Pinotti G, Rigacci L, Uhlmann C, Picozzi P, Vezzulli P, Ponzoni M, Zucca E, Caligaris-Cappio F, Cavalli F; International Extranodal Lymphoma Study Group (IELSG). High-dose cytarabine plus high-dose methotrexate versus high-dose methotrexate alone in patients with primary CNS lymphoma: A randomised phase 2 trial. *Lancet.* 2009; 374:1512-1520.

[11] Pels H, Juergens A, Glasmacher A, Schulz H, Engert A, Linnebank M, Schackert G, Reichmann H, Kroschinsky F, Vogt-Schaden M, Egerer G, Bode U, Schaller C, Lamprecht M, Hau P, Deckert M, Fimmers R, Bangard C, Schmidt-Wolf IG, Schlegel U. Early relapses in primary CNS lymphoma after response to polychemotherapy without intraventricular treatment: Results of a phase II study. *J. Neurooncol.* 2009;91:299-305.

[12] Thiel E, Korfel A, Martus P, Kanz L, Griesinger F, Rauch M, Röth A, Hertenstein B, von Toll T, Hundsberger T, Mergenthaler HG, Leithäuser M, Birnbaum T, Fischer L,

Jahnke K, Herrlinger U, Plasswilm L, Nägele T, Pietsch T, Bamberg M, Weller M. High-dose methotrexate with or without whole brain radiotherapy for primary CNS lymphoma (G-PCNSL-SG-1): a phase 3, randomised, non-inferiority trial. *Lancet Oncol.* 2010;11(11):1036-1047.

[13] Wieduwilt MJ, Valles F, Issa S, Behler CM, Hwang J, McDermott M, Treseler P, O'Brien J, Shuman MA, Cha S, Damon LE, Rubenstein JL. Immuno- chemotherapy with intensive consolidation for primary CNS lymphoma: A pilot study and prognostic assessment by diffusion-weighted MRI. *Clin. Cancer Res.* 2012; 18:1146-1155.

[14] Morris PG, Correa DD, Yahalom J, Raizer JJ, Schiff D, Grant B, Grimm S, Lai RK, Reiner AS, Panageas K, Karimi S, Curry R, Shah G, Abrey LE, DeAngelis LM, Omuro A. Rituximab, methotrexate, procarbazine, and vincristine followed by consolidation reduced-dose whole-brain radiotherapy and cytarabine in newly diagnosed primary CNS lymphoma: final results and long-term outcome. *J. Clin. Oncol.* 2013;31(31):3971-3979.

[15] Reni M, Ferreri AJ, Villa E. Second-line treatment for primary central nervous system lymphoma. *Br. J. Cancer.* 1999;79:530-534.

[16] Plotkin SR, Betensky RA, Hochberg FH, Grossman SA, Lesser GJ, Nabors LB, Chon B, Batchelor TT. Treatment of relapsed central nervous system lymphoma with high-dose methotrexate. *Clin. Cancer Res.* 2004;10:5643-5646.

[17] Pentsova E, Deangelis LM, Omuro A. Methotrexate re-challenge for recurrent primary central nervous system lymphoma. *J. Neurooncol.* 2014;117(1):161-165.

[18] Yamanaka R, Shinbo Y, Sano M, Homma J, Tsuchiya N, Yajima N, Tamura T, Hondoh H, Takahashi H, Morii K, Onda K, Tanaka R. Salvage therapy and late neurotoxicity in patients with recurrent primary CNS lymphoma treated with a modified ProMACE-MOPP hybrid regimen. *Leuk. Lymphoma.* 2007;48:1119-1126.

[19] Rubenstein JL, Combs D, Rosenberg J, Levy A, McDermott M, Damon L, Ignoffo R, Aldape K, Shen A, Lee D, Grillo-Lopez A, Shuman MA. Rituximab therapy for CNS lymphomas: targeting the leptomeningeal compartment. *Blood.* 2003;101:466-468.

[20] Coiffier B, Lepage E, Briere J, Herbrecht R, Tilly H, Bouabdallah R, Morel P, Van Den Neste E, Salles G, Gaulard P, Reyes F, Lederlin P, Gisselbrecht C. CHOP chemotherapy plus rituximab compared with CHOP alone in elderly patients with diffuse large-B-cell lymphoma. *N. Engl. J. Med.* 2002;346:235-242.

[21] Shenkier TN, Voss N, Chhanabhai M, Fairey R, Gascoyne RD, Hoskins P, Klasa R, Morris J, O'Reilly SE, Pickles T, Sehn L, Connors JM. The treatment of primary central nervous system lymphoma in 122 immunocompetent patients: a population-based study of successively treated cohorts from the British Colombia Cancer Agency. *Cancer.* 2005;103:1008-1017.

[22] Yamanaka R, Morii K, Shinbo Y, Homma J, Sano M, Tsuchiya N, Yajima N, Tamura T, Hondoh H, Takahashi H, Kakuma T, Tanaka R. Results of treatment of 112 cases of primary CNS lymphoma. *Jpn. J. Clin. Oncol.* 2008;38:373-380.

[23] Batchelor TT, Grossman SA, Mikkelsen T, Ye X, Desideri S, Lesser GJ. Rituximab monotherapy for patients with recurrent primary CNS lymphoma. *Neurology.* 2011;76(10):929-930.

[24] Shih C, Chen VJ, Gossett LS, Gates SB, MacKellar WC, Habeck LL, Shackelford KA, Mendelsohn LG, Soose DJ, Patel VF, Andis SL, Bewley JR, Rayl EA, Moroson BA, Beardsley GP, Kohler W, Ratnam M, Schultz RM. LY231514, a pyrrolo[2,3-

d]pyrimidine-based antifolate that inhibits multiple folate-requiring enzymes. *Cancer Res.* 1997;57(6):1116-1123.

[25] Stapleton SL, Reid JM, Thompson PA, Ames MM, McGovern RM, McGuffey L, Nuchtern J, Dauser R, Blaney SM. Plasma and cerebrospinal fluid pharmacokinetics of pemetrexed after intravenous administration in non-human primates. *Cancer Chemother. Pharmacol.* 2007;59(4):461-466.

[26] Raizer JJ, Rademaker A, Evens AM, Rice L, Schwartz M, Chandler JP, Getch CC, Tellez C, Grimm SA.Pemetrexed in the treatment of relapsed/refractory primary central nervous system lymphoma. *Cancer.* 2012;118(15):3743-3748.

[27] Zhang JP, Lee EQ, Nayak L, Doherty L, Kesari S, Muzikansky A, Norden AD, Chen H, Wen PY, Drappatz J.Retrospective study of pemetrexed as salvage therapy for central nervous system lymphoma. *J. Neurooncol.* 2013;115(1):71-77.

[28] Zhao HT, Chen J, Shi SB, Tian J, Tao RJ.Pemetrexed plus rituximab as second-line treatment for primary central nervous system lymphoma. *Med. Oncol.* 2015;32(1):351.

[29] Kancherla RR, Nair JS, Ahmed T, Durrani H, Seiter K, Mannancheril A, Tse-Dinh YC. Evaluation of topotecan and etoposide for non-Hodgkin lymphoma: correlation of topoisomerase-DNA complex formation with clinical response. *Cancer.* 2001;91:463-471.

[30] Herben VM, ten Bokkel Huinink WW, Beijnen JH. Clinical pharmacokinetics of topotecan. *Clin. Pharmacokinet.* 1996;31:85-102.

[31] Fischer L, Thiel E, Klasen HA, Birkmann J, Jahnke K, Martus P, Korfel A. Prospective trial on topotecan salvage therapy in primary CNS lymphoma. *Ann. Oncol.* 2006;17:1141-1145.

[32] Voloschin AD, Betensky R, Wen PY, Hochberg F, Batchelor T. Topotecan as salvage therapy for relapsed or refractory primary central nervous system lymphoma. *J Neurooncol.* 2008;86:211-215.

[33] Cheson BD, Rummel MJ.Bendamustine: rebirth of an old drug. *J. Clin. Oncol.* 2009;27(9):1492-1501.

[34] Chamberlain MC.Salvage therapy with bendamustine for methotrexate refractory recurrent primary CNS lymphoma: a retrospective case series. *J. Neurooncol.* 2014;118(1):155-162.

[35] Zhu D, Corral LG, Fleming YW, Stein B.Immunomodulatory drugs Revlimid (lenalidomide) and CC-4047 induce apoptosis of both hematological and solid tumor cells through NK cell activation. *Cancer Immunol. Immunother.* 2008;57(12):1849-1859.

[36] Houillier C, Choquet S, Touitou V, Martin-Duverneuil N, Navarro S, Mokhtari K, Soussain C, Hoang-Xuan K.Lenalidomide monotherapy as salvage treatment for recurrent primary CNS lymphoma. *Neurology.* 2015;84(3):325-326.

[37] Maza S, Kiewe P, Munz DL, Korfel A, Hamm B, Jahnke K, Thiel E. First report on a prospective trial with yttrium-90-labeled ibritumomab tiuxetan (ZevalinTM) in primary CNS lymphoma. *Neuro Oncol.* 2009;11(4):423-429.

[38] Herrlinger U, Brugger W, Bamberg M, Küker W, Dichgans J, Weller M. PCV salvage chemotherapy for recurrent primary CNS lymphoma. *Neurology.* 2000;54:1707-1708.

[39] Zelenetz AD, Hamlin P, Kewalramani T, Yahalom J, Nimer S, Moskowitz CH. Ifosfamide, carboplatin, etoposide (ICE)-based second-line chemotherapy for the

management of relapsed and refractory aggressive non-Hodgkin's lymphoma. *Ann. Oncol.* 2003;14 (Suppl 1):5-10.

[40] Kroll RA, Neuwelt EA. Outwitting the blood-brain barrier for therapeutic purposes: osmotic opening and other means. *Neurosurgery.* 1998;42:1083-1099.

[41] Neuwelt EA, Barnett PA, McCormick CI, Remsen LG, Kroll RA, Sexton G. Differential permeability of a human brain tumor xenograft in the nude rat: impact of tumor size and method of administration on optimizing delivery of biologically diverse agents. *Clin. Cancer Res.* 1998;4:1549-1555.

[42] Muldoon LL, Soussain C, Jahnke K, Johanson C, Siegal T, Smith QR, Hall WA, Hynynen K, Senter PD, Peereboom DM, Neuwelt EA. Chemotherapy delivery issues in central nervous system malignancy: a reality check. *J. Clin. Oncol.* 2007;25:2295-2305.

[43] Tyson RM, Siegal T, Doolittle ND, Lacy C, Kraemer DF, Neutwelt EA. Current status and future of relapsed primary central nervous system lymphoma (PCNSL). *Leuk. Lymphoma.* 2003;44:627-633.

[44] Kaijser GP, De Kraker J, Bult A, Underberg WJ, Beijnen JH. Pharmacokinetics of ifosfamide and some metabolites in children. *Anticancer Res.* 1998;18(3B):1941-1949.

[45] Relling MV, Mahmoud HH, Pui CH, Sandlund JT, Rivera GK, Ribeiro RC, Crist WM, Evans WE.Etoposide achieves potentially cytotoxic concentrations in CSF of children with acute lymphoblastic leukemia. *J. Clin. Oncol.* 1996;14(2):399-404.

[46] Mappa S, Marturano E, Licata G, Frezzato M, Frungillo N, Ilariucci F, Stelitano C, Ferrari A, Sorarù M, Vianello F, Baldini L, Proserpio I, Foppoli M, Assanelli A, Reni M, Caligaris-Cappio F, Ferreri AJ. Salvage chemoimmunotherapy with rituximab, ifosfamide and etoposide (R-IE regimen) in patients with primary CNS lymphoma relapsed or refractory to high-dose methotrexate-based chemotherapy. *Hematol. Oncol.* 2013;31(3):143-150.

[47] Soussain C, Choquet S, Fourme E, Delgadillo D, Bouabdallah K, Ghesquières H, Damaj G, Dupriez B, Vargaftig J, Gonzalez A, Houillier C, Taillandier L, Hoang-Xuan K, Leblond V. Intensive chemotherapy with thiotepa, busulfan and cyclophosphamide and hematopoietic stem cell rescue in relapsed or refractory primary central nervous system lymphoma and intraocular lymphoma: a retrospective study of 79 cases. *Haematologica.* 2012;97(11):1751-1756.

[48] Soussain C, Hoang-Xuan K, Taillandier L, Fourme E, Choquet S, Witz F, Casasnovas O, Dupriez B, Souleau B, Taksin AL, Gisselbrecht C, Jaccard A, Omuro A, Sanson M, Janvier M, Kolb B, Zini JM, Leblond V; Société Française de Greffe de Moëlle Osseuse-Thérapie Cellulaire. Intensive chemotherapy followed by hematopoietic stem-cell rescue for refractory and recurrent primary CNS and intraocular lymphoma. *J. Clin. Oncol.* 2008;26:2512-2518.

[49] Hoang-Xuan K, Bessell E, Bromberg J, Hottinger AF, Preusser M, Rudà R, Schlegel U, Siegal T, Soussain C, Abacioglu U, Cassoux N, Deckert M, Dirven CM, Ferreri AJ, Graus F, Henriksson R, Herrlinger U, Taphoorn M, Soffietti R, Weller M; European Association for Neuro-Oncology Task Force on Primary CNS Lymphoma.Diagnosis and treatment of primary CNS lymphoma in immunocompetent patients: guidelines from the European Association for Neuro-Oncology. *Lancet Oncol.* 2015;16(7):e322-332.

[50] Heideman RL, Cole DE, Balis F, Sato J, Reaman GH, Packer RJ, Singher LJ, Ettinger LJ, Gillespie A, Sam J, Poplack DG. Phase I and pharmacokinetic evaluation of

thiotepa in the cerebrospinal fluid and plasma of pediatric patients: evidence for dose-dependent plasma clearance of thiotepa. *Cancer Res.* 1989;49:736-741.

[51] Hassan M, Oberg G, Ericson K, Ehrsson H, Eriksson L, Ingvar M, Stone-Elander S, Thorell JO, Smedmyr B, Warne N, Widén L. In vivo distribution of [^{11}C]-busulfan in cynomolgus monkey and in the brain of a human patient. *Cancer Chemother. Pharmacol.* 1992;30:81-85.

[52] Soussain C, Patte C, Ostronoff M, Delmer A, Rigal-Huguet F, Cambier N, Leprisé PY, François S, Cony-Makhoul P, Harousseau JL, Small noncleaved cell lymphoma and leukemia in adults. A retrospective study of 65 adults treated with the LMB pediatric protocols. *Blood.* 1995;85:664-674.

[53] Nguyen PL, Chakravarti A, Finkelstein DM, Hochberg FH, Batchelor TT, Loeffler JS. Results of whole-brain radiation as salvage of methotrexate failure for immunocompetent patients with primary CNS lymphoma. *J. Clin. Oncol.* 2005;23:1507-1513.

[54] Hottinger AF, DeAngelis LM, Yahalom J, Abrey LE. Salvage whole brain radiotherapy for recurrent or refractory primary CNS lymphoma. *Neurology* 2007;69:1178-1182.

[55] Nelson DF, Martz KL, Bonner H, Nelson JS, Newall J, Kerman HD, Thomson JW, Murray KJ. Non-Hodgkin's lymphoma of the brain: can high dose, large volume radiation therapy improve survival? Report on a prospective trial by the Radiation Therapy Oncology Group (RTOG): RTOG 8315. *Int. J. Radiat. Oncol. Biol. Phys.* 1992;23:9-17.

[56] DeAngelis LM, Yahalom J, Thaler HT, and Kher U. Combined modality therapy for primary CNS lymphoma. *J Clin Oncol.* 1992;10: 635-643.

[57] Bessell EM, Graus F, Punt JA, Firth JL, Hope DT, Moloney AJ, Lopez-Guillermo A, Villa S. Primary non-Hodgkin's lymphoma of the CNS treated with BVAM or CHOD/BVAM chemotherapy before radiotherapy. *J. Clin. Oncol.*1996;14:945-954.

[58] Reni M, Ferreri AJ, Garancini MP, Villa E. Therapeutic management of primary central nervous system lymphoma in immunocompetent patients: results of a critical review of the literature. *Ann. Oncol.*1997;8:227-234.

In: Primary Central Nervous System Lymphoma (PCNSL) ISBN: 978-1-63485-322-4
Editor: Ryuya Yamanaka

Chapter 16

MOLECULAR TARGETED THERAPY FOR DLBCL

Keisuke Kawamoto and Jun Takizawa*
Department of Hematology, Endocrinology and Metabolism,
Faculty of Medicine, Niigata University, Niigata, Japan

ABSTRACT

Diffuse large B-cell lymphoma (DLBCL), an aggressive B-cell neoplasm, is the most common type of non-Hodgkin lymphoma affecting patients of all ages. Rituximab therapy combined with cyclophosphamide, vincristine, adriamycin, and prednisolone (R-CHOP) has drastically improved survival rates in these patients; however, about 30–40% of DLBCL patients die from disease progression. Currently, rituximab-based standard therapies are used as first line chemotherapy but patients who require salvage chemotherapy have a poor prognosis for survival. Studies performed on the biologic landscape of DLBCL and its subtypes reveal that a diverse range of oncogenic driver mutations and signaling pathways are essential for growth and survival of lymphoma cells. Since small molecule inhibitors can target these signaling pathways, DLBCL therapies are currently undergoing a paradigm shift away from conventional approaches toward targeted agents to improve the molecular knowledge of DLBCL subtypes. Well-conducted clinical trials will be essential to develop precision medicine and increase the number of DLBCL patients that can be cured. Specifically, ibrutinib (BTK inhibitor), idelalisib (PI3K inhibitor), and venetoclax (BCL-2 inhibitor) are suggested molecular targets for DLBCL treatment. This chapter will review the current therapies used for DLBCL treatment and suggest several drugs that could serve as novel therapeutic approaches for the treatment of this disease.

Keywords: DLBCL, MYC, ibrutinib, idelalisib, venetoclax

---

* *Correspondence to : Jun Takizawa
Email: juntaki@med.niigata-u.ac.jp.

Introduction

Diffuse large B-cell lymphoma (DLBCL) is a heterogeneous form of aggressive B-cell lymphoma and is the most common type of malignant lymphomas, accounting for approximately 30–35% of all non-Hodgkin lymphomas (NHLs) [1-3]. In 2012, it was estimated that approximately 19,000 people in the United States alone died of DLBCL [3].

DLBCL was first treated with anthracycline-based regimens (1970s) [4]. Combining chemotherapy with cyclophosphamide, vincristine, adriamycin, and prednisolone (CHOP) became standard for DLBCL patients since the randomized study performed by Fisher et al., 1993 [5]. Rituximab therapy combined with CHOP (R-CHOP) has drastically improved survival rates of patients from all DLBCL subtypes [6-9]; however, about 30–40% of DLBCL patients do not achieve remission with initial chemotherapy treatment or relapse after achieving remission, eventually dying from disease progression [10].

The most recent breakthrough in treatment for DLBCL patients has been the development of rituximab, a chimeric monoclonal antibody targeted against the CD20 receptor. The first study to show the benefits of rituximab for the treatment of advanced DLBCL was reported by the Groupe d'Etude des Lymphomes de l'Adulte (GELA). They performed a randomized study of CHOP and R-CHOP therapies in DLBCL patients that were 60 years or older [6]. The complete remission (CR) rate (63% versus 76%, $P = 0.005$) and the 2-year event-free survival (EFS) rate (39% versus 57%, $P < 0.001$) were improved with R-CHOP therapy [6]. In addition, R-CHOP therapy improved the 6-year EFS of younger DLBCL patients with good prognostic features, compared to CHOP therapy (74.3% versus 55.8%, $P < 0.001$) [11]. Based on these results, R-CHOP therapy has become the standard treatment for all DLBCL patients.

The standard salvage therapy for relapsed or refractory DLBCL is high dose chemotherapy combined with autologous stem cell transplantation (ASCT). However, the outcome is poor in DLBCL patients with relapses after rituximab-containing first line therapy [12]. Therefore, development of novel therapeutic approaches is essential for these patients, even though the development of a treatment superior to R-CHOP has been limited for over a decade. A randomized study using ASCT as therapy, compared CR and dose-dense strategies, and showed no improvement over R-CHOP [13, 14]. Although another randomized study from GELA showed that rituximab, doxorubicin, cyclophosphamide, vindesine, bleomycin, and prednisone (R-ACVBP) therapy was superior to R-CHOP in low risk DLBCL patients between 18-59 years (3 year EFS, 81% versus 67%, $P = 0.0035$; 3 year overall survival, 92% versus 84%, $P = 0.007$), the toxicity of this therapy limited its clinical use [15]. The dose-adjusted etoposide, doxorubicin, cyclophosphamide, vincristine, predonisone, and rituximab (DA-EPOCH-R) therapy has proved highly effective against a specific molecular subtype of DLBCL [16, 17]. DA-EPOCH-R therapy is currently being compared to R-CHOP therapy in a randomized study [16]. Ultimately, R-CHOP remains the current standard therapy for newly diagnosed DLBCL.

DLBCL is a heterogeneous disease with numerous genetic alterations, although it is characterized by morphologically indistinguishable tumors. In clinical aspects, the international prognostic index (IPI) is the most widely used term for risk stratification [18]. Several studies have performed risk stratification in order to isolate the group of DLBCL patients with poor prognosis. Conversely, in both biological and pathological aspects, gene expression profiling (GEP) of DLBCL has showed significant molecular heterogeneity among morphologically indistinguishable tumors [19]. DLBCL can be divided into three distinct molecular cell-of-origin subtypes: germinal center B (GCB) cell, activated B cell (ABC), and primary mediastinal B cell lymphoma (PMBL) types [19-23].

IPI is the most useful clinical tool to predict DLBCL prognosis; however, it does not reflect the genetic and molecular heterogeneity of the disease. The three cell-of-origin subtypes have distinct mechanisms of oncogenic activation and have different prognoses. For example, most patients with PMBL can be cured with DA-EPOCH-R without mediastinal radiotherapy (3 year PFS: 100%; 3-year OS: 97%) [17]. It was considered that patients with GCB-type DLBCL had a better prognosis than ABC-type DLBCL before the development of rituximab; however, its clinical significance has been controversial when combined with R-CHOP [24, 25]. On the other hand, it was shown that GCB-type patients treated with DA-EPOCH-R therapy had better prognosis than ABC-type (5-year PFS, 100% versus 67%, P = 0.008) [16]. The majority of patients who fail initial therapy are usually of the ABC type; therefore, identifying therapeutic targets for this DLBCL group has a high priority. In addition, *MYC* translocation (*MYC*+), which presents in approximately 10% of all DLBCL patients, has been reported to be a prognostic factor in DLBCL patients treated with R-CHOP therapy [26-30]. Although Burkitt lymphoma also has a *MYC* translocation, *MYC*+DLBCL is genetically distinct from this lymphoma [31]. Retrospective analyses have shown that *MYC*+DLBCL frequently had additional oncogenic translocations involving *BCL2*, *BCL6*, and *CCND1*. These double-hit lymphomas are associated with poor prognosis when treated with R-CHOP therapy [32-34]. However, it is unclear whether *MYC*+ is enough to indicate a poor prognosis, or if other additional genetic aberrations are also necessary. Previous research showed that DA-EPOCH-R might be effective for *MYC*+DLBCL treatment. Furthermore, there is an ongoing prospective study to determine if newly diagnosed *MYC*+DLBCL and Burkitt lymphoma patients can benefit from this therapy [35]. A CORAL study suggested that patients with *MYC*+DLBCL do not benefit from ASCT therapy [36]. Compared to patients without detectable *MYC* translocation, relapsed *MYC*+DLBCL patients had a worse PFS (18% versus 42%, P = 0.0322) and OS (29% versus 62%, P = 0.0113). Furthermore, double-expression of MYC and BCL2 proteins in DLBCL, which is called as double-expressor lymphoma (DEL), has also been suggested to be a prognostic factor. The cut-off expression values for MYC and BCL2 are different throughout studies [37-42]. In addition, it has not been demonstrated whether DLBCL patients with concomitant MYC and BCL2 expression are molecularly distinct groups.

The discovery of new signaling pathways through gene expression profiling (GEP), transcriptome sequencing, RNA interference screens, and DNA sequencing have identified an array of new therapeutic targets in DLBCL in the current era of molecular-based disease definition. Targeting specific oncogene addictions within DLBCL subtypes offers a more precise approach for the development of optimal therapies compared with previously standard chemotherapy-based approaches [43]. We describe the current molecular knowledge of each DLBCL subtype and discuss effective and promising molecular targets to develop therapies for each subtype.

NOVEL TARGETS FOR DLBCL TREATMENT

B-Cell Receptor Signaling Inhibition

The survival of normal B cells requires continuous signaling through the surface B-cell receptor (BCR), which engages downstream growth and survival signaling pathways, such as phosphoinositide 3-kinase (PI3K), protein kinase C β (PKC β), and mammalian target of rapamycin (mTOR). BCR signaling is mediated through a variety of protein kinases including spleen tyrosine kinase (SYK) and Lyn and Bruton's tyrosine kinase (BTK) [44]. Signaling through the BCR pathway can be independent of antigen stimulation because of somatic mutations to key components in the BCR signaling pathway such as CARD11, MYD88, and CD79A/B that engage in the NF-κB pathway. Susceptibility to BCR inhibition is explained by this continuous active BCR signaling, which is called "addicted to BCR signaling".

BTK is activated early in the BCR signaling cascade. Ibrutinib (PCI-32765), a selective tyrosine kinase inhibitor, is a small molecule that covalently and irreversibly binds to BTK and consequently blocks survival, proliferation, and migration of B-cell malignancies [46-48]. In DLBCL, knockdown of BTK, using short hairpin RNAs (shRNAs), was found to be highly toxic to an ABC type DLBCL cell line with wildtype CADR11, but not for one with mutant CARD11 [49].

A phase 1 clinical trial showed that ibrutinib treatment was able to decrease relapsed/refractory B cell malignancies with a 60% overall response rate [50]. Furthermore, a phase 2 clinical study using ibrutinib in 70 patients with relapsed/refractory DLBCL, showed a 40% overall survival rate in the first 25 patients. These patients suffered from ABC type DLBCL and were treated with daily doses of 560 mg of ibrutinib [51]. Only one out of 20 patients with GCB type DLBCL responded to ibrutinib treatment, supporting its selectivity for the ABC type DLBCL. Mutational analysis of pre-treatment and post-treatment biopsies showed that clinical responses were observed in ABC type DLBCL patients with wild type CD79B or mutated CD79B, suggesting that ibrutinib efficacy is not dependent upon a BCR mutation, and that there exists an alternative mechanism for BCR signaling. However, patients with a MYD88 mutation but without a CD79B mutation did not respond to ibrutinib treatment, whereas all patients who had both mutations responded, suggesting an alternative activation mechanism. These results suggest that BTK could be a target for ABC type DLBCL. A randomized phase 3 clinical trial of non-GCB type DLBCL patients has begun.

PI3K/Akt/mTOR Inhibition

The PI3K signaling pathway is associated with numerous cellular processes that are essential for cancer progression, including metabolism, growth, migration, survival, and angiogenesis. This pathway is activated by B-cell malignancies and somatic mutations of downstream effectors [21]. The functional consequences of PTEN inactivation were studied in 248 samples from newly diagnosed DLBCL patients. Loss of PTEN protein expression, assessed by immunohistochemistry (IHC), was presented in 55% of GCB type DLBCL cell lines and in only 14% of non-GCB type DLBCL cell lines. PTEN was inversely correlated to the PI3K/Akt pathway in GCB type DLBCL cell lines, suggesting that constitutive activation of this pathway and oncogenic addition characterized a specific DLBCL subtype [52]. Inhibition of PI3K showed selective toxicity in PTEN deficient GCB type DLBCL cell lines that was not observed in PTEN positive GCB type DLBCL [52]. These results strongly suggest that PTEN negative DLBCL will respond to PI3K/Akt pathway inhibition therapies.

Three classes (Class 1, 2 and 3) of PI3Ks have been investigated; however, Class 1A was the most clinically effective on cancer. Class 1A PI3Ks are activated by growth factors through various receptor tyrosine kinases and PI3K catalytic subunit isoforms. PI3K/Akt/mTOR pathway inhibitors have been used for clinical development [53]. For example, idelalisib (CAL-101) is a potent small-molecule inhibitor of the PI3K isoform, P110δ which blocks the constitutive activation of the PI3K/Akt/mTOR pathway [54]. This drug was used to treat nine DLBCL patients and was well tolerated; however, it did not result in a clinical response [55]. It is currently being studied for DLBCL management and as a treatment for indolent lymphomas. Evelorimus and temsirolimus are mTOR inhibitors that have showed modest activity (25-30%) across a variety of aggressive lymphoma subtypes: DLBCL, follicular lymphoma grade 3, mantle cell lymphoma, and transformed lymphoma. These inhibitors have also been studied to determine their molecular efficacy on different subtypes of lymphoma. Small-molecule inhibitors of Akt have been used in DLBCL cell lines and are currently undergoing early phase clinical trial as single agents for all subtypes of relapsed/refractory DLBCL [56, 57].

BCL2 Inhibition

The apoptosis regulator, BCL2, could represent a therapeutic target in GCB type DLBCL. *BCL2* is deregulated through various mechanisms in the different DLBCL subtypes. *BCL2* rearrangement with t(14;18) is found in 34% of GCB type DLBCL patients, and, furthermore, *BCL2* has been reported to be the most translocated and mutated gene in this subtype of DLBCL [58, 59].

Navitoclax (ABT-263) is a first generation BCL-2 inhibitor that showed clinical significance in chronic lymphocytic leukemia, however, severe hematological toxicity, such as thrombocytopenia, was produced due to co-inhibition of B-cell lymphoma-extra large (Bcl-xL) [56].

Venetoclax (ABT-199) is a second-generation inhibitor of BCL-2 that showed no significant binding to Bcl-xL but resulted in significant clinical effects in a variety of B-cell lymphomas, including DLBCL [57, 60]. In addition, it produced less thrombocytopenia than navitoclax.

Conclusion

DLBCL is a heterogeneous molecular disease with identifiable subtypes that are at high risk for treatment failure using standard immunochemotherapy. Although DLBCL remains treatable in advanced stages, up to 30–40% patients fail to respond to initial therapy, diminishing the effectiveness of salvage options. R-CHOP therapy has been an important breakthrough in the 2000s; however, since we are now able to define DLBCL subtypes with gene-expression profiling and/or mutation analyses, treatment options could include drugs aimed at specific signaling pathways.

Numerous small molecules and pathways inhibitors are now in advanced research stages and show high promise. Therefore, the next major breakthrough in DLBCL treatment is highly expected; however, clinical trials of novel therapies that do not account for the different DLBCL subtypes will not aid to identify an optimal treatment course for this disease. To achieve personalized precision therapy for DLBCL patients, novel targets based on patients with mutational profiles that respond poorly to standard treatment must be developed. Correlative research, such as pre-treatment and post-treatment biopsies, is also essential to understand both sensitivity and resistance to therapy.

REFERENCES

[1] Smith A., Roman E., Howell D., Jones R., Patmore R., Jack A., (2010). The Haematological Malignancy Research Network (HMRN): a new information strategy for population based epidemiology and health service research. *Br. J. Haematol.* 148, 739-753.

[2] Sabattini E., Bacci F., Sagramoso C., Pileri S.A., (2010). WHO classification of tumours of haematopoietic and lymphoid tissues in 2008: an overview. *Pathologica.* 102, 83-87.

[3] Siegel R., Naishadham D., Jemal A., (2013). Cancer statistics, 2013. *C.A. Cancer J. Clin.* 63, 11-30.

[4] DeVita V.T., Jr., Canellos G.P., Chabner B., Schein P., Hubbard S.P., Young R.C., (1975). Advanced diffuse histiocytic lymphoma, a potentially curable disease. *Lancet.* 1, 248-250.

[5] Fisher R.I., Gaynor E.R., Dahlberg S., Oken M.M., Grogan T.M., Mize E.M., Glick J.H., Coltman C.A. Jr, Miller T,P., (1993). Comparison of a standard regimen (CHOP) with three intensive chemotherapy regimens for advanced non-Hodgkin's lymphoma. *N. Engl. J. Med.* 328, 1002-1006.

[6] Coiffier B., Lepage E., Briere J., Herbrecht R., Tilly H., Bouabdallah R., Morel P., Van Den Neste E., Salles G., Gaulard P., Reyes F., Lederlin P., Gisselbrecht C., (2002). CHOP chemotherapy plus rituximab compared with CHOP alone in elderly patients with diffuse large-B-cell lymphoma. *N. Engl. J. Med.* 346, 235-242.

[7] Sehn L.H., Donaldson J., Chhanabhai M., Fitzgerald C., Gill K., Klasa R., MacPherson N., O'Reilly S., Spinelli J.J., Sutherland J., Wilson K.S., Gascoyne R.D., Connors J.M., (2005). Introduction of combined CHOP plus rituximab therapy dramatically improved outcome of diffuse large B-cell lymphoma in British Columbia. *J. Clin. Oncol.* 23, 5027-5033.

[8] Fu K., Weisenburger D.D., Choi W.W., Perry K.D., Smith L.M., Shi X., Hans C.P., Greiner T.C., Bierman P.J., Bociek R.G., Armitage J.O., Chan W.C., Vose J.M., (2008). Addition of rituximab to standard chemotherapy improves the survival of both the germinal center B-cell-like and non-germinal center B-cell-like subtypes of diffuse large B-cell lymphoma. *J. Clin. Oncol.* 26, 4587-4594.

[9] Jacobs S.A., Swerdlow S.H., Kant J., Foon K.A., Jankowitz R., Land S.R., DeMonaco N., Joyce J., Osborn J.L., Evans T.L., Schaefer P.M., Luong T.M., (2008). Phase II trial

of short-course CHOP-R followed by 90Y-ibritumomab tiuxetan and extended rituximab in previously untreated follicular lymphoma. *Clin. Cancer. Res.* 14, 7088-7094.

[10] Campo E., Swerdlow S.H., Harris N.L., Pileri S., Stein H., Jaffe E.S., (2011). The 2008 WHO classification of lymphoid neoplasms and beyond: evolving concepts and practical applications. *Blood.* 117, 5019-5032.

[11] Pfreundschuh M., Kuhnt E., Trumper L., Osterborg A., Trneny M., Shepherd L., Gill D.S., Walewski J., Pettengell R., Jaeger U., Zinzani P.L., Shpilberg O., Kvaloy S., de Nully Brown P., Stahel R., Milpied N., López-Guillermo A., Poeschel V., Grass S., Loeffler M., Murawski N., (2011). CHOP-like chemotherapy with or without rituximab in young patients with good-prognosis diffuse large-B-cell lymphoma: 6-year results of an open-label randomised study of the MabThera International Trial (MInT) Group. *Lancet. Oncol.* 12, 1013-1022.

[12] Gisselbrecht C., Glass B., Mounier N., Singh Gill D., Linch D.C., Trneny M., Bosly A., Ketterer N., Shpilberg O., Hagberg H., Ma D., Brière J., Moskowitz C.H., Schmitz N. (2010). Salvage regimens with autologous transplantation for relapsed large B-cell lymphoma in the rituximab era. *J. Clin. Oncol.* 28, 4184-4190.

[13] Schmitz N., Nickelsen M., Ziepert M., Haenel M., Borchmann P., Schmidt C., Viardot A., Bentz M., Peter N., Ehninger G., Doelken G., Ruebe C., Truemper L., Rosenwald A., Pfreundschuh M., Loeffler M., Glass B.; German High-Grade Lymphoma Study Group (DSHNHL), (2012). Conventional chemotherapy (CHOEP-14) with rituximab or high-dose chemotherapy (MegaCHOEP) with rituximab for young, high-risk patients with aggressive B-cell lymphoma: an open-label, randomised, phase 3 trial (DSHNHL 2002-1). *Lancet. Oncol.* 13, 1250-1259.

[14] Cunningham D., Hawkes E.A., Jack A., Qian W., Smith P., Mouncey P., Pocock C., Ardeshna K.M., Radford J.A., McMillan A., Davies J., Turner D., Kruger A., Johnson P., Gambell J., Linch D., (2013). Rituximab plus cyclophosphamide, doxorubicin, vincristine, and prednisolone in patients with newly diagnosed diffuse large B-cell non-Hodgkin lymphoma: a phase 3 comparison of dose intensification with 14-day versus 21-day cycles. *Lancet* 381, 1817-1826.

[15] Recher C., Coiffier B., Haioun C., Molina T.J., Ferme C., Casasnovas O., Thiéblemont C., Bosly A., Laurent G., Morschhauser F., Ghesquières H., Jardin F., Bologna S., Fruchart C., Corront B., Gabarre J., Bonnet C., Janvier M., Canioni D , Jais J.P., Salles G., Tilly H.; Groupe d'Etude des Lymphomes de l'Adulte, (2011). Intensified chemotherapy with ACVBP plus rituximab versus standard CHOP plus rituximab for the treatment of diffuse large B-cell lymphoma (LNH03-2B): an open-label randomised phase 3 trial. *Lancet* 378, 1858-1867.

[16] Wilson W.H., Jung S.H., Porcu P., Hurd D., Johnson J., Martin S.E., Czuczman M., Lai R., Said J., Chadburn A., Jones D., Dunleavy K., Canellos G., Zelenetz A.D., Cheson B.D., Hsi E.D., (2012). A Cancer and Leukemia Group B multi-center study of DA-EPOCH-rituximab in untreated diffuse large B-cell lymphoma with analysis of outcome by molecular subtype. *Haematologica.* 97, 758-765.

[17] Dunleavy K., Pittaluga S., Maeda L.S., Advani R., Chen C.C., Hessler J., Steinberg S.M., Grant C., Wright G., Varma G., Staudt L.M., Jaffe E.S., Wilson W.H., (2013). Dose-adjusted EPOCH-rituximab therapy in primary mediastinal B-cell lymphoma. *N. Engl. J. Med.* 368, 1408-1416.

[18] The International Non-Hodgkin's Lymphoma Prognostic Factors Project. (1993). A predictive model for aggressive non-Hodgkin's lymphoma. *N. Engl. J. Med.* 329, 987-994.

[19] Alizadeh A.A., Eisen M.B., Davis R.E., Ma C., Lossos I.S., Rosenwald A., Boldrick J.C., Sabet H., Tran T., Yu X., Powell J.I., Yang L., Marti G.E., Moore T., Hudson J. Jr, Lu L., Lewis D.B., Tibshirani R., Sherlock G., Chan W.C., Greiner T.C., Weisenburger D.D., Armitage J.O., Warnke R., Levy R., Wilson W., Grever M.R., Byrd J.C., Botstein D., Brown P.O., Staudt L.M., (2000). Distinct types of diffuse large B-cell lymphoma identified by gene expression profiling. *Nature.* 403, 503-511.

[20] Rosenwald A., Wright G., Chan W.C., Connors J.M., Campo E., Fisher R.I., Gascoyne R.D., Muller-Hermelink H.K., Smeland E.B., Giltnane J.M., Hurt E.M., Zhao H., Averett L., Yang L., Wilson W.H., Jaffe E.S., Simon R., Klausner R.D., Powell J., Duffey P.L., Longo D.L., Greiner T.C., Weisenburger D.D., Sanger W.G., Dave B.J., Lynch J.C., Vose J., Armitage J.O., Montserrat E., López-Guillermo A., Grogan T.M., Miller T.P., LeBlanc M., Ott G., Kvaloy S., Delabie J., Holte H., Krajci P., Stokke T., Staudt L.M.; Lymphoma/Leukemia Molecular Profiling Project (2002). The use of molecular profiling to predict survival after chemotherapy for diffuse large-B-cell lymphoma. *N. Engl. J. Med.* 346, 1937-1947.

[21] Lenz G., Wright G.W., Emre N.C., Kohlhammer H., Dave S.S., Davis R.E., Carty S., Lam L.T., Shaffer A.L., Xiao W., Powell J., Rosenwald A., Ott G., Muller-Hermelink H.K., Gascoyne R.D., Connors J.M., Campo E., Jaffe E.S., Delabie J., Smeland E.B., Rimsza L.M., Fisher R.I., Weisenburger D.D., Chan W.C., Staudt L.M., (2008). Molecular subtypes of diffuse large B-cell lymphoma arise by distinct genetic pathways. *Proc. Natl. Acad. Sci. U S A.* 105, 13520-13525.

[22] Wright G., Tan B., Rosenwald A., Hurt E.H., Wiestner A., Staudt L.M., (2003). A gene expression-based method to diagnose clinically distinct subgroups of diffuse large B cell lymphoma. *Proc. Natl. Acad. Sci. U. S. A.* 100, 9991-9996.

[23] Rosenwald A., Wright G., Leroy K., Yu X., Gaulard P., Gascoyne R.D., Chan W.C., Zhao T., Haioun C., Greiner T.C., Weisenburger D.D., Lynch J.C., Vose J., Armitage J.O., Smeland E.B., Kvaloy S., Holte H., Delabie J., Campo E., Montserrat E., Lopez-Guillermo A., Ott G., Muller-Hermelink H.K., Connors J.M., Braziel R., Grogan T.M., Fisher R.I., Miller T.P., LeBlanc M., Chiorazzi M., Zhao H., Yang L., Powell J., Wilson W.H., Jaffe E.S., Simon R., Klausner R.D., Staudt L.M. (2003) Molecular diagnosis of primary mediastinal B cell lymphoma identifies a clinically favorable subgroup of diffuse large B cell lymphoma related to Hodgkin lymphoma. *J Exp Med.* 198, 851-862.

[24] Lenz G., Wright G., Dave S.S., Xiao W., Powell J., Zhao H., Xu W., Tan B., Goldschmidt N., Iqbal J., Vose J., Bast M., Fu K., Weisenburger D.D., Greiner T.C., Armitage J.O., Kyle A., May L., Gascoyne R.D., Connors J.M., Troen G., Holte H., Kvaloy S., Dierickx D., Verhoef G., Delabie J., Smeland E.B., Jares P., Martinez A., Lopez-Guillermo A., Montserrat E., Campo E., Braziel R.M., Miller T.P., Rimsza L.M., Cook J.R., Pohlman B., Sweetenham J., Tubbs R.R., Fisher R.I., Hartmann E., Rosenwald A., Ott G., Muller-Hermelink H.K., Wrench D., Lister T.A., Jaffe E.S., Wilson W.H., Chan W.C., Staudt L.M.; Lymphoma/Leukemia Molecular Profiling Project 2008. Stromal gene signatures in large-B-cell lymphomas. *N. Engl. J. Med.* 359, 2313-2323.

[25] Nyman H., Adde M., Karjalainen-Lindsberg M.L., Taskinen M., Berglund M., Amini R.M., Blomqvist C., Enblad G., Leppä S., (2007). Prognostic impact of immunohistochemically defined germinal center phenotype in diffuse large B-cell lymphoma patients treated with immunochemotherapy. *Blood.* 109, 4930-4935.

[26] Barrans S., Crouch S., Smith A., Turner K., Owen R., Patmore R., Roman E/, Jack A., (2010). Rearrangement of MYC is associated with poor prognosis in patients with diffuse large B-cell lymphoma treated in the era of rituximab. *J. Clin. Oncol.* 28, 3360-3365.

[27] Klapper W., Stoecklein H., Zeynalova S., Ott G., Kosari F., Rosenwald A., Loeffler M., Trümper L., Pfreundschuh M., Siebert R., (2008). Structural aberrations affecting the MYC locus indicate a poor prognosis independent of clinical risk factors in diffuse large B-cell lymphomas treated within randomized trials of the German High-Grade Non-Hodgkin's Lymphoma Study Group (DSHNHL). *Leukemia.* 22, 2226-2229.

[28] Kojima M., Nishikii H., Takizawa J., Aoki S., Noguchi M., Chiba S., Chiba S., Ando K., Nakamura N., (2013). MYC rearrangements are useful for predicting outcomes following rituximab and chemotherapy: multicenter analysis of Japanese patients with diffuse large B-cell lymphoma. *Leuk. Lymphoma.* 54, 2149-2154.

[29] Yoon S.O., Jeon Y.K., Paik J.H., Kim W.Y., Kim Y.A., Kim J.E., Kim C.W., (2008). MYC translocation and an increased copy number predict poor prognosis in adult diffuse large B-cell lymphoma (DLBCL), especially in germinal centre-like B cell (GCB) type. *Histopathology.* 53, 205-217.

[30] Savage K.J., Johnson N.A., Ben-Neriah S., Connors J.M., Sehn L.H., Farinha P., Horsman D.E., Gascoyne R.D., (2009). MYC gene rearrangements are associated with a poor prognosis in diffuse large B-cell lymphoma patients treated with R-CHOP chemotherapy. *Blood.* 114, 3533-3537.

[31] Jaffe E.S., Pittaluga S., (2011). Aggressive B-cell lymphomas: a review of new and old entities in the WHO classification. *Hematology Am. Soc. Hematol. Educ. Program.* 2011, 506-514.

[32] Johnson N.A., Savage K.J., Ludkovski O., Ben-Neriah S., Woods R., Steidl C., Dyer M.J., Siebert R., Kuruvilla J., Klasa R., Connors J.M., Gascoyne R.D., Horsman D.E., (2009). Lymphomas with concurrent BCL2 and MYC translocations: the critical factors associated with survival. *Blood.* 114, 2273-2279.

[33] Aukema S.M., Siebert R., Schuuring E., van Imhoff G.W., Kluin-Nelemans H.C., Boerma E.J., Kluin P.M., (2011). Double-hit B-cell lymphomas. *Blood.* 117, 2319-2331.

[34] Snuderl M., Kolman O.K., Chen Y.B., Hsu J.J., Ackerman A.M., Dal Cin P., Ferry J.A., Harris N.L., Hasserjian R.P., Zukerberg L.R., Abramson J.S., Hochberg E.P., Lee H., Lee A.I., Toomey C.E., Sohani A.R., (2010). B-cell lymphomas with concurrent IGH-BCL2 and MYC rearrangements are aggressive neoplasms with clinical and pathologic features distinct from Burkitt lymphoma and diffuse large B-cell lymphoma. *Am. J. Surg, Pathol.* 34, 327-340.

[35] Dunleavy K., (2015). Aggressive B cell Lymphoma: Optimal Therapy for MYC-positive, Double-Hit, and Triple-Hit DLBCL. *Curr. Treat. Options. Oncol.* 16, 58.

[36] Cuccuini W., Briere J., Mounier N., Voelker H.U., Rosenwald A., Sundstrom C., Cogliatti S., Hirchaud E., Ysebaert L., Bron D., Soulier J., Gaulard P., Houlgatte R., Gisselbrecht C., Thieblemont C., (2012). MYC+ diffuse large B-cell lymphoma is not

salvaged by classical R-ICE or R-DHAP followed by BEAM plus autologous stem cell transplantation. *Blood.* 119, 4619-4624.

[37] Green T.M., Young K.H., Visco C., Xu-Monette Z.Y., Orazi A., Go R.S., Nielsen O., Gadeberg O.V., Mourits-Andersen T., Frederiksen M., Pedersen L.M., Møller M.B., (2012). Immunohistochemical double-hit score is a strong predictor of outcome in patients with diffuse large B-cell lymphoma treated with rituximab plus cyclophosphamide, doxorubicin, vincristine, and prednisone. *J. Clin. Oncol.* 30, 3460-3467.

[38] Hu S., Xu-Monette Z.Y., Tzankov A., Green T., Wu L., Balasubramanyam A., Liu W.M., Visco C., Li Y., Miranda R.N., Montes-Moreno S., Dybkaer K., Chiu A., Orazi A., Zu Y., Bhagat G., Richards K.L., Hsi E.D., Choi W.W., Zhao X., van Krieken J.H., Huang Q., Huh J., Ai W., Ponzoni M., Ferreri A.J., Zhou F., Slack G.W., Gascoyne R.D., Tu M., Variakojis D., Chen W., Go R.S., Piris M.A., Møller M.B., Medeiros L.J., Young K.H., (2013). MYC/BCL2 protein coexpression contributes to the inferior survival of activated B-cell subtype of diffuse large B-cell lymphoma and demonstrates high-risk gene expression signatures: a report from The International DLBCL Rituximab-CHOP Consortium Program. *Blood.* 121, 4021-4031.

[39] Johnson N.A., Slack G.W., Savage K.J., Connors J.M., Ben-Neriah S., Rogic S., Scott D.W., Tan K.L., Steidl C., Sehn L.H., Chan W.C., Iqbal J., Meyer P.N., Lenz G., Wright G., Rimsza L.M., Valentino C., Brunhoeber P., Grogan T.M., Braziel R.M., Cook J.R., Tubbs R.R., Weisenburger D..D., Campo E., Rosenwald A., Ott G., Delabie J., Holcroft C., Jaffe E.S., Staudt L.M., Gascoyne R.D., (2012). Concurrent expression of MYC and BCL2 in diffuse large B-cell lymphoma treated with rituximab plus cyclophosphamide, doxorubicin, vincristine, and prednisone. *J. Clin. Oncol.* 30, 3452-3459.

[40] Perry A.M., Alvarado-Bernal Y., Laurini J.A., Smith L.M., Slack G.W., Tan K.L., Sehn L.H., Fu K., Aoun P., Greiner T.C., Chan W.C., Bierman P.J., Bociek R.G., Armitage J.O., Vose J.M., Gascoyne R.D., Weisenburger D.D., (2014). MYC and BCL2 protein expression predicts survival in patients with diffuse large B-cell lymphoma treated with rituximab. *Br. J. Haematol.* 165, 382-391.

[41] Dunleavy K., Grant C., Wilson W.H., (2013). Using biologic predictive factors to direct therapy of diffuse large B-cell lymphoma. *Ther. Adv. Hematol.* 4, 43-57.

[42] Horn H., Ziepert M., Becher C., Barth T.F., Bernd H.W., Feller A.C., Klapper W., Hummel M., Stein H., Hansmann M.L., Schmelter C., Möller P., Cogliatti S., Pfreundschuh M., Schmitz N., Trümper L., Siebert R., Loeffler M., Rosenwald A., Ott G.; German High-Grade Non-Hodgkin Lymphoma Study Group., (2013)., MYC status in concert with BCL2 and BCL6 expression predicts outcome in diffuse large B-cell lymphoma. *Blood.* 121, 2253-2263.

[43] Steinhardt J.J., Gartenhaus R.B., (2012). Promising personalized therapeutic options for diffuse large B-cell Lymphoma Subtypes with oncogene addictions. *Clin. Cancer. Res.* 18, 4538-4548.

[44] Gauld S.B., Dal Porto J.M., Cambier J.C., (2002). B cell antigen receptor signaling: roles in cell development and disease. *Science* 296, 1641-1642.

[45] Weniger M.A., Wiestner A., (2011). Molecular targeted approaches in mantle cell lymphoma. *Semin. Hematol.* 48, 214-226.

[46] Young R.M., Shaffer A.L. 3rd, Phelan J.D., Staudt L.M., (2015). B-cell receptor signaling in diffuse large B-cell lymphoma. *Semin. Hematol.* 52, 77-85.

[47] Zhou M., Wang J., Ouyang J., Xu J.Y., Chen B., Zhang Q.G., Zhou R.F., Yang Y.G., Shao X.Y., Xu Y., Chen Y.M., Fan X.S., Wu H.Y., (2014). MYC protein expression is associated with poor prognosis in diffuse large B cell lymphoma patients treated with RCHOP chemotherapy. *Tumour Biol.* 35, 6757-6762.

[48] Honigberg L.A., Smith A.M., Sirisawad M., Verner E., Loury D., Chang B., Li S., Pan Z., Thamm D.H., Miller R.A., Buggy J.J., (2010). The Bruton tyrosine kinase inhibitor PCI-32765 blocks B-cell activation and is efficacious in models of autoimmune disease and B-cell malignancy. *Proc. Natl. Acad. Sci. U S A.* 107, 13075-13080.

[49] Davis R.E., Ngo V.N., Lenz G., Tolar P., Young R.M., Romesser P.B., Kohlhammer H., Lamy L., Zhao H., Yang Y., Xu W., Shaffer A.L., Wright G., Xiao W., Powell J., Jiang J.K., Thomas C.J., Rosenwald A., Ott G., Muller-Hermelink H.K., Gascoyne R.D., Connors J.M., Johnson N.A., Rimsza L.M., Campo E., Jaffe E.S., Wilson W.H., Delabie J., Smeland E.B., Fisher R.I., Braziel R.M., Tubbs R.R., Cook J.R., Weisenburger D.D., Chan W.C., Pierce S.K., Staudt L.M., (2010). Chronic active B-cell-receptor signalling in diffuse large B-cell lymphoma. *Nature* 463, 88-92.

[50] Kenkre V.P., Kahl B.S., (2012). The future of B-cell lymphoma therapy: the B-cell receptor and its downstream pathways. *Curr. Hematol. Malig. Rep.* 7, 216-220.

[51] Chang B.Y., Francesco M., De Rooij M.F., Magadala P., Steggerda S.M., Huang M.M., Kuil A., Herman S.E., Chang S., Pals S.T., Wilson W., Wiestner A. Spaargaren M., Buggy J.J., Elias L., (2013). Egress of CD19(+)CD5(+) cells into peripheral blood following treatment with the Bruton tyrosine kinase inhibitor ibrutinib in mantle cell lymphoma patients. *Blood.* 122, 2412-2424.

[52] Pfeifer M., Grau M., Lenze D., Wenzel S.S., Wolf A., Wollert-Wulf B., Dietze K., Nogai H., Storek B., Madle H., Dörken B., Janz M., Dirnhofer S., Lenz P., Hummel M., Tzankov A., Lenz G., (2013). PTEN loss defines a PI3K/AKT pathway-dependent germinal center subtype of diffuse large B-cell lymphoma. *Proc. Natl. Acad. Sci. U S A.* 110, 12420-12425.

[53] Rodon J., Dienstmann R., Serra V., Tabernero J., (2013). Development of PI3K inhibitors: lessons learned from early clinical trials. *Nat. Rev. Clin. Oncol.* 10, 143-153.

[54] Lannutti B.J., Meadows S.A., Herman S.E., Kashishian A., Steiner B., Johnson A.J., Byrd J.C., Tyner J.W., Loriaux M.M., Deininger M., Druker B.J., Puri K.D., Ulrich R.G., Giese N.A., (2011). CAL-101, a p110delta selective phosphatidylinositol-3-kinase inhibitor for the treatment of B-cell malignancies, inhibits PI3K signaling and cellular viability. *Blood.* 117, 591-594.

[55] Castillo J.J., Furman M., Winer E.S., (2012). CAL-101: a phosphatidylinositol-3-kinase p110-delta inhibitor for the treatment of lymphoid malignancies. *Expert. Opin. Investig. Drugs.* 21, 15-22.

[56] Wilson W.H., O'Connor O.A., Czuczman M.S., LaCasce A.S., Gerecitano J.F., Leonard J.P., Tulpule A., Dunleavy K., Xiong H., Chiu Y.L., Cui Y., Busman T., Elmore S.W., Rosenberg S.H., Krivoshik A.P., Enschede S.H., Humerickhouse R.A., (2010). Navitoclax, a targeted high-affinity inhibitor of BCL-2, in lymphoid malignancies: a phase 1 dose-escalation study of safety, pharmacokinetics, pharmacodynamics, and antitumour activity. *Lancet Oncol.* 11, 1149-1159.

[57] Souers A.J., Leverson J.D., Boghaert E.R., Ackler S.L., Catron N.D. Chen J., Dayton B.D., Ding H., Enschede S.H., Fairbrother W.J., Huang D.C., Hymowitz S.G., Jin S., Khaw S.L., Kovar P.J., Lam L.T., Lee J., Maecker H.L., Marsh K.C., Mason K.D.,

Mitten M.J., Nimmer P.M., Oleksijew A., Park C.H., Park C.M., Phillips D.C., Roberts A.W., Sampath D., Seymour J.F., Smith M.L., Sullivan G.M., Tahir S.K., Tse C., Wendt M.D., Xiao Y., Xue J.C., Zhang H., Humerickhouse R.A., Rosenberg S.H., Elmore S.W., (2013). ABT-199, a potent and selective BCL-2 inhibitor, achieves antitumor activity while sparing platelets. *Nat. Med.* 19, 202-208.

[58] Schuetz J.M., Johnson N.A., Morin R.D., Scott D.W., Tan K., Ben-Nierah S., Boyle M., Slack G.W., Marra M.A., Connors J.M., Brooks-Wilson A.R., Gascoyne R.D., (2012)., BCL2 mutations in diffuse large B-cell lymphoma. *Leukemia.* 26, 1383-1390.

[59] Iqbal J., Sanger W.G., Horsman D.E., Rosenwald A., Pickering D.L., Dave B., Dave S., Xiao L., Cao K., Zhu Q., Sherman S., Hans C.P., Weisenburger D.D., Greiner T.C., Gascoyne R.D., Ott G., Müller-Hermelink H.K., Delabie J., Braziel R.M., Jaffe E.S., Campo E., Lynch J.C., Connors J.M., Vose J.M., Armitage J.O., Grogan T.M., Staudt L.M., Chan W.C., (2004). BCL2 translocation defines a unique tumor subset within the germinal center B-cell-like diffuse large B-cell lymphoma. *Am.J. Pathol.* 165, 159-166.

[60] Davids M.S., Letai A., (2013). ABT-199: taking dead aim at BCL-2. *Cancer Cell.* 23, 139-141.

IV. SPECIFIC SUBTYPE

In: Primary Central Nervous System Lymphoma (PCNSL) ISBN: 978-1-63485-322-4
Editor: Ryuya Yamanaka

Chapter 17

Intraocular Lymphoma (Vitreoretinal Lymphoma)

Tokuhide Oyama*, MD, PhD
Division of Ophthalmology and Visual Sciences,
Graduate School of Medical and Dental Sciences,
Niigata University, Niigata, Japan

Abstract

Primary intraocular lymphoma (PIOL) is an ocular malignancy that is a subset of primary central nervous system lymphoma. Secondary intraocular lymphoma is an ocular involvement of systemic lymphoma. The majority of PIOL is diffuse large B-cell lymphoma as well as primary central nervous system lymphoma. PIOL can masquerade as uveitis, white dot syndromes, or occasionally as other neoplasms such as metastatic cancers. Use of several tests such as cytokine concentration measurements in the aqueous or vitreous humor, immuno-histopathological examinations, vitreoretinal biopsy and ocular coherence tomography improve the diagnostic yield. Although several systemic chemotherapies and radiotherapy have been performed, use of intravitreal chemotherapy recently tried, prognosis remains poor. The optimal treatment approach for PIOL remains controversial and, as a result, there is currently no established treatment.

Keywords: intraocular lymphoma, vitreoretinal lymphoma, radiotherapy, intravitreal chemotherapy, systemic chemotherapy

* Corresponding Author address: Tokuhide Oyama, M.D., Ph.D, Division of Ophthalmology, Niigata University Graduate School Medical and Dental Sciences, Ashahimachi-dori, Niigata 951-8510, Japan, Phone: +81-25-227-2296; Fax: +81-25-227-0785, Email: manjyu@med.niigata-u.ac.jp (T. Oyama).

INTRODUCTION

Terminology

Although a few cases of intraocular "reticulum cell sarcoma" were reported in the 1950s and early 1960s [1, 2], these handful of cases did not demonstrate lymphoma cells in the retina, vitreous, optic nerve, and/or central nervous system (CNS). In the late 1970s and early 1980s the term "reticulum cell sarcoma" became a misnomer as researchers demonstrated the origin of the tumor cells to be transformed lymphoid cells(malignant B-and T-cell), not histiocytes [3]. The "reticulum cell sarcoma in the eye" was changed to "primary intraocular lymphoma" or "tumor that involves both the globe and the CNS [4]. Several researchers have recommend the term "primary intraocular lymphomas" should represent lymphomas originating from all ocular tissues, and since lymphomas originating from the retina-vitreous, choroid are distinctive, "primary vitreoretinal lymphoma" should be proposed and used [5, 6]. The term intraocular lymphoma is used as the standard term throughout this chapter.

Intraocular lymphoma is broadly divided into primary and secondary types. Primary intraocular lymphoma (PIOL) was originally defined as a subset of primary central nervous system lymphoma (PCNSL) that presents exclusively as lymphoma affecting ocular tissues without systemic nodal or extranodal malignant lymphoma lesions or as lesions within the cranium or cerebrospinal fluid [7, 8]. In the majority of cases of PIOL, lesions are observed within the vitreous humor and retina. This condition is also commonly referred to as primary vitreoretinal lymphoma.

Secondary intraocular lymphoma is characterized by ocular migration of lymphoma cells from systemic nodal or extranodal malignant lesions not involving the central nervous system. Intraocular lesions generally affect the uvea or choroid and often manifest as malignant lymphoma of the testes [9] or systemic T-cell lymphoma; [10] however, these conditions are rare. Systemic T-cell lymphomas and lymphomas of the testes with intraocular involvement share many clinical features typical of B-cell PIOL.

PCNSL is a rare disease that comprises 1–2% of non-Hodgkin's lymphoma and less than 5% of intracranial tumors. PIOL is observed in fewer than 1% of primary intraocular malignant tumors [2, 11]. However, in recent years, the incidence of PCNSL and PIOL has increased in developed countries, such as the United States, the EU, and regions of Asia, with the US experiencing an increased incidence of approximately three-fold during the first decade of the 21st century [14]. In the US, approximately 300–380 new cases of PIOL are reported each year [15]. Large-scale studies have demonstrated that PCNSL accounts for 4–6% of primary brain tumors and that 15–25% of PCNSL patients have intraocular lymphoma. These studies further demonstrated that approximately 60–90% of PIOL patients develop lymphoma cell invasion in the CNS several years after the initial presentation of PIOL, with both eyes affected in approximately 80% of cases [4, 7, 8, 13-18].

A variety of explanations have been offered for the increasing incidence of these diseases; however, worldwide trends toward aging populations, improvements in diagnostic technologies, and increased awareness of these disease among physicians and medical professional may all have contributed to an increase in the number of cases diagnosed. This change may also be partly attributable to increases in the number of patients with iatrogenic immunosuppression [6, 8, 12-24].

Pathogenesis

The World Health Organization Classification of Tumors of the Central Nervous System, 4th edition, emphasizes an approach whereby clinical features are correlated with the distinct morphology, immunophenotype, and genotype of specific neoplasm types. Accordingly, PIOL is categorized as a subset of primary diffuse large B-cell lymphomas (DLBCL) of the CNS [25, 26].

Many of the mechanisms underlying the pathogenesis of PCNSL and PIOL, which is the subset of PCNSL remain unknown, although a range of hypotheses have been posited. Infection by a variety of pathogens has been suggested to play a role in the pathogenesis of many human malignancies. For example, human herpes-8 virus infection has been associated with the development of Kaposi's sarcoma and other malignancies, the human papilloma virus with uterocervical cancer and cervical neck cancer, the human T-lymphotropic virus-1 with adult T-cell lymphoma, and Helicobacter pylori and Chlamydia trachomatis with mucosa-associated lymphoid tissue (MALT) lymphoma [27-29].

On the other hand, although it has been suggested that the Epstein–Barr (EB) virus is involved in the development of PCNSL, with a significantly higher morbidity rate related to PCNSL observed in immunocompromised patients compared to patients with normal immune systems, this observation is thought to be largely attributable to latent infection EB virus in B-cells. This hypothesis was partially suggested in response to the observation that most patients with acquired immune deficiency syndrome (AIDS) who develop PCNSL are found to be infected with EB virus, and that these patients have a particularly poor prognosis due to the aggressive nature of PCNSL. However, the low rate of EB virus infection in cases of PIOL argues against this hypothesis [7, 30-33]. Interestingly, human herpes-8 virus and Toxoplasma gondii have been posited as involved in the pathogenesis of PIOL in immunocompetent individuals [30, 34].

The observation that malignant lymphomas arise in structures related to the CNS, such as the brain and eyes, in which immunological lymphatic tissues are not present has yet to be convincingly explained. Based on reports that the lymphoma cells isolated from PCNSL patients have the same DNA rearrangement clonality as corresponding cells isolated from the blood and bone marrow has led to the hypothesis that lymphoma cells migrate hematogenously from systemic nodal and extranodal sites to eyes and the CNS, where no lymphoid tissue is normally present [35].

The potential involvement of chemokines has also been reported. Chemokines represent important molecules that function in cell recruitment to a variety of tissues in the body. PIOL cells have been shown to express the B-cell chemokine receptors CXCR4 and CXCR5 with their corresponding ligands CXCL12 and CXCL13 shown to be expressed by retinal pigment epithelium (RPE) cells adjacent to PIOL cells rather than by PIOL cells that have directly invaded the RPE cells. The expression of these molecules may facilitate lymphocyte migration from the choroid to the RPE [36, 45].

Immunophenotype and Molecular Biology

Normally, malignant lymphoma cells are observed as large, discohesive, pleomorphic cells with a large nucleocytoplasmic ratio and a clear nucleolus. Their size is typically 2–5-

fold that of small lymphocytes, with a nuclear morphology that ranges from circular to elliptical and is often folded. Sometimes, these cells are shaped like clover leaves. However, only a small amount of samples of PIOL can be taken by pars plana vitrectomy and vitreous aspiration, and reactive lymphocytes, histiocytes, and necrotic debris are present on glass slides of those samples. Therefore, an accurate diagnosis based solely on histochemical analyses using Wright–Giemsa and Papanicolaou stains is usually challenging (Figure 1), with diagnostic coverage varying from 9.9% to 83% [13, 37-41].

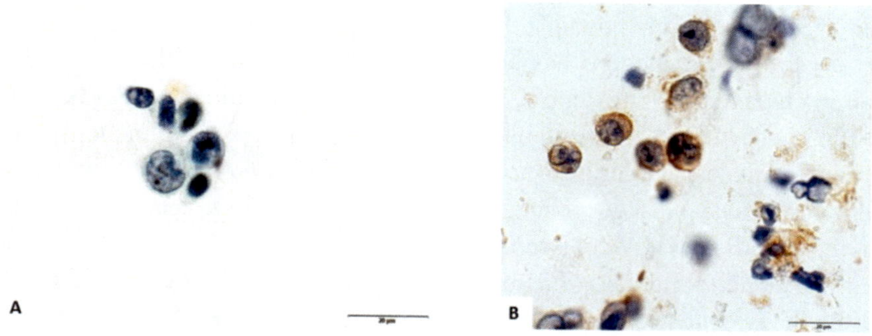

Figure 1. This photomicrograph showing several cells collected via diagnostic pars plana vitrectomy (PIOL, B-cell type). A) Large cells approximately 3 times the size of small lymphocytes with a high nuclear-cytoplasmic ratio and 2 or 3 of large nucleolus. Nuclei are variously elliptical to horseshoe-shaped and folded (Papanicolaou staining). B) Malignant lymphoma cells with membranous CD20 expression are shown to be CD20 antigen-positive (3,3′-Diaminobenzidine, tetrahydrochloride staining).

Studies evaluating the immunophenotype of malignant PIOL lymphoma cells have demonstrated that 98% of PCNSL/PIOL are derived from B-cell lineages that express CD20 and 2% are derived from T-cell lineages [13, 37-41]. Flow cytometry and immunohistochemical studies have demonstrated that PIOL lymphoma cells express CD10, 19, 20, 22, 79a, the 5′ -untranslated region of B-cell lymphoma 6 (BCL-6), interferon regulatory factor 4 (IRF4 or MUM1), and PAX-5 to varying degrees. Further, light chain (κ , λ) restriction of immunoglobulin heavy chain (IgH) genes has demonstrated utility in contributing to the diagnosis of PIOL [42, 44-46]. Light chain restriction of IgH allows evaluation of monoclonal B-cell populations, with high κ/λ ratios of 3–0.6 indicating the presence of malignant lymphoma cells.[45].

The rearrangement of immunoglobulin genes allows B-cells to produce a varied antigen repertoire during the differentiated mature stage. It is possible to investigate B-cell clonality by utilizing this diversity.

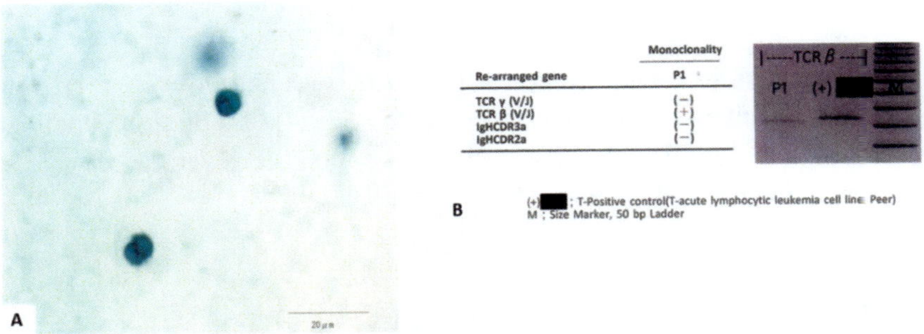

Figure 2. This photomicrograph showing several cells collected via diagnostic pars plana vitrectomy (PIOL, T-cell type). A) Medium-sized cells with large nuclear-cytoplasmic ratios and lobe-shaped nuclei. B) Polymerase chain reaction amplification products demonstrating monoclonal rearrangement of the T-cell receptor (TCR) β gene (P1).

Rearrangement begins with the selection of a fragment from the DH and JH gene clusters among the many VH, DH, and JH gene clusters in the variable region of IgH genes. Next, one fragment from a VH gene cluster and the combined DH-JH gene are rearranged. An exceedingly wide variety of antigens are produced via VH gene rearrangement during somatic mutation in response to antigenic stimulation. In the early 1990s, polymerase chain reaction (PCR) was used to investigate whether B-cell IgH gene rearrangement followed a single pattern or not; this resulted in its use in diagnosing B-cell lymphoma, a type of neoplastic proliferation. PCR allows testing of small samples and is currently used in microdissection, as well as multiplex PCR and other tests that utilize a variety of primers [46]. Studies of systemic non-Hodgkin lymphomas have identified the third complementarity-determining region (CDR3) as the IgH gene rearrangement region where variable region rearrangement takes place. Primers such as FR2, FR3, and CDR3 are commonly used to determine B-cell monoclonality [46]. As T-cells become able to recognize various antigens during the process of differentiation in the same manner as B-cells, T-cell receptors (TCRs) are commonly observed to have undergone rearrangement (e.g., TCR-β, γ gene) in rare cases of T-cell PIOL. This allows PCR to be used for investigation [10, 47, 48] (Figure 2).

Gene expression profiling (GEP) has continued to be developed for the investigation of molecular abnormalities, such as systemic DLBCL. DNA array analysis allows the classification of DLBCL into germinal center B-cell-like (GCB) type and activated B-cell-like (ABC) types. Subsequently, a category known as "unclassified" was added. Studies have evaluated the prognosis and treatments of GCB cases versus non-GCB cases (comprised of ABC cases and unclassified cases); they demonstrated that GCB cases have a relatively good prognosis, whereas non-GCB cases have a poor prognosis. [49] CD10, BCL-6, and MUM1 immunohistochemistry reportedly allows the simple determination of GCB or non-GCB without the use of GEP. PIOL typically has a IRF4/MUM1+, BCL6+/− and CD10+ immunophenotype and also shows similar phenotype to DLBCL in non-GCB cases [50]. However, a recent study [51] reported the presence of a unique BCL2+ BCL-6+ BCL-10+ immunophenotype, indicating cases in the GCB group may also resemble DLBCL.

Age

The peak age of PIOL incidence ranges from 50 to 70 years; however, very rarely, cases have been reported in children and adolescents [45, 52-54]. Studies of small groups of patients have reported that PIOL is more common in women; however, large scale studies of PIOL have observed no gender difference [15, 55-58].

Ocular Manifestations and Clinical Symptoms

The classical symptoms of PIOL are visual distortions, including blurred vision and floaters, and painless reduced visual acuity (observed in 80–90% of cases). However, there have been cases without loss of visual acuity. These symptoms are thought to be predominantly because of vitreous clouding—the most commonly observed finding in PIOL (70%–90% of cases)[7, 52, 56, 67]. Thus, patients often present with loss of visual acuity; however, a few patients whose vitreous clouding exists out of the collimation axis complain of reductions in visual acuity, which is an important distinguishing factor from uveitis [59, 63]. Conjunctival or ciliary hyperemia, photopsia, and palpebral sebum are very rarely reported in PIOL cases, unlike in uveitis cases. [45, 58] PIOL presents characteristically with clinical findings that mimic uveitis except for these findings [6-9, 15-17, 43, 45, 57, 58]. In recent years, as the incidence of PCNSL and PIOL has increased in many countries, the ratio of PIOL to all uveitis cases is increasing annually [15, 60, 61]. PIOL patients do not have systemic symptoms such as cachexia or lymphadenopathy. PCNSL and PIOL patients present with similar systemic symptoms, and B symptoms that are often observed in non-Hodgkin lymphoma, such as weight loss, fever, and perspiration, are almost never observed [61]. A retrospective study conducted in Europe reported an incidence of B symptoms in cases of PCNSL at approximately 7% [62].

The classic presentation of PIOL is advanced age and steroid-resistant chronic uveitis. However, initial steroid administration may occasionally result in improvements in clinical findings in cases of PIOL. The efficacy of steroid therapy may then gradually reduce, with cell invasion into the anterior chamber and vitreous clouding recurring in the majority of cases [45, 63-65]. Although it is not possible to make a definitive clinical diagnosis of PIOL based solely on the presence of intraocular inflammation refractory to steroid therapy, PIOL should be considered as a differential diagnosis in cases of heavy vitreous clouding with intraretinal and subretinal yellow-white lesions [8, 45, 66-72].

PIOL progresses relatively gradually, with diagnosis often delayed due to a similar clinical presentation to uveitis. Previous reports indicate an average delay of 12 and 24 months between the appearance of ophthalmological symptoms and definitive diagnosis; however, this has recently reduced to 6–12 months [52, 57, 69-72]. Factors contributing to reducing the time to diagnosis include the following: increased awareness of PIOL among neurosurgeons, hematologists, and ophthalmologists and the improved ease and speed of tests and diagnostic tools such as vitreoretinal biopsy, immunohistological tests, flow cytometry, and PCR [45-47, 56-57, 59, 63-64, 68-73].

OCULAR EXAMINATIONS AND DIAGNOSIS

When examining middle-aged and elderly patients with uveitis, ophthalmologists must routinely perform the following tests to accurately diagnose PIOL [45, 55-57, 59, 63-66, 68-72]. Based on clinical progression of patients, the cause of the uveitis should be carefully investigated using slit lamp microscopy, funduscopy, ultrasonography, fluorescein angiography of the fundus, and serological testing, including for the presence of antibodies (e.g., Toxoplasma, Histoplasma, cat scratch titers, tuberculin skin tests, angiotensin converting enzyme, and HLA-typing) [67].

The following differential diagnoses are particularly important to consider when PIOL is suspected: varicella zoster virus (VZV) or herpes simplex virus causing acute retinal necrosis [74], or cytomegalovirus (CMV) retinitis due to CMV [70, 75], viral infectious uveitis such as chorioretinitis due to Toxoplasma gondii infection [76]. Bacterial diseases such as Treponema pallidum [77]. Leading to syphilis and Bartonella henselae [78] causing cat scratch disease as well as birdshot choroidopathy, which is non-infectious uveitis, causing bilateral posterior uveitis need to be considered [56]. Sarcoidosis, [79, 80] Bechet disease [81], and Vogt–Koyanagi–Harada disease [82] are also mentioned as systemic ocular inflammatory diseases.

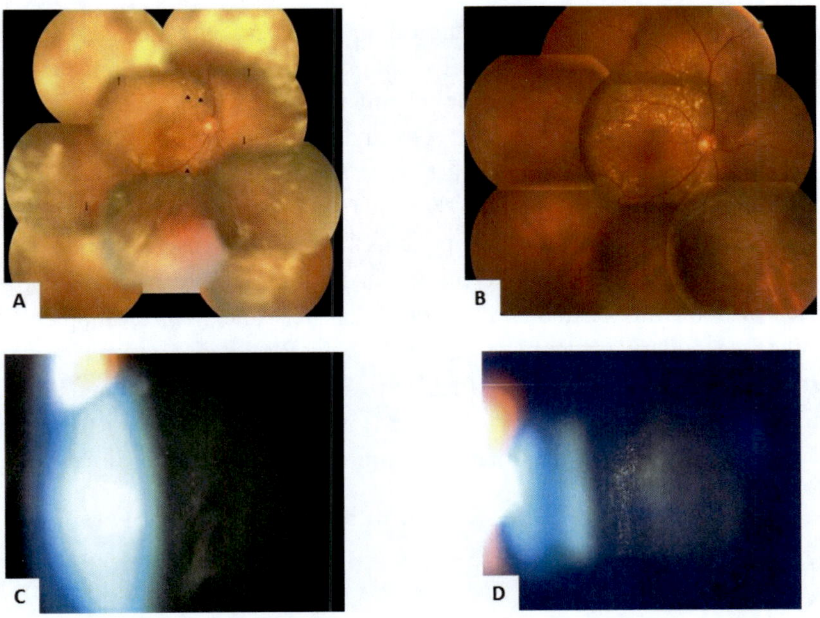

Figure 3. Typical vitreous clouding. A) Typical aurora borealis-like vitreous clouding surrounding the fundus (black arrows) and spotted yellowish subretinal lesions (black arrow heads). B) Local ocular therapy and systemic chemotherapy resulted in the resolution of ocular lesions. C) Aurora borealis-like vitreous clouding and large tumor cells arranged in clumps. D) Large cells atypical of uveitis cases.

Sarcoidosis should be excluded using plain chest radiography and CT imaging. PIOL should be considered in cases where a definitive diagnosis cannot be reached despite the use of the above tests and steroid therapy fails to lead to satisfactory clinical improvements [79, 80]. In cases where PIOL is suspected, additional head MRI, whole spine MRI, and cerebrospinal fluid testing should be performed [56]. Mandatory ophthalmological imaging tests include full field fundus photography, which allows the intermittent evaluation of small changes in fundus findings discussed in the following sections (Figure 3a, b). Ultrasound, fluorescein, indocyanine green fluorescein angiogram, fundus autofluorescence, and ocular coherence tomography are not necessary but are often performed as required [45].

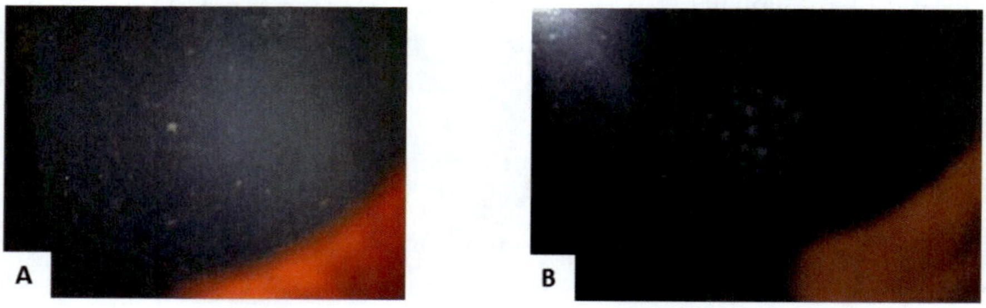

Figure 4. Keratic precipitates (KP) in the anterior chamber. (A) Unlike KP observed in uveitis, KP in PIOL are asteroid or starfish-shaped and are observed with relative frequency in cases of recurrence. (B) Mutton-fat KP observed in normal granulomatous uveitis cases.

Slit Lamp Microscopy

Slit lamp microscopy represents the simplest and quickest outpatient test. First, it allows inspection of the anterior chamber for cells and keratic precipitates. In cases of uveitis, "inflammatory cells" within the anterior chamber typically include lymphocytes and leukocytes; however, malignant lymphoma cells and reactive inflammatory cells are present in cases of PIOL. Anterior chamber cells are a less frequent finding than uveitis; however, previous studies have reported that 20%–40% of patients present with anterior chamber cells [4, 12, 17, 45, 52, 56, 68]. In rare cases, patients present with pseudohypopyon, in which PIOL cells build up within the anterior chamber leading to elevated intraocular pressure due to the occlusion of Schlemm's canal and the trabecular network by infiltrating cells, which in turn may lead to secondary glaucoma [12, 83, 84]. In PIOL, keratic precipitates are star-shaped rather than the mutton-fat KP of variable sizes often observed in uveitis (Figure 4a, b). KP are relatively frequently observed during PIOL recurrences following treatment [12, 17, 52, 56, 68]. Posterior synechiae are relatively rare in PIOL compared to uveitis, as PIOL rarely causes lesions in the iris [83, 84].

Fundus Examinations

Outpatient fundus examinations can be performed quickly and simply. Although the finding of widespread vitreous clouding is suggestive of uveitis, it is also a characteristic finding in PIOL cases known as vitritis (vitreous cells and haze) [4, 7, 45, 52, 56, 64, 68, 84]. Occasionally described as "aurora borealis-like," malignant lymphoma cells are larger than the inflammatory cells observed in uveitis and other conditions and form sheets and clumps occasionally organizing into strand-like cell clusters that can be seen on slit lamp microscopy (Figure 3a).

Retinal and subretinal lesions are considered the most important fundus findings in cases of PIOL. These lesions appear as fluffy white, yellow, and slightly orange lesions with either clear or unclear and "vague" margins often presenting as single or multiple lobed lesions (Figure 5a) [45, 64, 68, 86]. These lesions are often observed fused together and atrophied. Because vitreous clouding often prevents the identification of such lesions, larger numbers of cases are thought to exist than are actually observed [45, 64]. As confirmed by autopsy studies, which allow histopathological analyses, malignant lymphoma cells invade between the retinal pigment epithelium (RPE) and Bruch's membrane during the early stage of the disease before expanding beyond the RPE into the retina, which causes RPE atrophy, RPE detachment, retinal detachment, and retinal necrosis [37, 71, 87, 88].

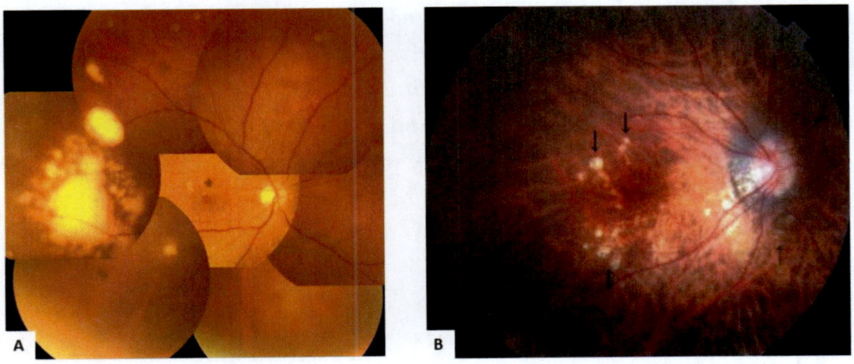

Figure 5. Typical retinal and subretinal lesions in the right eye of a PIOL patient. A) Several representative yellowish and lobe-shaped formations are shown. B) White and yellow choroidal lesions with clear margin differ from typical PIOL (black arrows).

Choroid and scleral lesions are extremely rare in cases of PIOL. These lesions differ from classic PIOL clear marginal lesions that are white, yellow, and slightly orange (Figure 5b). Previous studies have reported the scattered presence of grayish-white lesions and small punctate lesions that expand by gradual fusion. These lesions are not considered vitreoretinal lesions [1, 37, 45]. Retinal vessel occlusion and optic disc invasion are also rare, but careful observation is required as these conditions do occasionally occur in case of PIOL (Figure 6a, b) [89-91].

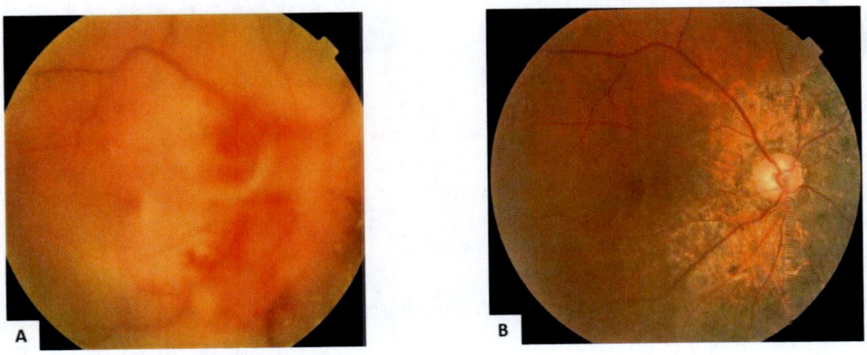

Figure 6. Optic nerve head invasion and retinal vascular occlusion in the right eye of a PIOL patient. A) Although the image is blurry due to vitreous clouding, hemorrhaging due to widespread optic nerve head invasion and retinal vascular occlusion can be seen. Corrected visual acuity was 20/1000 at the time of imaging. B) Local ocular therapy and systemic chemotherapy resulted in alleviation of ocular lesions. Corrected visual acuity had improved to 20/30 at the time of imaging.

Fluorescein, Indocyanine Green Fluorescein Angiogram

Fluorescein angiography (FA) has demonstrated utility in cases with retinal lesions that cannot be clearly viewed by ophthalmoscopy. In the field of ophthalmology, FA is frequently used to diagnose diabetic retinopathy, age-related macular degeneration (AMD), and uveitis. For example, hyperfluorescent lesions, known as "leopard spots," that are a characteristic finding of ocular syphilis may also indicate the presence of RPE disorders [77]. FA has demonstrated utility in the diagnosis of RPE and vascular wall disorders, and may allow visualization of the condition of the RPE and Bruch's membrane where PIOL tumor cells are observed [92-94]. RPE disorders are characterized by granular and punctate staining patterns on the latter half of FA imaging (Figure 7a, b). Vascular wall disorders are observed as various degrees of fluorescein dye leaking from areas adjacent to vascular walls. Although FA may also demonstrate vascular occlusion and vascular wall disorders in cases of PIOL [92, 93], these findings are not as commonly observed as in cases of uveitis or other inflammatory diseases. Nevertheless, viable tumor cells may be observed as hypofluorescent due to an inability to uptake fluorescein dye. And the cell membrane of these cells are not easily penetrated by fluorescein dye [92-94]. In a relatively large case study, Cassoux et al. reported window defects and hypofluorescent lesions as the commonest FA patterns in PIOL cases, observed in approximately 60% of patients. A round hyperfluorescent pattern was observed in approximately 40% of patients. However, a relatively small proportion of PIOL patients present with vasculitis [52]. Although there are no definitive FA findings for PIOL, FA may have substantial clinical utility in supporting a preliminary diagnosis.

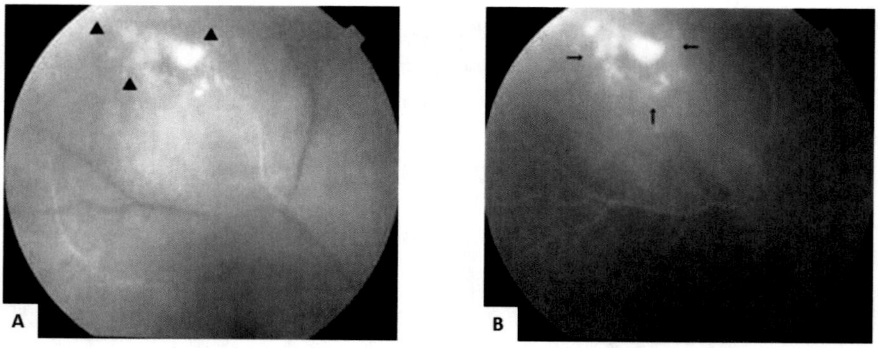

Figure 7. Peri-retinal fluorescein angiography findings in the right eye of a PIOL patient. A) Contrast at the beginning of the imaging demonstrates highly luminescent lesions that correspond to atrophy of the retinal pigment epithelium and pale-spotted hyperfluorescent lesions (black arrow heads). B) Contrast at the latter half of imaging demonstrates granular and spotted staining patterns over a wider area than seen in low-contrast images (black arrows).

Indocyanine green (ICG) fluorescein angiography allows evaluation of choroidal circulation. In addition to conventional FA, ICG is frequently used in cases of age-related macular degeneration and has excellent utility in identifying choroidal neovascularization. ICG and FA may also be used to depict and diagnose choroidal tumors, such as choroidal melanoma and hemangioma. Small, hypofluorescent lesions on contrast imaging at the early stage have been shown to be associated with PIOL and become gradually invisible on the latter half of the ICG imaging. Hypofluorescent lesions are frequently observed on FA imaging. However, to our knowledge, there are no previous studies describing the characteristic ICG FA findings of PIOL [92].

Fundus Autofluorescence

In recent years, fundus autofluorescence (FAF), a non-invasive test unlike FA or ICG, has come to be used in the diagnosis of a variety of retinochoroidal diseases. For example, studies have reported the characteristic findings of Best disease, Stargardt disease, pigmentary degeneration of the retina, cone-rod dystrophy, AMD, and other diseases. Further, the autofluorescence of FAF depends on the presence of lipofuscin in RPE cells [95, 96]. Lipofuscin accumulates as a result of aging and reduced RPE function. As FAF findings reflect RPE cell function, hypopigmented lesions indicate reduced function and hyperpigmented lesions indicate functional activation that may an increase the risk of future reductions in RPE cell function. The absence of FAF findings indicates that photoreceptors and RPE are functioning normally.

Although a variety of FAF findings may be observed in cases of PIOL, Casady et al. reported a "granular autofluorescence pattern (hyper-, hypo-)" as the most commonly observed finding, seen when tumor cells are active [97]. A granular pattern with hyper autofluorescent spots enveloped by a hypo-autofluorescent ring is observed in many cases of PIOL. However, the hyper-/hypo- autofluorescent pattern is reversed in some cases, which has led to the assumption that hypo autofluorescence occurs when malignant lymphoma cells are present in the RPE [98]. These lesions may not necessarily correspond with the "leopard spots" observed on FA [99]. Although FAF findings may indicate the presence of PIOL, the absence of FAF findings does not necessarily indicate the absence of PIOL or PIOL recurrence. As PIOL malignant lymphoma cells invade the RPE and Bruch's membrane during early-stage disease [37, 64, 71, 87, 93, 88, 100]. RPE cells may be observed as directly damaged by this process. However, FAF findings may not represent the actual pathology of PIOL as FAF simply reflects RPE cell functionality due to its reliance on lipofuscin metabolism by RPE cells.

Ocular Coherence Tomography

Fundus examination instruments have undergone remarkable recent advances, which have allowed retinal tomography to be performed simply on an outpatient basis. The use of ocular coherence tomography (OCT) has facilitated the imaging and observation of the structures of the retinal layers, such as the retinal ganglion cell layer and the neuroepithelial layer as well as the suprachoroidal layer, which used to be observed using histopathological slides. OCT also allows identification of lesions of the RPE and Bruch's membrane, which are early indicators of PIOL (Figure 8a, b). Recently, many intraocular tumors, posterior uveitis, and myelin nerve fiver can be differentiated from PIOL based on the evaluation of using OCT [101, 102].

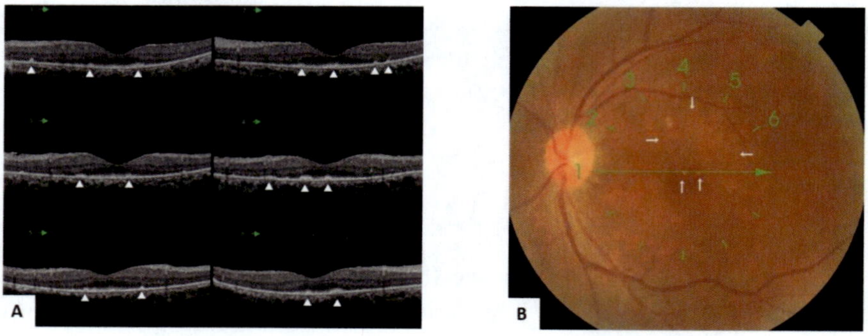

Figure 8. Early diagnosis of PIOL using ocular coherence tomography(OCT). (A) Multiple hyper-reflective nodules at the level between the sub-RPE and Bruch's membrane (white arrow heads). (B) Pale white lesions (white arrows) can barely be observed on the fundus image, and the lesions are unclear. OCT images shown are in the direction of the arrows on the corresponding fundus image (A).

Hyper-reflective bands and nodules at the level of the RPE, and separation of the RPE and Bruch's membrane, are characteristic imaging findings in cases of PIOL. Recently, the use of spectral-domain OCT (SD-OCT) has allowed the creation of detailed images. The use of SD-OCT also allows identification of rupture of the ellipsoid zone, previously known as the inner segment/outer segment (IS/OS) line, which may indicate injury to the RPE and resultant damage to the photoreceptor outer segment [98, 103]. These developments in diagnostic technologies allowing imaging at almost the cellular level may facilitate treatment that preserves good visual acuity through the early identification of lesions in the macular area of the retina that have the greatest effect on visual acuity.

Diagnostic Pars Plana Vitrectomy

Pars plana vitrectomy involves the surgical resection of vitreous humor, along with invasive tumor cells and reactive inflammatory cells, which manifest as the vitreous clouding observed in the majority of PIOL cases. Histopathological tests, cytokine measurements, and PCR (to confirm IgH rearrangement) are then performed.

Pars plana vitrectomy is a commonly performed surgical procedure in ophthalmology. An infusion port, light guide port, and vitreous cutter port are created in the anterior portion of the vitreous cavity, with samples collected by performing three port 20-, 23-, and 25-gauge pars plana vitrectomy [45, 104-109]. The collection method that we recommend involves resecting and suctioning the vitreous gel from the vitreous cavity using an undiluted light guide and a vitreous cutter. A total of 1.5–2 ml of vitreous gel is able to be suctioned (dry tapping) [37-42, 45, 104]. The use of irrigating solution, which is routine during vitreous surgery, may cause necrosis of tumor cells, leading to inaccurate cytokine concentration measurements. Care is required during dry taping as it may lead to hypotony, expulsive hemorrhaging, and other complications. Thus, some authors have suggested air, perfluoron infusion, or digital pressure to the eye wall in order to prevent such complications by maintaining intraocular pressure. Specimens collected using dry tapping are used for cytodiagnosis, histopathological examinations, cytokine concentration measurements, and PCR for IgH rearrangement. However, as malignant lymphoma cells undergo morphological changes after approximately 60 minutes, samples must be processed carefully and quickly [37, 105-107]. In normal cytodiagnosis, determination of the structure of cell clusters may be difficult and apoptosis and necrosis of tumor cells may also be observed; thus, analysis using cytodiagnosis alone is challenging [105, 109].

Accordingly, centrifugal separation has recently become used for the isolation of cells with generating a cell block prior to paraffin embedding for histological analyses. Recently, histological images constituted of thin slices of consecutive cells using histological techniques have been operated using centrifugal separation for the isolation of malignant cells prior to blocking the generation of cells following paraffin embedding.

In addition, immunostaining and PCR have been performing to increase diagnostic sensitivity [45, 47, 107-109].

Intraocular irrigation is typically initiated after dry tapping is completed, and vitrectomy is then completed. Cytodiagnosis, flow cytometry [104] and PCR can be performed if at least 3 ml of vitreous humor can be collected. After vitrectomy of periocular structures, such as the vitreous base and pars plana, collected samples are placed in the cassette of a vitreous machine and subjected to centrifugal separation for use in cytodiagnosis and cell culture techniques, which further increase diagnostic sensitivity.

Diagnostic Chorioretinal Biopsy

Diagnostic chorioretinal biopsy is often performed in the following cases: the absence of vitreous clouding observed in the majority of PIOL cases; failure to detect tumor cells in collected samples of cerebrospinal fluid or vitreous humor from pars plana vitrectomy; and the presence of chorioretinal lesions only on ophthalmoscopy (slit lamp microscopy, fundus examinations). As this is a highly invasive procedure, care should be taken to prevent or minimize any loss of visual acuity. Diagnostic chorioretinal biopsy can be performed using an endoretinal biopsy approach or a transscleral biopsy approach. When performed posterior to the equator of the eye, the endoretinal biopsy approach is easier to perform however, when performed anterior to the equator of the eye, the transscleral biopsy approach is more likely to be easier to perform [45, 110-113].

When utilizing the endoretinal biopsy approach, either retinal photocoagulation around the biopsy site 1 week to several days prior to the biopsy or the use of diathermy to coagulate the retina and choroid during vitrectomy should be performed in order to prevent retinal detachment or vitreous hemorrhage during or after biopsy. Samples are then collected using either scissors or microforceps. After biopsy completion, silicon oil injection and gas tamponade are performed with great care in order to avoid retinal detachment or vitreous hemorrhage [45, 110, 114, 115].

When utilizing the transscleral biopsy approach, a Flieringa's ring is used to prevent collapse of the eye. A full-thickness or near-full-thickness scleral flap is created at the biopsy site, and the biopsy is performed with diathermal coagulation in order to prevent choroidal hemorrhage [111-113]. Since vitreous prolapse is unavoidable, the scleral flap is securely sutured following the conclusion of the biopsy. An infusion port, light guide port, and vitreous cutter port are created in the anterior of the vitreous cavity, as is routine in the field of ophthalmology, and 3-port 20-, 23-, and 25-gauge pars plana vitrectomy is performed followed by intraocular vitreous processing.

The Role of Cytokines

Cytokine concentration measurements using enzyme-linked immunosorbent assay (ELISA) and other methods are extremely important in differentiating uveitis from PIOL. In the 1990s, it was reported that there were higher concentrations of interleukin (IL)-10 in the vitreous humor and cerebrospinal fluid of patients with PIOL and PCNSL [116-118]. IL-10 is a cytokine that is produced predominantly by type II helper T cells (Th2 cells) in addition to a variety of other cells, such as B-cells, monocytes, and keratinocytes. IL-10 predominantly acts to suppress lymphocytes and macrophages [119]. Although serum IL-10 levels are elevated in patients with autoimmune diseases, IL-6 and interferon (IFN)-γ may be elevated in addition to IL-10 in cases of PIOL, as seen in uveitis [123]. IL-6 is a cytokine that plays an important role in hematogenesis and the inflammatory response. IL-6 has been the subject of a large number of studies over several decades and is known to be produced by T-cells, macrophages, endothelial cells, fibroblasts, among other cells. IL-6 induces the migration of monocytes to sites of inflammation. Anterior chamber fluid concentrations of IL-6 have been shown to be elevated in cases of uveitis [120]. However, despite several reports of the utility of IL-10/IL-6 ratio and IL-10/IFN-γ ratio measurements in differentiating uveitis from PIOL, IL-6 and IL-10 measurements are unable to provide a definitive diagnosis of PIOL [13, 39, 121, 123]. The limitation of IL-6 and IL-10 measurements is predominantly attributable to measurement error and occasional overlapping of numerical ranges. As a result, cytodiagnosis and immunohistopathological examinations remain the most important tests for the diagnosis of PIOL.

An IL-10/IL-6 ratio of 1 or above is extremely suggestive of B-cell PIOL (positive predictive value, 70–80%); however, ratios of 1 or higher may also be observed in cases of T-cell PIOL [48, 116, 118, 122]. In addition, there is no difference in the IL-10/IL-6 and IL-10/IFN-γ ratios between cases of PCNSL with ocular lesions and cases of PIOL without CNS lesions. On the other hand, the IL-10/IFN-γ ratio in cases PIOL and PCNSL with ocular lesions differs substantially from that of uveitis [123].

In rare cases of T-cell PIOL, IL-10 levels may be elevated compared to IL-6 levels, although several studies have reported low levels [48, 122]. In addition, IL-10 and TGF-β levels may be elevated as in cases of cutaneous T-cell lymphoma [124].

Treatment of PIOL often results in decreased anterior chamber and vitreous cavity IL-10 levels, indicating measurements of IL-10 levels may have utility in determining therapeutic efficacy.

Therapeutic Management

The prompt initiation of treatment is important following a definitive diagnosis of PIOL; however, MRI imaging to determine the presence of other lesions in the CNS (intracranial, whole spinal column; Figure 9) is also important. Secondary IOL, a type of systemic lymphoma with CNS invasion, should also be excluded.

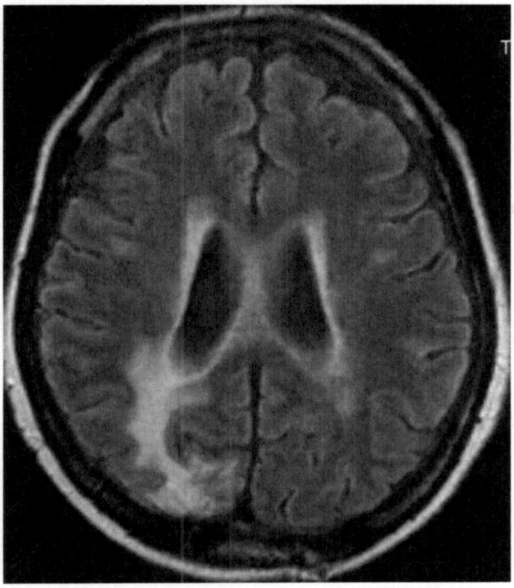

Figure 9. A PIOL case complicated with intracranial lesions. As approximately half of PIOL cases involve lymphoma cell invasion into the central nervous system (CNS), detailed examination of the CNS should be periodically performed.

PIOL is a type of malignant lymphoma that responds well to radiotherapy and chemotherapy; however, the prognosis of PIOL has yet to be fully elucidated. The optimal treatment approach for PIOL remains controversial and, as a result, there is currently no established treatment.

Radiotherapy

As malignant PIOL and PCNSL lymphoma cells are radiosensitive, radiotherapy represents an extremely important treatment method. Previously, radiation therapy alone for PIOL was utilized; [4, 8, 37, 134] however, combined radiation and chemotherapy is currently recommended for PIOL from the result of high cerebral relapse rate [69, 125-128]. Radiation monotherapy for stage I systemic DLBCL has demonstrated very positive treatment outcomes, with a 5-year survival rate of 94%. However, the 5-year survival rate following radiation monotherapy for stage IE PCNSL remains extremely poor at only 4% [129, 131].

A prospective phase II study of PCNSL conducted by the US Radiation Therapy Oncology Group (RTOG) found that when 40 Gy whole brain radiation with local 20 Gy boosts was performed, the response rate was relatively good at 81%, with a median survival period of 12.2 months. Subsequent clinical trials indicated that increasing the radiation dose to 45 Gy or more does not increase survival [129, 132]. Autopsy studies of PCNSL patients have indicated that areas considered normal on MRI or imaging had in fact been invaded by malignant lymphoma cells. As a result, radiation therapy for PCNSL has been standardized to whole brain irradiation at a dose of 40–45 Gy.

In studies to date, radiotherapy for PIOL has most often been performed at a minimum dose of 30 Gy and maximum dose of 50 Gy at 1.5–2.0 Gy per fraction, with an average of 40

Gy [4, 37, 57, 65, 130, 133, 134]. Irradiation of the eye with a dose of 40 Gy produces a high response rate of at least 70%; however, radiation monotherapy is not recommended due to the high risk of subsequent recurrence. Radiotherapy cannot be performed an unlimited number of times and its utilization is limited by the risks of complications, such as radiation retinopathy, radiation cataract, and severe dry eye [57, 130, 133, 134]. Recently, systemic chemotherapy has been frequently administered in conjunction with localized eye chemotherapy [128, 135-138].

Systemic Chemotherapy

The current standard treatment for PCNSL is high-dose methotrexate (HD-MTX), used as systemic chemotherapy for the treatment of PIOL. CHOP therapy, the standard therapy for diffuse large B-cell lymphoma comprised of doxorubicin, cyclophosphamide, vincristine, and prednisolone, has been shown to be ineffective in cases of PCNSL in multi-institution phase II clinical studies [139, 140]. The inability of these drugs to pass the blood-brain barrier (BBB) has been posited as the major reason for the lack of efficacy of the CHOP regime in treating PCNSL. Thus, the key to the efficacy of chemotherapy for the treatment of PCNSL is the ability of the drugs utilized to pass the BBB. The eye has a barrier similar to the BBB, known as the blood-ocular barrier system (BOB). The BOB consists of two major barriers: the blood aqueous barrier; and the blood retinal barrier (BRB). The BRB is a particularly impermeable and restrictive physiological barrier that regulates ion, protein, and water flux into and out of the retina [141-143].

Standard doses of methotrexate (MTX) are unable to pass the BBB; however, large doses of 1 g/m^2 or greater are able to pass the BBB. In addition, PCNSL lymphoma cells are sensitive to the MTX. MTX inhibits enzymes synthesizing folic acid, resulting in inhibition of synthesis and repair of DNA and amino acids. A study by DeAngelis et al. and subsequent phase II trials and multi-institution trials have reported the efficacy of HD-MTX in the treatment of PCNSL. Currently, MTX has demonstrated the greatest improvements in long-term survival when used in combination therapy with radiotherapy [144-147].

In their study of systemic chemotherapy for PIOL, Batchelor et al. administered HD-MTX intravenously (8 g/m^2) to nine PIOL patients and reported extremely poor intraocular distribution of MTX due to the BOB [142]. Even at large doses of 8 g/m^2, vitreous MTX levels were only one-one hundredth of serum MTX levels, with extremely low vitreous concentrations of approximately 1μM. As a result, five patients required additional radiotherapy. As large doses of MTX result in systemic adverse drug effects, intraocular drug distribution is poor, and systemic chemotherapy normally results in recurrence in the long term, MTX levels in the vitreous cavity may currently be insufficient. Mason et al. reported that MTX administration directly into the cerebrospinal fluid may be more effective than intravenous infusions [148]. However, it has subsequently been suggested that vitreous MTX concentrations are also insufficient with this administration route [149]. Currently, the direct administration of MTX and rituximab (human-murine chimeric monoclonal antibody specific to CD20) into the vitreous cavity, described in a subsequent section, is utilized in order to avoid systemic adverse drug effects and ensure sufficient vitreous cavity drug levels.

Other drugs that are able to pass the BBB and BOB include cytosine arabinoside (ARA-C) at high doses, which has been reported to have efficacy in the treatment of PIOL [150,

151]. However, the ARA-C has been found to have poor efficacy in a proportion of patients, thereby requiring radiotherapy. These findings indicate poor intraocular drug distribution remains a substantial clinical issue.

Alkylating agents, which have good BBB and BOB permeability, are expected to have efficacy in the treatment of PIOL. Alkylating agents are representative cytotoxic anticancer agents that were developed as a result of mustard gas research. They have multiple alkyl group sites that form covalent bonds with DNA bases. By binding with two DNA chains (chain cross-links), they interfere with DNA replication. Previously, Sullivan et al. reported that procarbazine, other nitrosourea drugs, and vincristine, have efficacy in the treatment of PIOL [143]. Alkylating agents such as Ifosfamide and trofosmide have also been shown to have efficacy in the treatment of PCNSL and PIOL; [152-155] however, monotherapy did not produce high response rates.

Local Chemotherapy (Intravitreal Chemotherapy)

Methotrexate (MTX)

Although radiotherapy has a substantial cytotoxic effect on PIOL tumor cells, its use is limited by the high risk of recurrence and eye complications that restrict its safe use to a single course. Local intraocular chemotherapy has been long considered because systemic chemotherapy is unable to achieve the intraocular local drug levels required for a substantial cytotoxic effect on PIOL tumor cells [155]. Fishburne et al. were the first to inject MTX (400 μg/0.1 ml) directly into the vitreous cavity [156]. A subsequent relatively large-scale case series conducted by Smith et al. indicated that this treatment was effective in all studied cases [157]. The treatment protocol comprised twice weekly injections for 1 month once per week for the next 2 months, and then once per month for 9 months for a total of 1 year. Frenkel et al. used the same protocol to treat 26 patients (44 eyes) and reported that local treatment alone was effective, with no systemic adverse drug effects, and over 90% of patients had complete remission over 10 years. Thirteen injections, on an average, were required to achieve complete remission [158].

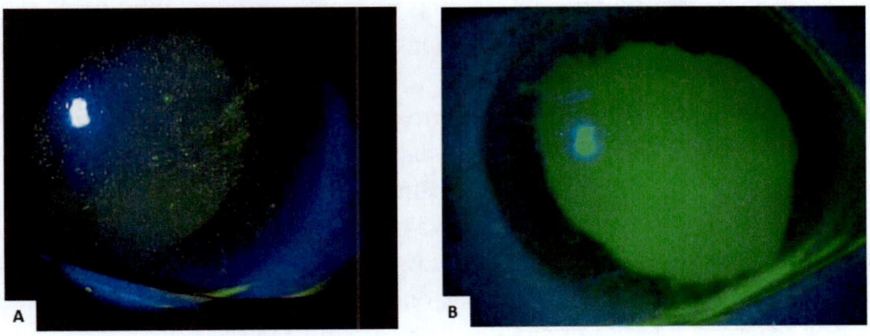

Figure 10. Corneal epitheliopathy caused by several MTX intravitreal injections. A) Fluorescein staining demonstrating the presence of corneal epitheliopathy ranging from yellow-green spotting to hurricane keratopathy. B) Severe corneal erosion caused visual acuity loss and severe eye pain.

An intraocular MTX concentration of 1 μmol/l was required for a cytotoxic effect on malignant lymphoma cells, and a single intravitreal injection of MTX was maintained within the vitreous for approximately 5 days. Thus, several studies have reported good local intraocular control rates, even in studies of protocols that deviated from that reported by Frenkel et al. [156-159]. However, CNS and systemic recurrence currently remains a clinical issue when utilizing local intraocular treatment, the prognosis of PIOL remains poor, and the prevention of recurrence in locations other than the eye remains an important issue.

Adverse intraocular local drug effects resulting from intravitreal injection of MTX reportedly include cataracts (73% of cases), corneal epithelial disorders (58%; Figure 10), maculopathy (42%), vitreous hemorrhage (8%), atrophy of the optic nerve (4%), and aseptic endophthalmitis (4%) [157]. Such effects are usually temporary; severe complications are extremely rare as long as intravitreal injection is carefully performed.

Recently, Sen et al. reported PIOL cases resistant to MTX therapy. The CD20 antibody rituximab, which is discussed below, may have efficacy in such cases [160].

Rituximab

Rituximab (Rituxan®; Genentech, Inc, South San Francisco, CA, and IDEC Pharmaceuticals, San Diego, CA) is a molecularly targeted drug that was approved for clinical use by the US Food and Drug Administration in 1997. Rituximab is a monoclonal anti-human CD20 human/mouse chimera antibody that has clinical utility in the treatment of CD20 antibody-positive malignant lymphoma, rheumatism, and a wide range of autoimmune diseases. CD20 antibody-positive B-cell lymphoma is identified in over 90% of PIOL cases, indicating cell-selective therapy likely protects CD20 antibody-negative normal stem cells, neurons, glial cells, and others [161].

Rituximab intravitreal injection therapy is often used in cases where MTX intravitreal injection is ineffective or has only a weak effect or where MTX intravitreal injection results in serious intraocular adverse effects [162, 163]. Kim et al. were the first to report animal studies of rituximab and observed a half-life of intraocular rituximab of 4.7 days [164, 165]. Their investigation of ocular toxicity in rabbit eyes demonstrated no effects on the optical microscopic level by Kitzmann et al. Further, there have been no reports indicating that rituximab has definite ocular toxicity in humans.[166]. Rituximab is similar to bevacizumab (and has an equivalent molecular weight), a drug frequently used in intravitreal injections for AMD. Results from rabbit, studies have demonstrated that rituximab penetrates all retinal layers [164-168].

Larkin et al. conducted a study of long-term progress outcomes of rituximab therapy in 48 eyes (34 patients) and reported complete remission in 31 eyes (approximately 65% of patients) with an average of 3.5 intravitreal injections; however, remission occurred in 7 eyes. Adverse drug effects were observed in 25% of cases, but serious effects, such as loss of visual acuity, were few [169]. Ohguro et al. reported two cases that demonstrated good clinical progress after intravitreal rituximab injections once per week, but they did not describe the visual acuity or electroretinogram findings of these patients [163].

Many studies have evaluated intravitreal injections of rituximab (1 mg/ 0.1 ml), with many using weekly intravitreal injections conducted continuously over several months [162, 163, 165, 169]. Fewer local intraocular adverse drug effects were observed with intravitreal injection of rituximab than with MTX, though there have been many reports of the development of cataracts following intravitreal injections of rituximab. Most adverse events are related to intravitreal injection technique, indicating that serious adverse events are extremely rare as long as the procedure is performed carefully. The majority of reported studies have been case studies and short-term observational studies. Therefore, multicenter long-term observational studies with large numbers of cases are required in order to determine the optimum dose, optimum number of injections, and the efficacy of rituximab intravitreal therapy in addition to systemic chemotherapy.

OUTCOME

PIOL frequently recurs in the CNS following local therapy (radiotherapy and intravitreal chemotherapy) alone, which contributes to the poor prognosis of PIOL. A study by the Japanese Intraocular Lymphoma Study Group reported a 5-year survival rate of 61.1% [13], and a report issued by an international PCNSL collaborative group reported a median progression-free survival of 18 months and overall survival (OS) of 31 months [125]. A separate study reported a median OS of 57 months in cases of PIOL alone without CNS lesions; however, a median OS of 12–20 months and a 2-year survival rate of 39% in cases with CNS lesions [69] indicating favorable prognosis is dependent on the absence of CNS lesions [125, 147]. In a recent study of the risk factors for CNS invasion, Cho et al. reported no association between age, sex, length of observation period, cerebrospinal fluid invasion, or bone marrow invasion with CNS invasion in cases of PIOL, with malignant lymphoma cells with a high Ki-67 index, a measure of cell proliferation, the only risk factor for CNS invasion identified. Ki-67 is a nucleoprotein related to the cell cycle that is expressed during cell proliferation, which allows it to be used as a marker of cell proliferation and activation of the cell cycle. A high Ki67 index is positively correlated with tumor malignancy, advanced disease stage, and low survival rates [170].

The optimal treatment for PIOL remains controversial, with agreed guidelines for the treatment of PIOL yet to be established. The use of systemic chemotherapy in PIOL cases reportedly increases median progression-free survival from 5.5 months to 12 months, thereby underscoring the necessity of systemic therapy [126].

However, in a multi-institution joint study of 83 PIOL patients, Grimm et al. reported no differences in progression-free survival or OS between a group of 23 patients (focal treatment alone) that received intraocular methotrexate and ocular radiation and a group of 53 patients (extensive treatment) that received systemic chemotherapy with or without whole brain radiotherapy, focal treatments [69]. Accordingly, the necessity of systemic chemotherapy in PIOL patients remains controversial.

In 2011, an international PCNSL collaborative group released recommendations for PIOL treatment methods. Local ocular therapy (intravitreal MTX, intravitreal rituximab, or ocular radiation with 30–35-Gy external beam) was recommended for cases of PIOL affecting one eye with no CNS lesions. In cases of PIOL affecting both eyes with no CNS lesions, local ocular therapy or local ocular therapy with concurrent systemic chemotherapy (HD-MTX with the addition of rituximab when possible) was recommended. The report recommends systemic chemotherapy (described above) in combination with local ocular therapy in cases of PIOL with CNS lesions. [15] The British Neuro-Oncology Society guidelines recommend systemic chemotherapy (with HD-MTX) in combination with ocular radiation for both eye, even in cases of PIOL affecting one eye. Intravitreal chemotherapy is listed as an option in cases of recurrence. [66, 128] The National Comprehensive Cancer Network recommends local ocular therapy, intravitreal chemotherapy, or ocular radiation with concurrent systemic chemotherapy (with HD-MTX) [66]. [http://www.nccn.org]

The use of hematopoietic stem cell rescue with intense chemotherapy (combined with thiotepa, busulfan, and cyclophosphamide) has been reported to improve the median survival time, although this therapy resulted in partial response or relapse in most of the patients [171]. However, powerful systemic chemotherapy cannot be administered to all patients due to the high frequency of severe systemic adverse effects.

After MTX intravitreal injections were commenced, reports from Japan indicated that its early use in combination systemic therapy, known as R-MPV (rituximab, HD-MTX, procarbazine, and vincristine) with whole brain radiotherapy at a dose of 23.4 Gy was effective [127]. A study of five treatment-naïve PIOL patients reported that all five patients achieved complete remission during the median observation period of 32 months and currently remain remission-free. Currently, the efficacy of R-MPV with MTX intravitreal injections is being evaluated by a prospective study.

A recent multicenter study of 78 PIOL cases conducted in Europe by Riemens et al. evaluated in patients in three groups: a local ocular therapy only group (n = 31); a systemic chemotherapy only group (n = 21); and a local ocular and systemic chemotherapy combination therapy group (n = 23) [172]. The results of this study demonstrated almost identical 5-year survival rates among the groups, with no significant difference in the rate of progression to CNS lesions. Current treatments are unable to prevent the development of CNS lesions; however, the authors concluded that systemic chemotherapy is associated with significant side effects despite demonstrating lack of superiority to local treatment. This was a surprising report that indicated the mere presence of adverse drug effects prevents improvement of survival rates when systemic therapy is used in cases of PIOL. Specifically, HD-MTX-based systemic therapy administered with whole brain radiotherapy in elderly patients is associated with neurotoxicity (ataxia, dementia, leuko-encephalopathy, etc.), which leads to decreased post-therapy quality of life.

PIOL is a relatively rare disease. Treatment options for PIOL should be considered by specialists from a number of fields, including ophthalmology, oncology, hematology, radiology, and pathology. PCNSL treatments cannot be simply re-purposed for the treatment of PIOL [173]. Randomized-controlled clinical trials have not been performed for PIOL and are unlikely. However, previous multicenter studies of standard therapies have provided valuable data. The development of novel techniques, such as the use of transscleral therapy instead of intraocular chemotherapy and individualized targeted therapies through the use of genetic profiling, may improve the prognosis of PIOL in the near future.

REFERENCES

[1] Vogel MH, Font RL, Zimmerman LE, Levine RA, (1968). Reticulum cell sarcoma of the retina and uvea. Report of six cases and review of the literature. *Am J Ophthalmol.* 66, 205-215.

[2] Givner I, (1955). Malignant lymphoma with ocular involvement; a clinico-pathologic report. *Am J Ophthalmol.* 39, 29-32.

[3] Klingele TG, Hogan MJ, (1975). Ocular reticulum cell sarcoma. *Am J Ophthalmol.* 79, 39-47.

[4] Char DH, Ljung BM, Miller T, Phillips T, (1988). Primary intraocular lymphoma (ocular reticulum cell sarcoma) diagnosis and management. *Ophthalmology.* 95, 625-630.

[5] Coupland SE, Chan CC, Smith J, (2009). Pathophysiology of retinal lymphoma. *Ocul Immunol Inflamm.* 17, 227-237.

[6] Chan CC, Sen HN, (2013). Current concepts in diagnosing and managing primary vitreoretinal (intraocular) lymphoma. *Discov Med.* 15, 93-100.

[7] Chan CC, Buggage RR, Nussenblatt RB, (2002). Intraocular lymphoma. *Curr Opin Ophthalmol.* 13, 411-418.

[8] Buggage RR, Chan CC, Nussenblatt RB, (2001). Ocular manifestations of central nervous system lymphoma. *Curr Opin Oncol.* 13, 137-142.

[9] Wallace DJ, Altemare CR, Shen DF, deSmet MD, Buggage RR, Nussenblatt RB, Chan CC, (2006). Primary testicular and intraocular lymphomas: two case reports and a review of the literature. *Surv Ophthalmol.* 51, 41-50.

[10] Levy-Clarke GA, Greenman D, Sieving PC, Byrnes G, Shen D, Nussenblatt RB, Chan CC, (2008). Ophthalmic manifestations, cytology, immunohistochemistry, and molecular analysis of intraocular metastatic T-cell lymphoma: report of a case and review of the literature. *Surv Ophthalmol.* 53, 285-295.

[11] DeAngelis LM, (2001). Brain tumors. *N Engl J Med.* 344, 114-123.

[12] Freeman LN, Schachat AP, Knox DL, Michels RG, Green WR, (1987). Clinical features, laboratory investigations, and survival in ocular reticulum cell sarcoma. *Ophthalmology.* 94, 1631-1639.

[13] Kimura K, Usui Y, Goto H; Japanese Intraocular Lymphoma Study Group, (2012). Clinical features and diagnostic significance of the intraocular fluid of 217 patients with intraocular lymphoma. *Jpn J Ophthalmol.* 56, 383-389.

[14] Schabet M, (1999). Epidemiology of primary CNS lymphoma. *J Neurooncol.* 43, 199-201.

[15] Chan CC, Rubenstein JL, Coupland SE, Davis JL, Harbour JW, Johnston PB, Cassoux N, Touitou V, Smith JR, Batchelor TT, Pulido JS, (2011). Primary vitreoretinal lymphoma: a report from an International Primary Central Nervous System Lymphoma Collaborative Group symposium. *Oncologist.* 16, 1589-1599.

[16] Chan CC, Sen HN, (2013). Current concepts in diagnosing and managing primary vitreoretinal (intraocular) lymphoma. *Discov Med.* 15, 93-100.

[17] Peterson K, Gordon KB, Heinemann MH, DeAngelis LM, (1993). The clinical spectrum of ocular lymphoma. *Cancer.* 72, 843-849.

[18] Rockwood EJ, Zakov ZN, Bay JW, (1984). Combined malignant lymphoma of the eye and CNS (reticulum-cell sarcoma). Report of three cases. *J Neurosurg.* 61, 369-374.

[19] Nasir S, DeAngelis LM, (2000). Update on the management of primary CNS lymphoma. *Oncology* (Williston Park). 14, 228-234.

[20] Rivero ME, Kuppermann BD, Wiley CA, Garcia CR, Smith MD, Dreilinger A, Freeman WR, (1999). Acquired immunodeficiency syndrome-related intraocular B-cell lymphoma. *Arch Ophthalmol.* 117, 616-622.

[21] Chan SM, Hutnik CM, Heathcote JG, Orton RB, Banerjee D, (2000). Iris lymphoma in a pediatric cardiac transplant recipient: clinicopathologic findings. *Ophthalmology*. 107, 1479-82.

[22] Coskuncan NM, Jabs DA, Dunn JP, Haller JA, Green WR, Vogelsang GB, Santos GW, (1994). The eye in bone marrow transplantation. VI. Retinal complications. *Arch Ophthalmol.* 112, 372-379.

[23] Kheterpal S, Kirkby GR, Neuberger JM, Rosenthal AR, Murray PI, (1993). Intraocular lymphoma after liver transplantation. *Am J Ophthalmol.* 116, 507-508.

[24] Rizkalla K, Rodrigues S, Proulx A, Tingey DP, Heathcote JG, (2005). Primary intraocular lymphoma arising during methotrexate treatment of temporal arteritis. *Can J Ophthalmol.* 40, 585-592.

[25] Harris NL, Jaffe ES, Diebold J, Flandrin G, Muller-Hermelink HK, Vardiman J, Lister TA, Bloomfield CD, (1999). The World Health Organization classification of neoplastic diseases of the hematopoietic and lymphoid tissues. Report of the Clinical Advisory Committee meeting, Airlie House, Virginia, November, (1997). *Ann Oncol.* 10, 1419-1432.

[26] Swerdlow SH, Campo E, Harris NL, Jaffe ES, Pileri SA, Stein H, Thiele J, Vardiman, JW. WHO Classification of Tumours of Haematopoietic and Lymphoid Tissues, Fourth Edition WHO Classification of Tumours, Volume 2

[27] Isaacson PG, Du MQ, (2004). MALT lymphoma: from morphology to molecules. *Nat Rev Cancer.* 4, 644-653.

[28] Pinzone MR, Berretta M, Cacopardo B, Nunnari G, (2015). Epstein-barr virus- and Kaposi sarcoma-associated herpesvirus-related malignancies in the setting of human immunodeficiency virus infection. *Semin Oncol.* 42, 258-271.

[29] Nevens D, Nuyts S, (2015). HPV-positive head and neck tumours, a distinct clinical entity. *B-ENT.* 11, 81-87.

[30] Chan CC, Shen DF, Whitcup SM, Nussenblatt RB, (1999). Detection of human herpesvirus-8 and Epstein-Barr virus DNA in primary intraocular lymphomas. *Blood.* 93, 2749-2751.

[31] Coté TR, Manns A, Hardy CR, Yellin FJ, Hartge P, (1996). Epidemiology of brain lymphoma among people with or without acquired immunodeficiency syndrome. AIDS/Cancer Study Group. J *Natl Cancer Inst.* 88, 675-679.

[32] Utsuki S, Oka H, Miyajima Y, Kijima C, Yasui Y, Fujii K, (2011). Epstein-Barr virus (EBV)-associated primary central nervous system lymphoma: is incidence of EBV expression associated with median survival time? *Brain Tumor Pathol.* 28, 145-149.

[33] Kuze T, Nakamura N, Hashimoto Y, Sasaki Y, Abe M, (2000). The characteristics of Epstein-Barr virus (EBV)-positive diffuse large B-cell lymphoma: comparison between EBV(+) and EBV(-) cases in Japanese population. *Jpn J Cancer Res.* 91, 1233-1240.

[34] Shen DF, Herbort CP, Tuaillon N, Buggage RR, Egwuagu CE, Chan CC, (2001). Detection of Toxoplasma gondii DNA in primary intraocular B-cell lymphoma. *Mod Pathol.* 14, 995-999.

[35] McCann KJ, Ashton-Key M, Smith K, Stevenson FK, Ottensmeier CH, (2009). Primary central nervous system lymphoma: tumor-related clones exist in the blood and bone marrow with evidence for separate development. *Blood.* 113, 4677-4680.

[36] Chan CC, Shen D, Hackett JJ, Buggage RR, Tuaillon N, (2003). Expression of chemokine receptors, CXCR4 and CXCR5, and chemokines, BLC and SDF-1, in the eyes of patients with primary intraocular lymphoma. *Ophthalmology.* 110, 421-426.
[37] Char DH, Ljung BM, Deschênes J, Miller TR, (1988). Intraocular lymphoma: immunological and cytological analysis. *Br J Ophthalmol.* 72, 905-911
[38] Mruthyunjaya P, Jumper JM, McCallum R, Patel DJ, Cox TA, Jaffe GJ, (2002). Diagnostic yield of vitrectomy in eyes with suspected posterior segment infection or malignancy. *Ophthalmology.* 109, 1123-1129.
[39] Liu K, Klintworth GK, Dodd LG, (1999). Cytologic findings in vitreous fluids. Analysis of 74 specimens. *Acta Cytol.* 43, 201-206.
[40] Kanavi MR, Soheilian M, Hosseini SB, Azari AA, (2014). 25-gauge transconjunctival diagnostic vitrectomy in suspected cases of intraocular lymphoma: a case series and review of the literature. *Int J Ophthalmol.* 7, 577-581.
[41] Wittenberg LA, Maberley DA, Ma PE, Wade NK, Gill H, White VA, (2008). Contribution of vitreous cytology to final clinical diagnosis fifteen-year review of vitreous cytology specimens from one institution. *Ophthalmology.* 115, 1944-1950.
[42] Davis JL, Viciana AL, Ruiz P, (1997). Diagnosis of intraocular lymphoma by flow cytometry. *Am J Ophthalmol.* 124, 362-372.
[43] Rothova A, Ooijman F, Kerkhoff F, Van Der Lelij A, Lokhorst HM, (2001). Uveitis masquerade syndromes. *Ophthalmology.* 108, 386-399.
[44] Coupland SE, Loddenkemper C, Smith JR, Braziel RM, Charlotte F, Anagnostopoulos I, Stein H, (2005). Expression of immunoglobulin transcription factors in primary intraocular lymphoma and primary central nervous system lymphoma. *Invest Ophthalmol Vis Sci.* 46, 3957-3964.
[45] Chan CC, Gonzalez JA, (2007). *Primary Intraocular Lymphoma.* Hackensack, NJ:World Scientific Publishing Co Pte Ltd.
[46] Coupland SE, Hummel M, Müller HH, Stein H, (2005). Molecular analysis of immunoglobulin genes in primary intraocular lymphoma. *Invest Ophthalmol Vis Sci.* 46, 3507-3514.
[47] White VA, Gascoyne RD, Paton KE, (1999). Use of the polymerase chain reaction to detect B- and T-cell gene rearrangements in vitreous specimens from patients with intraocular lymphoma. *Arch Ophthalmol.* 117, 761-765.
[48] Coupland SE, Anastassiou G, Bornfeld N, Hummel M, Stein H, (2005). Primary intraocular lymphoma of T-cell type: report of a case and review of the literature. *Graefes Arch Clin Exp Ophthalmol.* 243, 189-197.
[49] Muris JJ, Meijer CJ, Vos W, van Krieken JH, Jiwa NM, Ossenkoppele GJ, Oudejans JJ, (2006). Immunohistochemical profiling based on Bcl-2, CD10 and MUM1 expression improves risk stratification in patients with primary nodal diffuse large B cell lymphoma. *J Pathol.* 208, 714-723.
[50] Hans CP, Weisenburger DD, Greiner TC, Gascoyne RD, Delabie J, Ott G, Müller-Hermelink HK, Campo E, Braziel RM, Jaffe ES, Pan Z, Farinha P, Smith LM, Falini B, Banham AH, Rosenwald A, Staudt LM, Connors JM, Armitage JO, Chan WC, (2004). Confirmation of the molecular classification of diffuse large B-cell lymphoma by immunohistochemistry using a tissue microarray. *Blood.* 103, 275-282
[51] Wallace DJ, Shen D, Reed GF, Miyanaga M, Mochizuki M, Sen HN, Dahr SS, Buggage RR, Nussenblatt RB, Chan CC, (2006). Detection of the bcl-2 t(14;18)

translocation and proto-oncogene expression in primary intraocular lymphoma. *Invest Ophthalmol Vis Sci.* 47, 2750-2756.

[52] Cassoux N, Merle-Beral H, Leblond V, Bodaghi B, Miléa D, Gerber S, Fardeau C, Reux I, Xuan KH, Chan CC, LeHoang P, (2000). Ocular and central nervous system lymphoma: clinical features and diagnosis. *Ocul Immunol Inflamm.* 8, 243-250.

[53] Wender A, Adar A, Maor E, Yassur Y, (1994). Primary B-cell lymphoma of the eyes and brain in a 3-year-old boy. *Arch Ophthalmol.* 112, 450-451.

[54] Sobrin L, Dubovy SR, Davis JL, Murray TG, (2005). Isolated,bilateralintraocular lymphoma in a 15-year-old girl. *Retina.* 25,370-373.

[55] Qualman SJ, Mendelsohn G, Mann RB, Green WR, (1983). Intraocular lymphomas. Natural history based on a clinicopathologic study of eight cases and review of the literature. *Cancer.* 52, 878-886.

[56] Whitcup SM, de Smet MD, Rubin BI, Palestine AG, Martin DF, Burnier M Jr, Chan CC, Nussenblatt RB, (1993). Intraocular lymphoma. Clinical and histopathologic diagnosis. *Ophthalmology.* 100, 1399-1406.

[57] Hoffman PM, McKelvie P, Hall AJ, Stawell RJ, Santamaria JD, (2003). Intraocular lymphoma: a series of 14 patients with clinicopathological features and treatment outcomes. *Eye* (Lond). 7, 13-21.

[58] Chan H, Bolling JP, (1993). Intravitreal large-cell lymphoma. *Mayo Clin Proc.* 68, 1011-1015.

[59] Sagoo MS, Mehta H, Swampillai AJ, Cohen VM, Amin SZ, Plowman PN, Lightman S, (2014). Primary intraocular lymphoma. *Surv Ophthalmol.* 59, 503-516.

[60] Nakahara H, Kaburaki T, Takamoto M, Okinaga K, Matsuda J, Konno Y, Kawashima H, Numaga J, Fujino Y, Amano S, (2014). Statistical analyses of Endogenous Uveitis Patients (2007-2009) in central Tokyo area and Comparison with Previous Studies (1963-2006). *Ocul Immunol* Inflamm. 25, 1-6.

[61] Touitou V, LeHoang P, Bodaghi B, (2015). Primary CNS lymphoma. *Curr Opin Ophthalmol.* 26, 526-533.

[62] Bataille B, Delwail V, Menet E, Vandermarcq P, Ingrand P, Wager M, Guy G, Lapierre F, (2000). Primary intracerebral malignant lymphoma: report of 248 cases. *J Neurosurg.* 92, 261-266.

[63] Hwang CS, Yeh S, Bergstrom CS, (2014). Diagnostic vitrectomy for primary intraocular lymphoma: when, why, how? *Int Ophthalmol Clin.* 54, 155-171.

[64] Chan CC, Wallace DJ, (2004). Intraocular lymphoma: update on diagnosis and management. *Cancer Control.* 11, 285-295.

[65] Hormigo A, Abrey L, Heinemann MH, DeAngelis LM, (2004). Ocular presentation of primary central nervous system lymphoma: diagnosis and treatment. *Br J Haematol.* 126, 202-208.

[66] Davis JL, (2013). Intraocular lymphoma: a clinical perspective. *Eye* (Lond). 27, 153-162.

[67] Sen HN, Bodaghi B, Hoang PL, Nussenblatt RB, (2009). Primary intraocular lymphoma: diagnosis and differential diagnosis. *Ocul Immunol Inflamm.* 17, 133-141.

[68] Levy-Clarke GA, Chan CC, Nussenblatt RB, (2005). Diagnosis and management of primary intraocular lymphoma. *Hematol Oncol Clin North Am.* 19, 739-749.

[69] Grimm SA, Pulido JS, Jahnke K, Schiff D, Hall AJ, Shenkier TN, Siegal T, Doolittle ND, Batchelor T, Herrlinger U, Neuwelt EA, Laperriere N, Chamberlain MC, Blay JY,

Ferreri AJ, Omuro AM, Thiel E, Abrey LE, (2007). Primary intraocular lymphoma: an International Primary Central Nervous System Lymphoma Collaborative Group Report. *Ann Oncol* 18, 1851-1855.

[70] Akpek EK, Ahmed I, Hochberg FH, Soheilian M, Dryja TP, Jakobiec FA, Foster CS, (1999). Intraocular-central nervous system lymphoma: clinical features, diagnosis, and outcomes. *Ophthalmology.* 106, 1805-1810.

[71] Barr CC, Green WR, Payne JW, Knox DL, Jensen AD, Thompson RL, (1975). Intraocular reticulum-cell sarcoma: clinico-pathologic study of four cases and review of the literature. *Surv Ophthalmol.* 19, 224-239.

[72] Jahnke K, Thiel E, Abrey LE, Neuwelt EA, Korfel A, (2007). Diagnosis and management of primary intraocular lymphoma: an update. *Clin Ophthalmol.* 1, 247-258.

[73] Chan CC, (2003). Molecular pathology of primary intraocular lymphoma. *Trans Am Ophthalmol Soc.* 101, 275-292.

[74] Garweg J, Böhnke M, (1997). Varicella-zoster virus is strongly associated with atypical necrotizing herpetic retinopathies. *Clin Infect* Dis. 24, 603-608.

[75] de Smet MD, Nussenblatt RB, Davis JL, Palestine AG, (1990). Large cell lymphoma masquerading as a viral retinitis. *Int Ophthalmol.* 14, 413-417.

[76] Davis JL, Solomon D, Nussenblatt RB, Palestine AG, Chan CC, (1992). Immunocytochemical staining of vitreous cells. Indications, techniques, and results. *Ophthalmology.* 99, 250-256.

[77] Margo CE, Hamed LM, (1992). Ocular syphilis. *Surv Ophthalmol.* 37, 203-220.

[78] Roe RH, Michael Jumper J, Fu AD, Johnson RN, Richard McDonald H, Cunningham ET, (2008). Ocular bartonella infections. *Int Ophthalmol Clin.* 48, 93-105.

[79] Birnbaum AD, Huang W, Sahin O, Tessler HH, Goldstein DA, (2012). Ocular sarcoidosis misdiagnosed as primary intraocular lymphoma. *Retina.* 30, 310-316.

[80] Govender P, Berman JS, (2015). The Diagnosis of Sarcoidosis. *Clin Chest Med.* 36, 585-602.

[81] Tugal-Tutkun I, Onal S, Altan-Yaycioglu R, Huseyin Altunbas H, Urgancioglu M, (2004). Uveitis in Behçet disease: an analysis of 880 patients. *Am J Ophthalmol.* 138, 373-380.

[82] Rubsamen PE, Gass JD, (1991). Vogt-Koyanagi-Harada syndrome. Clinical course, therapy, and long-term visual outcome. *Arch Ophthalmol.* 109, 682-687.

[83] Matsuo T, Yamaoka A, Shiraga F, Matsuo N, (1998). Two types of initial ocular manifestations in intraocular-central nervous system lymphoma. *Retina.* 18, 301-307.

[84] Velez G, de Smet MD, Whitcup SM, Robinson M, Nussenblatt RB, Chan CC, (2000). Iris involvement in primary intraocular lymphoma: report of two cases and review of the literature. *Surv Ophthalmol.* 44, 518-526.

[85] van Oterendorp C, Ness T, Illerhaus G, Neuburger M, Jordan JF, (2014). The trabectome as treatment option in secondary glaucoma due to intraocular lymphoma. *J Glaucoma.* 23, 482-484.

[86] Coupland SE, Heimann H, Bechrakis NE, (2004). Primary intraocular lymphoma: a review of the clinical, histopathological and molecular biological features. *Graefes Arch Clin Exp Ophthalmol.* 242, 901-913.

[87] Wagoner MD, Gonder JR, Albert DM, Canny CL, (1980). Ocular pathology for clinicians: 3. Intraocular reticulum cell sarcoma. *Ophthalmology.* 87, 724-727.

[88] Tuaillon N, Chan CC, (2001). Molecular analysis of primary central nervous system and primary intraocular lymphomas. *Curr Mol Med.* 1, 259-272.

[89] Gill MK, Jampol LM, (2001). Variations in the presentation of primary intraocular lymphoma: case reports and a review. *Surv Ophthalmol.* 45, 463-471.

[90] Hedayatfar A, Phaik Chee S, (2012). Presumptive primary intraocular lymphoma presented as an intraocular mass involving the optic nerve head. *J Ophthalmic Inflamm Infect.* 2, 49-51.

[91] Gass JD, Trattler HL, (1991). Retinal artery obstruction and atheromas associated with non-Hodgkin's large cell lymphoma (reticulum cell sarcoma). *Arch Ophthalmol.* 109, 1134-1139.

[92] Fardeau C, Lee CP, Merle-Béral H, Cassoux N, Bodaghi B, Davi F, Lehoang P, (2009). Retinal fluorescein, indocyanine green angiography, and optic coherence tomography in non-Hodgkin primary intraocular lymphoma. *Am J Ophthalmol.* 147,886-894.

[93] Velez G, Chan CC, Csaky KG, (2002). Fluorescein angiographic findings in primary intraocular lymphoma. *Retina.* 22, 37-43.

[94] Gass JD, (1972). Fluorescein angiography. An aid in the differential diagnosis of intraocular tumors. *Int Ophthalmol Clin.* 12, 85-120.

[95] Schmitz-Valckenberg S, Holz FG, Bird AC, Spaide RF, (2008). Fundus autofluorescence imaging: review and perspectives. *Retina.* 28, 385-409.

[96] Yeh S, Forooghian F, Wong WT, Faia LJ, Cukras C, Lew JC, Wroblewski K, Weichel ED, Meyerle CB, Sen HN, Chew EY, Nussenblatt RB, (2010). Fundus autofluorescence imaging of the white dot syndromes. *Arch Ophthalmol.* 128, 46-56.

[97] Casady M, Faia L, Nazemzadeh M, Nussenblatt R, Chan CC, Sen HN, (2014). Fundus autofluorescence patterns in primary intraocular lymphoma. *Retina.* 34, 366-372.

[98] Egawa M, Mitamura Y, Hayashi Y, Naito T, (2014). Spectral-domain optical coherence tomographic and fundus autofluorescence findings in eyes with primary intraocular lymphoma. *Clin Ophthalmol.* 31, 335-341.

[99] Ishida T, Ohno-Matsui K, Kaneko Y, Tobita H, Shimada N, Takase H, Mochizuki M, (2010). Fundus autofluorescence patterns in eyes with primary intraocular lymphoma. *Retina.* 30, 23-32.

[100] Gass JD, Sever RJ, Grizzard WS, Clarkson JG, Blumenkranz M, Wind CA, Shugarman R, (2003). Multifocal pigment epithelial detachments by reticulum cell sarcoma: a characteristic funduscopic picture. *Retina.* 23, 135-143.

[101] Shields CL, Materin MA, Shields JA, (2005). Review of optical coherence tomography for intraocular tumors. *Curr Opin Ophthalmol.* 16, 141-154.

[102] Gallagher MJ, Yilmaz T, Cervantes-Castañeda RA, Foster CS, (2007). The characteristic features of optical coherence tomography in posterior uveitis. *Br J Ophthalmol.* 91, 1680-1685.

[103] Jang HS, Sepah YJ, Sophie R, Bittencourt MG, Ferraz D, Hanout M, Liu H, Do DV, Nguyen QD, (2013). Longitudinal spectral domain optical coherence tomography changes in eyes with intraocular lymphoma. J Ophthalmic *Inflamm Infect.* 3, 59.

[104] Zaldivar RA, Martin DF, Holden JT, Grossniklaus HE, (2004). Primary intraocular lymphoma: clinical, cytologic, and flow cytometric analysis. *Ophthalmology.* 111, 1762-1767.

[105] Char DH, Kemlitz AE, Miller T, (2005). Intraocular biopsy. *Ophthalmol Clin* 18, 177-185.

[106] Coupland SE, Bechrakis NE, Anastassiou G, Foerster AM, Heiligenhaus A, Pleyer U, Hummel M, Stein H, (2003). Evaluation of vitrectomy specimens and chorioretinal biopsies in the diagnosis of primary intraocular lymphoma in patients with Masquerade syndrome. *Graefes Arch Clin Exp Ophthalmol.* 241, 860-870.

[107] Whitcup SM, Chan CC, Buggage RR, Nussenblatt RB, Byrnes GA, Rubin BI, (2000). Improving the diagnostic yield of vitrectomy for intraocular lymphoma. *Arch Ophthalmol.* 118, 446.

[108] Intzedy L, Teoh SC, Hogan A, Mangwana S, Mayer EJ, Dick AD, Pawade J, (2008). Cytopathological analysis of vitreous in intraocular lymphoma. *Eye* (Lond). 22, 289-293.

[109] Gonzales JA, Chan CC, (2007). Biopsy techniques and yields in diagnosing primary intraocular lymphoma. *Int Ophthalmol.* 27, 241-250.

[110] Johnston RL, Tufail A, Lightman S, Luthert PJ, Pavesio CE, Cooling RJ, Charteris D, (2004). Retinal and choroidal biopsies are helpful in unclear uveitis of suspected infectious or malignant origin. *Ophthalmology.* 111, 522-528.

[111] Peyman GA, Dodich NA, (1972). Full-thickness eye wall resection: an experimental approach for treatment of choroidal melanoma. I. Dacron-graft. *Invest Ophthalmol.* 11, 115-121.

[112] Peyman GA, Meisels HI, Batko KA, Vlchek JK, (1975). Full-thickness eye wall biopsy. I. An experimental approach to the tissue diagnosis and study of choroidal and retinal lesions. *Invest Ophthalmol.* 14, 484-487.

[113] Peyman GA, Juarez CP, Raichand M, (1981). Full-thickness eye-wall biopsy: long-term results in 9 patients. *Br J Ophthalmol.* 65, 723-726.

[114] Martin DF, Chan CC, de Smet MD, Palestine AG, Davis JL, Whitcup SM, Burnier MN Jr, Nussenblatt RB, (1993). The role of chorioretinal biopsy in the management of posterior uveitis. *Ophthalmology.* 100, 705-714.

[115] Cassoux N, Charlotte F, Rao NA, Bodaghi B, Merle-Beral H, Lehoang P, (2005). Endoretinal biopsy in establishing the diagnosis of uveitis: a clinicopathologic report of three cases. *Ocul Immunol Inflamm.* 13, 79-83.

[116] Blay JY, Burdin N, Rousset F, Lenoir G, Biron P, Philip T, Banchereau J, Favrot MC, (1993). Serum interleukin-10 in non-Hodgkin's lymphoma: a prognostic factor. *Blood.* 82, 2169-2174.

[117] Whitcup SM, Stark-Vancs V, Wittes RE, Solomon D, Podgor MJ, Nussenblatt RB, Chan CC, (1997). Association of interleukin 10 in the vitreous and cerebrospinal fluid and primary central nervous system lymphoma. *Arch Ophthalmol.* 115, 1157-1160.

[118] Chan CC, Whitcup SM, Solomon D, Nussenblatt RB, (1995). Interleukin-10 in the vitreous of patients with primary intraocular lymphoma. *Am J Ophthalmol.* 120, 671-673.

[119] Bogdan C, Vodovotz Y, Nathan C, (1991). Macrophage deactivation by interleukin 10. *J Exp Med.* 174, 1549-1555.

[120] Murray PI, Hoekzema R, van Haren MA, de Hon FD, Kijlstra A, (1990). Aqueous humor interleukin-6 levels in uveitis. *Invest Ophthalmol Vis Sci.* 31, 917-920.

[121] Wolf LA, Reed GF, Buggage RR, Nussenblatt RB, Chan CC, (2003). Vitreous cytokine levels. *Ophthalmology.* 110, 1671-1672.

[122] Wang Y, Shen D, Wang VM, Sen HN, Chan CC, (2011). Molecular biomarkers for the diagnosis of primary vitreoretinal lymphoma. *Int J Mol Sci.* 12, 5684-5697.

[123] Fisson S, Ouakrim H, Touitou V, Baudet S, Ben Abdelwahed R, Donnou S, Miloudi A, Galand C, Bodaghi B, Lehoang P, Brissard M, Le Garff-Tavernier M, Fridman WH, Sautès-Fridman C, Cassoux N, Merle-Béral H, (2013). Cytokine profile in human eyes: contribution of a new cytokine combination for differential diagnosis between intraocular lymphoma or uveitis. *PLoS One*. 8(2): e52385.

[124] Chang TP, Poltoratsky V, Vancurova I, (2015). Bortezomib inhibits expression of TGF-β1, IL-10, and CXCR4, resulting in decreased survival and migration of cutaneous T cell lymphoma cells. *J Immunol*. 194, 2942-2953.

[125] Grimm SA, McCannel CA, Omuro AM, Ferreri AJ, Blay JY, Neuwelt EA, Siegal T, Batchelor T, Jahnke K, Shenkier TN, Hall AJ, Graus F, Herrlinger U, Schiff D, Raizer J, Rubenstein J, Laperriere N, Thiel E, Doolittle N, Iwamoto FM, Abrey LE, (2008). Primary CNS lymphoma with intraocular involvement: International PCNSL Collaborative Group Report. *Neurology*. 71, 1355-1360.

[126] Jahnke K, Korfel A, Komm J, Bechrakis NE, Stein H, Thiel E, Coupland SE, (2006). Intraocular lymphoma 2000-2005: results of a retrospective multicentre trial. *Graefes Arch Clin Exp Ophthalmol*. 244, 663-669.

[127] Taoka K, Yamamoto G, Kaburaki T, Takahashi T, Araie M, Kurokawa M, (2012). Treatment of primary intraocular lymphoma with rituximab, high dose methotrexate, procarbazine, and vincristine chemotherapy, reduced whole-brain radiotherapy, and local ocular therapy. *Br J Haematol*. 57, 252-254.

[128] British Neuro-Oncology Society/NCAT Rare Tumor Guidelines (June 2011). Available at http://www.bnos.org.uk.

[129] Nelson DF, Martz KL, Bonner H, Nelson JS, Newall J, Kerman HD, Thomson JW, Murray KJ, (1992). Non-Hodgkin's lymphoma of the brain: can high dose, large volume radiation therapy improve survival? Report on a prospective trial by the Radiation Therapy Oncology Group (RTOG): RTOG 8315. *Int J Radiat Oncol Biol Phys* 23, 9-17.

[130] Isobe K, Ejima Y, Tokumaru S, Shikama N, Suzuki G, Takemoto M, Tsuchida E, Nomura M, Shibamoto Y, Hayabuchi N, (2006). Treatment of primary intraocular lymphoma with radiation therapy: a multi-institutional survey in Japan. *Leuk Lymphoma*. 47, 1800-1805.

[131] Deangelis LM, Yahalom J, Rosenblum M, Posner JB, (1987). Primary CNS lymphoma: managing patients with spontaneous and AIDS-related disease. *Oncology* (Williston Park). 1, 52-62.

[132] Corry J, Smith JG, Wirth A, Quong G, Liew KH, (1988). Primary central nervous system lymphoma: age and performance status are more important than treatment modality. *Int J Radiat Oncol Biol Phys*. 41, 615-620.

[133] Berenbom A, Davila RM, Lin HS, Harbour JW, (2007). Treatment outcomes for primary intraocular lymphoma: implications for external beam radiotherapy. *Eye* (Lond).21, 1198-1201.

[134] Margolis L, Fraser R, Lichter A, Char DH, (1980). The role of radiation therapy in the management of ocular reticulum cell sarcoma. *Cancer*. 45, 688-692.

[135] Sandor V, Stark-Vancs V, Pearson D, Nussenblat R, Whitcup SM, Brouwers P, Patronas N, Heiss J, Jaffe E, de Smet M, Kohler D, Simon R, Wittes R, (1998). Phase II trial of chemotherapy alone for primary CNS and intraocular lymphoma. *J Clin Oncol*. 16, 3000-3006.

[136] Hoang-Xuan K, Bessell E, Bromberg J, Hottinger AF, Preusser M, Rucà R, Schlegel U, Siegal T, Soussain C, Abacioglu U, Cassoux N, Deckert M, Dirven CM, Ferreri AJ, Graus F, Henriksson R, Herrlinger U, Taphoorn M, Soffietti R, Weller M; European Association for Neuro-Oncology Task Force on Primary CNS Lymphoma. (2015). Diagnosis and treatment of primary CNS lymphoma in immunocompetent patients: guidelines from the European Association for Neuro-Oncology. *Lancet Oncol,* 16, 322-332.

[137] Ferreri AJ, Blay JY, Reni M, Pasini F, Gubkin A, Tirelli U, Calderoni A, Zucca E, Cortelazzo S, Chassagne C, Tinguely M, Borisch B, Berger F, Ponzoni M, Cavalli F; International Extranodal Lymphoma Study Group (IELSG).,(2002). Relevance of intraocular involvement in the management of primary central nervous system lymphomas. *Ann Oncol.* 13, 531-538.

[138] Kim SK, Chan CC, Wallace DJ, (2005). Management of primary intraocular lymphoma. *Curr Oncol Rep.* 7, 74-79.

[139] O'Neill BP., O'Fallon JR, Earle JD, Colgan JP, Brown LD, Krigel RL. (1995). Primary central nervous system non-Hodgkin's lymphoma: survival advantages with combined initial therapy? *Int J Radiat Oncol* Biol Phys 33, 663-673.

[140] Schultz C, Scott C, Sherman W, Donahue B, Fields J, Murray K, Fisher B, Abrams R, Meis-Kindblom J, (1996). Preirradiation chemotherapy with cyclophosphamide, doxorubicin, vincristine, and dexamethasone for primary CNS lymphomas: initial report of radiation therapy oncology group protocol 88-06. *J Clin Oncol* 14, 556-564.

[141] Henson JW, Yang J, Batchelor T, (1999). Intraocular methotrexate level after high-dose intravenous infusion. *J Clin Oncol.* 17, 1329.

[142] Batchelor TT, Kolak G, Ciordia R, Foster CS, Henson JW, (2003). High-dose methotrexate for intraocular lymphoma. *Clin Cancer Res.* 9, 711-715.

[143] Sullivan SF, Dallow RI, (1977). Intraocular reticulum cell sarcoma: its dramatic response to systemic chemotherapy and its angiogenic potential. *Ann Ophthalmol.* 9, 401-406.

[144] DeAngelis LM, Seiferheld W, Schold SC, Fisher B, Schultz CJ, (2002). Combination chemotherapy and radiotherapy for primary central nervous system lymphoma: Radiation Therapy Oncology Group Study 93-10. *J Clin Oncol.* 20, 4643-4648.

[145] Abrey LE, Yahalom J, DeAngelis LM, (2000). Treatment for primary CNS lymphoma: the next step. *J Clin Oncol.* 18, 3144-3150.

[146] Hiraga S, Arita N, Ohnishi T, Kohmura E, Yamamoto K, Oku Y, Taki T, Sato M, Aozasa K, Yoshimine T, (1999). Rapid infusion of high-dose methotrexate resulting in enhanced penetration into cerebrospinal fluid and intensified tumor response in primary central nervous system lymphomas. *J Neurosurg.* 91, 221-230.

[147] Ferreri AJ, Reni M, Pasini F, Calderoni A, Tirelli U, Pivnik A, Aondio GM, Ferrarese F, Gomez H, Ponzoni M, Borisch B, Berger F, Chassagne C, Iuzzolino P, Carbone A, Weis J, Pedrinis E, Motta T, Jouvet A, Barbui T, Cavalli F, Blay JY, (2002). A multicenter study of treatment of primary CNS lymphoma. *Neurology.* 58, 1513-1520.

[148] Mason JO, Fischer DH, (2003). Intrathecal chemotherapy for recurrent central nervous system intraocular lymphoma. *Ophthalmology.* 110, 1241-1244.

[149] de Smet MD, Stark-Vancs V, Kohler DR, Smith J, Wittes R, Nussenblatt RB, (1996). Intraocular levels of methotrexate after intravenous administration. *Am J Ophthalmol.* 121, 442-444.

[150] Baumann MA, Ritch PS, Hande KR, Williams GA, Topping TM, Anderson T, (1986). Treatment of intraocular lymphoma with high-dose Ara-C. *Cancer.* 57, 1273-1275.
[151] Strauchen JA, Dalton J, Friedman AH, (1989). Chemotherapy in the management of intraocular lymphoma. *Cancer.* 63, 1918-1921.
[152] Jahnke K, Bechrakis NE, Coupland SE, Schmittel A, Foerster MH, Fischer L, Thiel E, Korfel A, (2004). Treatment of primary intraocular lymphoma with oral trofosfamide: report of two cases and review of the literature. *Graefes Arch Clin Exp Ophthalmol.* 242, 771-776.
[153] Jahnke K, Wagner T, Bechrakis NE, Willerding G, Coupland SE, Fischer L, Thiel E, Korfel A, (2005). Pharmacokinetics and efficacy of ifosfamide or trofosfamide in patients with intraocular lymphoma. *Ann Oncol.* 16, 1974-1978.
[154] Jahnke K, Thiel E, Bechrakis NE, Willerding G, Kraemer DF, Fischer L, Korfel A, (2009). Ifosfamide or trofosfamide in patients with intraocular lymphoma. *J Neurooncol.* 93, 213-217.
[155] Ericson L, Karlberg B, Rosengren BH, (1964). Trials of intravitreal injections of chemotherapeutic agents in rabbits. *Acta Ophthalmol* (Copenh). 42, 721-726.
[156] Fishburne BC, Wilson DJ, Rosenbaum JT, Neuwelt EA, (1997). Intravitreal methotrexate as an adjunctive treatment of intraocular lymphoma. *Arch Ophthalmol.* 115, 1152-1156.
[157] Smith JR, Rosenbaum JT, Wilson DJ, Doolittle ND, Siegal T, Neuwelt EA, Pe'er J, (2002). Role of intravitreal methotrexate in the management of primary central nervous system lymphoma with ocular involvement. *Ophthalmology.* 109, 1709-1716.
[158] Frenkel S, Hendler K, Siegal T, Shalom E, Pe'er J, (2008). Intravitreal methotrexate for treating vitreoretinal lymphoma: 10 years of experience. *Br J Ophthalmol.* 92, 383-388.
[159] de Smet MD,(2001). Management of non-Hodgkin's intraocular lymphoma with intravitreal methotrexate. *Bull Soc Belge Ophtalmol.* 279, 91-95.
[160] Sen HN, Chan CC, Byrnes G, Fariss RN, Nussenblatt RB, Buggage RR, (2008). Intravitreal methotrexate resistance in a patient with primary intraocular lymphoma. *Ocul Immunol Inflamm.* 16, 29-33.
[161] Maloney DG, Smith B, Rose A, (2002). Rituximab: mechanism of action and resistance. *Semin Oncol.* 29, 2-9.
[162] Yeh S, Wilson DJ, (2010). Combination intravitreal rituximab and methotrexate for massive subretinal lymphoma. *Eye* (Lond). 24, 1625-1627.
[163] Ohguro N, Hashida N, Tano Y, (2008). Effect of intravitreous rituximab injections in patients with recurrent ocular lesions associated with central nervous system lymphoma. *Arch Ophthalmol.* 126, 1002-1003.
[164] Kim H, Csaky KG, Chan CC, Bungay PM, Lutz RJ, Dedrick RL, Yuan P, Rosenberg J, Grillo-Lopez AJ, Wilson WH, Robinson MR, (2006). The pharmacokinetics of rituximab following an intravitreal injection. *Exp Eye Res.* 82, 760-766.
[165] Kitzmann AS, Pulido JS, Mohney BG, Baratz KH, Grube T, Marler RJ, Donaldson MJ, O'Neill BP, Johnston PB, Johnson KM, Dixon LE, Salomao DR, Cameron JD, (2007). Intraocular use of rituximab. *Eye* (Lond). 21, 1524-1527.
[166] Bakri SJ, Cameron JD, McCannel CA, Pulido JS, Marler RJ, (2006). Absence of histologic retinal toxicity of intravitreal bevacizumab in a rabbit model. *Am J Ophthalmol.* 142, 162-164.

[167] Pulido JS, Bakri SJ, Valyi-Nagy T, Shukla D, (2007). Rituximab penetrates full-thickness retina in contrast to tissue plasminogen activator control. *Retina*. 27, 1071-1073.

[168] Shahar J, Avery RL, Heilweil G, Barak A, Zemel E, Lewis GP, Johnson PT, Fisher SK, Perlman I, Loewenstein A, (2006). Electrophysiologic and retinal penetration studies following intravitreal injection of bevacizumab (Avastin). *Retina*. 26, 262-269.

[169] Larkin KL, Saboo US, Comer GM, Forooghian F, Mackensen F, Merrill P, Sen HN, Singh A, Essex RW, Lake S, Lim LL, Vasconcelos-Santos DV, Foster CS, Wilson DJ, Smith JR, (2014). Use of intravitreal rituximab for treatment of vitreoretinal lymphoma. *Br J Ophthalmol*. 98, 99-103.

[170] Gerdes J, (1990). Ki-67 and other proliferation markers useful for immunohistological diagnostic and prognostic evaluations in human malignancies. Review. *Semin Cancer Biol*. 1, 199-206.

[171] Soussain C, Choquet S, Fourme E, Delgadillo D, Bouabdallah K, Ghesquières H, Damaj G, Dupriez B, Vargaftig J, Gonzalez A, Houillier C, Taillandier L, Hoang-Xuan K, Leblond V, (2012). Intensive chemotherapy with thiotepa, busulfan and cyclophosphamide and hematopoietic stem cell rescue in relapsed or refractory primary central nervous system lymphoma and intraocular lymphoma: a retrospective study of 79 cases. *Haematologica*.97, 1751-1756.

[172] Riemens A, Bromberg J, Touitou V, Sobolewska B, Missotten T, Baarsma S, Hoyng C, Cordero-Coma M, Tomkins-Netzer O, Rozalski A, Tugal-Tutkun I, Guex-Crosier Y, Los LI, Bollemeijer JG, Nolan A, Pawade J, Willermain F, Bodaghi B, ten Dam-van Loon N, Dick A, Zierhut M, Lightman S, Mackensen F, Moulin A, Errkens R, Wensing B, le Hoang P, Lokhorst H, Rothova A, (2015). Treatment strategies in primary vitreoretinal lymphoma: a 17-center European collaborative study. *JAMA Ophthalmol*. 133, 191-197.

[173] Choi JY, Kafkala C, Foster CS, (2006). Primary intraocular lymphoma: A review. *Semin Ophthalmol*. 21, 125-133.

In: Primary Central Nervous System Lymphoma (PCNSL) ISBN: 978-1-63485-322-4
Editor: Ryuya Yamanaka

Chapter 18

INTRAVASCULAR LYMPHOMA

Shigeru Koyano*[*]*, Hiroshi Doi and Fumiaki Tanaka
Department of Neurology and Stroke Medicine,
Yokohama City University, Graduate School of Medicine,
Yokohama, Japan

ABSTRACT

Intravascular lymphoma (IVL) is a rare diffuse large B-cell lymphoma characterized by the proliferation of clonal lymphocytes within the lumina of small vessels of various organs with relative sparing of the surrounding tissue. IVL displays aggressive clinical behavior and usually disseminated disease, resulting in a delay in timely and accurate diagnosis and fatal complications. The diagnosis is almost exclusively made by surgical biopsy of a suspected site of involvement; the brain and skin are the most commonly involved sites. Although some patients with this disease may be cured with anti-CD20 monoclonal antibody (rituximab) therapy, the foundation of treatment is early diagnosis and treatment.

Keywords: intravascular lymphoma, diffuse large B-cell lymphoma, skin biopsy, rituximab

INTRODUCTION

Intravascular lymphoma (IVL) was first described in 1959 by Pfleger and Tappeiner in Germany [1]. In the 2001 WHO classification of hematopoietic tumors, IVL was defined as a rare type of non-Hodgkin's lymphoma (NHL) characterized by the selective growth of neoplastic cells within blood vessel lumina. Subsequently intravascular large B-cell lymphoma (IVLBCL) was defined as a rare subtype of extranodal diffuse large B-cell lymphoma according to the WHO classification in 2008, and, in the recent revision of tumor classifications, it was classified as an independent disease entity [2]. IVL is characterized by

* Corresponding Author address: 3-9 Fukuura, Kanazawa-ku, Yokohama 236-0004, Japan. Email: koya77@yokohama-cu.ac.jp.

the proliferation of lymphoma cells within the lumina of small blood vessels, particularly capillaries and post-capillary venules, without an obvious extravascular tumor mass or detectable circulating lymphoma cells in the peripheral blood. The clinical features are various and most clinical and biological properties are largely unknown. Previously, approximately half of IVL cases were diagnosed only after autopsy because of the lack of remarkable lymphadenopathy and non-specific clinical abnormalities. However, the diagnosis has been recently facilitated by random skin biopsy and FDG-PET. IVL has been called by the following various names:

Tappeiner – Pfleger disease

- Angioendotheliomatosis proliferans systemisata
- Intravascular endothelioma
- (Malignant) angioendothelioma (tosis)
- Neoplastic angioendotheliosis (endotheliomatosis)
- Proliferating angioendotheliomatosis
- Systemic endotheliomatosis
- Angio-endotheliotropic (intravascular) lymphoma (Kiel Classification)
- Angiotropic (intravascular) (large-cell) lymphoma (Lukes-Collins Classification)
- Diffuse large B-cell lymphoma (REAL Classification)
- Intravascular (malignant) lymphoma (tosis)
- Intravascular large B-cell lymphoma (tosis)

EPIDEMIOLOGY

IVL is a rare disease with an estimated incidence of less than one person per million based on its rate of appearance in the literature from Western countries [3-10]; however, it is different in the frequency according to the reports from Asia. The frequency of IVL among non-Hodgkin lymphoma was reported as 0.24% in Asia, and that previously reported from Japan, Hong Kong, and Thailand was 0.1%, 0.31%, and 0.91%, respectively [11]. IVL has been described in patients with ages ranging from 13–90 years at onset, with a median age in the sixth to seventh decades. It occurs almost equally in men and women (sex ratio: men/women =1.2:1).

There are two clinical classifications of IVL. In Western countries, isolated cutaneous involvement without systemic disease have been reported and this type has been classified as the cutaneous variant of IVL. The Asian variant, which has been reported in the majority of Japanese patients, rarely involves the skin but usually shows hemophagocytosis, with multiple hematolymphoid organ involvement, and displays a higher clinical stage at diagnosis.

There are no known risk factors for IVL; however, there are several factors that influence IVL such as diabetes mellitus, tumor, and pleural effusion.

The prognosis of IVL is poor and the mortality rate is higher than 80%. Poor prognostic factors include advanced age, high fever, high value of LDH, impaired performance status, and thrombocytopenia. On the other hand, a good prognostic factor is the cutaneous variant of the classical IVL type, which is localized in the skin [12-14].

Pathophysiology

IVL is a rare subtype of extranodal diffuse large B-cell lymphoma characterized by the proliferation of clonal lymphocytes within the lumina of small vessels of various organs, particularly capillaries and post-capillary venules, without an obvious extravascular tumor mass formation or detectable circulating lymphoma cells in a large blood vessel or a lymph node. The predilection of the tumor cells of IVL for capillary endothelium is likely related to the expression of molecules on the surface of lymphocytes.

Thus, aberrant expression of CD11a and CD49d (VLA-4) on IVL cells has been proposed as a possible mechanism for this mechanism because these adhesion molecules would enable B- cells to bind to CD54 (CD11a ligand) and CD106 (CD49d ligand), which are expressed on endothelial cell surfaces [15]. B-cells in IVL may be able to adhere, at least in part, to capillary endothelial cells; however, they seem to lack some molecules, such as CD29 (β1 integrin subunit) and CD54 (ICAM-1), which are critical for extravasation [16]. In this way, the mechanism of IVL may be associated with a disorder of cell docking at the secondary locking stage of the interaction of a tumor cell with an endothelial cell. It is likely that multiple defects are involved in this mechanism and future studies on this topic are warranted.

Clinical Features

Although IVL is commonly a fatal disease characterized by an aggressive course and poor outcome, some exceptions with long-term survivors have been reported. The clinical manifestations of IVL are extremely heterogeneous and most of the signs and symptoms are related to the numerous preferentially involved organs. Presenting symptoms at initial diagnosis, clinical features, laboratory findings, and other organ involvement in a previous cohort series of patients with IVL are summarized in Table 1 [4, 6, 10, 12, 17-29].

Overview of Clinical Features

The clinical manifestations of IVL are the systemic symptoms such as fever of unknown origin and general fatigue; skin symptoms such as rash and erythema; and progressive neurological symptoms such as unconsciousness and cognitive deficits. The most common systemic symptom is fever (30-100%), and the prevalence of fever in IVL is much more common than that in other aggressive extranodal lymphomas. In some cases, a persistent fever of unknown origin prompts us to perform bone marrow biopsy, and ultimately the diagnosis of IVL [7]. Fever is associated with other B symptoms (B symptoms refer to systemic symptoms of fever, night sweats, and weight loss which can be associated with lymphoma) in half of cases, while weight loss without fever is present only in 10% of cases.

Table 1. Clinical features in IVL

	Kitagawa M (17)	Dimizio P (4)	Stroup RM (18)	Glass J (19)	Bergmann M (20)	Demirer T (22)	DiGiuseppe JA (21)	Calami KT (23)	Murase T (24)	Baehring JM (25)	Ferreri AJM (6)	Sukpanichnant S (26)	Sukpanichnant S (26)	Murase T (12)	Ferreri AJM (27)	Ferreri AJM (27)	Shimada K (28)	Matsue K (29)
geographical origin	Asia	Western	Western	Western	Western	Western	Western	Western	Asia	Western	Western	Western +Asia		Asia	Western	Asia	Asia	Asia
Number of cases	3	86	7	7	5	4	10	10	25	7	38	20	102	96	50	123	106	13
Age at diagnosis (years)	64.3 (50-77)	56.4 (13-84)	68.6 (59–78)	63.4 (58-75)	62.2 (54-72)	67.7 (58-77)	69.1 (53-85)		66 (44-84)	60.7 (39-79)	70 (34-90)	62.2 (34-77)		67 (41-85)	68 (34-90)	67 (44-78)	67 (34-84)	69 (64-84)
Sex (M/F)	2/1	39/45	5/2	5/2	4/1	3/1	6/4		13/25	4/3	18/20	8/12		50/46	23/19		59/47	5/8
Clinical features (%)																		
fever	33	30	43	30	60	100	60	70	100	43	45	70	84	76	42	87	84	92.3
Neurological symptoms	100	32	14	100	100	50	60	100	16	100	34	25	78	27	42	21	24.5	38.5
Skin lesions	0	15	14	14		50	40		0	14	39	10	53	15	38	3	17	
Weight loss		21		14					16	14	35			76			84	
General fatigue		0		14					64	29	16							
Abdominal symptoms	33	3		14					20		5							
Respiratory symptoms	33	0			20		20		0		3			34			33	
Urinary disturbance	33	1		43			20				8							
Edema		0								14	5							
Lymphadenopathy		1																
Laboratory Findings (%)																		
Anemia	66			14	80	75	30	90	88	43	63	70	83	66	66	84	67.9	69.2
Leukocytopenia	0			14					88	14	24	5		27	22	29	27.4	

	Kitagawa M (17)	Dimizio P (4)	Stroup RM (18)	Glass J (19)	Bergmann M (20)	Demirer T (22)	DiGiuseppe JA (21)	Calami KT (23)	Murase T (24)	Baehring JM (25)	Ferreri AJM (6)	Sukpanichnant S (26)	Sukpanichnant S (26)	Murase T (12)	Ferreri AJM (27)	Ferreri AJM (27)	Shimada K (28)	Matsue K (29)
geographical origin	Asia	Western	Western	Western	Western	Western	Western	Western	Asia	Western	Western	Western +Asia		Asia	Western	Asia	Asia	Asia
Thrombocytopenia	33			43		25		20			29	60		58	32	74	58.5	69.2
Serum LDH level	100			14	80			100	96		86	85	93		85	100	98.1	92.3
Serum sL2-R level									100					69			65.6	
Hemophagocytosis									100					61				
Hepato-splenomegaly				14						14				77			65.1	
Organ involvement (%)																		
Brain	100			14	100						43			2.5				
Skin	100							60		71	39			7.4				53.8
Liver	100			14	80						26	20		33.4	26	77		76.9
Spleen	0				40						26							
Kidney					80						21							
Bone marrow	33							0	76		32	20		66.7	30	74		7.7
Lymph Node	33										11				8	5		
Lung	0										19							

The clinical presentation, behavior and therapeutic outcome are extremely variable; in particular, it has been suggested that there exist some differences in clinical and histopathological characteristics between patients diagnosed in Western and Asian countries. In Western countries, a 'cutaneous variant' of IVL, which only involves single or multiple lesions of the skin and the neurological system without systemic involvement, was recently proposed [6, 21, 30-34].

Conversely, in Asian countries, the cutaneous variant of IVL seems to be extremely rare, and the patients presented with fever, anemia, thrombocytopenia, hepatosplenomegaly, hemophagocytosis, bone marrow invasion, respiratory disturbance, and disseminated intravascular coagulopathy, but usually lacked lymphadenopathy, mass formation, neurological abnormalities, and skin lesions [12, 24, 27, 34-39]. The reported percentage of patients with these various symptoms in the two IVL variants are as follows:

Initial symptoms in Western variant (6, 40): neurological symptoms (39%) and skin symptoms (39%) are the main symptoms. Other organ involvements are bone marrow (32%), spleen (26%), and liver (26%).

Initial symptoms in Asian variant (12, 24): neurological symptoms (15%) and skin symptoms (27%) are fewer than in the Western variant. Conversely, anemia (63%), thrombocytopenia (29%), leukocytopenia (24%), hypoalbuminaemia (18%), and hemophagocytosis (59%) are the main symptoms. Other organ involvements are bone marrow (75%), spleen (67%), and liver (55%).

Skin Symptoms [7, 10, 41]

Cutaneous lesions in IVL encompass a widespread morphology and distribution, including painful indurate erythematous eruption and poorly circumscribed plaques. Lesions are single or multiple and are more commonly situated in the upper arms, thighs and legs, the lower abdomen, breast, and submammary region. When accompanied by capillary telangiectasia, edema, and vascular pain, it is difficult to distinguish cutaneous lesions in IVL from inflammatory skin diseases such as thrombophlebitis and nodular erythema.

Various skin characteristics are as follows:

erythematous eruptions, poorly circumscribed violaceous plaques, large solitary plaques, erythematous and desquamative plaques, peau d'orange change, cellulitis, painful blue-red palpable nodular discolorations, ulcerated nodules, palpable purpura, and small red palpable spots.

Neurological Symptoms [19, 20, 25, 42-44]

In IVL, neurological symptoms are noted in 25% of patients at initial diagnosis and 75–85% of IVL patients present with extremely heterogeneous neurological symptoms at final diagnosis. Symptoms attributable to central nervous system (CNS) involvement in IVL are diverse, with sensory and motor deficits, meningoradiculitis, paresthesias, hypostenia, aphasia, dysarthria, hemiparesis, seizures, myoclonus, transient visual loss, and vertigo. Additionally, peripheral nervous system (PNS) manifestations such as sensory neuropathy are also observed.

In particular, the following four neurological symptoms have been reported.

1) progressive, multifocal cerebrovascular events
2) subacute encephalopathy
3) spinal cord and nerve root vascular syndromes
4) peripheral or cranial neuropathies

Progressive, Multifocal Cerebrovascular Events [45-52]

In IVL with CNS involvement, most of the common symptoms observed are related to ischemia and infarction due to small vessel occlusion by the tumor cells. Ischemic strokes are the prominent clinical condition, which hide the diagnosis of the underlying IVL for a considerably long period of time. Multiple acute and subacute strokes prompt the performance of a brain biopsy in case IVL is present.

Macroscopically, multiple, sometimes hemorrhagic, infarcts are distributed within the brain and spinal cord. Microscopically, the characteristic sign is the distension and occlusion of small blood vessels in the brain by the tumor cells. IVL initially presents with disseminated intravascular coagulation (DIC) complicated by intracerebral hemorrhage.

Subacute Encephalopathy [51, 53, 54]

In subacute encephalopathy of IVL, alterations in the levels of consciousness occur in most patients. In some patients, localizing signs are absent, but such signs are more often accompanied by paraparesis, seizure, or other symptoms. Since progression of a rapidly developing dementia and myoclonus without additional focal neurological signs has been reported, differential diagnosis includes Creutzfeld–Jakob–Disease (CJD), acute disseminated encephalomyelitis (ADEM), progressive multifocal leucoencephalopathy (PML), and autoimmune mediated encephalopathy.

Spinal Cord and Nerve Root Vascular Syndromes [54-65]

In IVL, although spinal cord lesions are a common complication, it is rare that the initial central nervous system involvement is limited to the spinal cord. The lumbosacral spinal cord is a favored site in the spinal cord. The latest progress in neuroimaging techniques have indicated that the most recent IVL cases with myelopathy often show a cauda equina-conus medullaris syndrome with ascending subacute sensorimotor deficits and sacral autonomic involvement, which is an unusual site for myelitis. These symptoms are explained by spinal cord and cauda equina invasion by this particular form of lymphoma. Pathological studies of a similar form have also demonstrated both arterial and venous involvements of the lower spinal cord and roots.

Peripheral or Cranial Neuropathies [66-72]

In rare cases IVL is initially presented with peripheral neuropathy that mimics Guillain–Barre´ Syndrome (GBS) [73] or mononeuropathy multiplex [74]. On the basis of ascending weakness and sensory abnormality, elevated CSF protein, and absent F waves on electrodiagnostic testing, a clinical diagnosis becomes more consistent with GBS. Subsequent clinical examinations and repeats of nerve conduction study indicate a closer resemblance to mononeuropathy multiplex.

B-cell lymphomas infiltrate the nervous systems, and an estimated 10% of these infiltrations involve the peripheral nervous system on the diagnosis of neurolymphomatosis (NL) [75]. NL is a rare manifestation of IVL in which lymphoma cells infiltrate the peripheral nerves. NL is characterized clinically by a painful polyneuropathy or polyradiculopathy, cranial neuropathy, painless polyneuropathy, and peripheral mononeuropathy. Unfortunately, the diagnosis of NL is often difficult and requires histological confirmation of the affected nerve, which may not be feasible and is often not diagnostic.

These neurological symptoms are indicated in Table 2.

Table 2. Neurological findings in IVL

	Smadja D (42)	Glass J (19)	Liszka U (43)	Bergmann M (20)	Beristain X (44)	Baehring JM (25)
Number of cases	39	114	68	5	8	5
Neurological symptoms (%)	100	63	60.3	100	100	100
disconsciousness	49			80		
dementia			45.3	40	87.5	40
epilepsy	28		13.2		75	
headache	15			20		20
psychiatric disability			20.6	60		
paraplegia				60		
spinal cord disorder	38	38	20.6	20	25	40
ataxia				20		20
urinary disturbance						20
eye movement disorder		16				20
peripheral neuropathy		5	3			
cranial nerve dysfunction		21				
cognitive dysfunction				20		20

DIAGNOSIS [3, 24, 25, 76]

According to the WHO classification in 2008(2), IVL is defined as an extranodal B-cell lymphoma characterized by tumor involvement in the lumina of vessels, especially capillaries, with the exception of larger arteries and veins.

It is indispensable for the diagnosis of IVL to confirm the fact that tumor involvement can occur in any organ. Identification of tumor cells is relatively easy from pathological specimens, and the organs selected by the physician for biopsy are key to accurate diagnosis. Accurate diagnosis includes symptoms such as fever, neurological symptoms, and skin symptoms but not lymphadenopathy, increased serum lactate dehydrogenase, or IL-2 receptor concentration. Immunophenotyping has shown that 85% to 90% of IVL cases have their origin in B cells and that 10% to 15% of IVL cases have their origin in T cells; natural killer cells are rarely the origin [77].

Criteria for the Asian variant

There are no standard criteria for IVL due to its rarity and its non-specific symptoms. There are, however, established criteria for the Asian variant, and these criteria are indicated in Table 3 [24].

Table 3. Improved diagnostic criteria for the Asian variant of intravascular lymphoma (AIVL)

1	Clinical and laboratory criteria (at least two out of three are required)
	a. Cytopaenia (not caused by hypoplastic or dysplastic marrow), affecting at least one of the two lineages, i.e., erythrocytes and platelets. Leucocytes are not included. It is prescribed by haemoglobin (<11 g/dl) or RBC ($<3.5 \times 10^{12}$/l), and/or platelet count ($<100 \times 10^{9}$/l)
	b. Hepatomegaly and/or splenomegaly, identified by computerized tomography, ultra sonography or physical examination
	c. Absence of overt lymphadenopathy and tumour formation
2	Histopathological criteria (all three terms are required)
	a. Erythrocyte-haemophagocytosis; usually seen mildly or moderately in haemopoietic system
	b. Immunophenotypical evidence of proliferating neoplastic B cells with large cell morphology
	c. Pathological findings of intravascular proliferation and/or sinusoidal involvement of lymphoma cells

Criteria 1 and 2 are required for the diagnosis of AIVL.

Random Skin Biopsy [78-89]

IVL was previously checked by skin biopsy, especially for the Western variant; however, skin biopsy was not performed for the Asian variant without skin symptoms. In 2003, the diagnosis of IVL was established by random skin biopsies in patients who presented with fever of unknown origin and who did not have clinically evident skin involvement. By 2007, the clinical usefulness of random skin biopsy for the histological diagnosis of IVL in patients with no skin lesions, but whose clinical and laboratory data were suggestive of IVL, was becoming clear. However, some patients present with negative findings from random skin biopsies. Further large-scale studies are needed to clarify the significance of random skin biopsies for diagnosis of IVL, because the number of studies on this new diagnostic procedure is currently too small to confirm its usefulness.

LABORATORY FINDINGS

Most IVL patients display a pathological hemogram (Table 4). Anemia and elevated lactate dehydrogenase, erythrocyte sedimentation rate, IL-2 receptor, and β2 microglobulin are the most common laboratory abnormalities seen in IVL. Leukocytopenia and thrombocytopenia are seen less often [7]. The majority of studies have shown IVL to be absent in peripheral blood by histological examination of a peripheral smear. Some tumor markers have been reported for IVL and serum prostatic acid phosphatase (PAP) is a useful tumor marker. The sensitivity and specificity of PAP are 100% and 91%, respectively, in the diagnosis of IVL [90, 91]. The serum levels of PAP are closely associated with disease status. Among other reported markers, LR11, which is a type I membrane protein that releases serum soluble LR11 by proteolytic shedding, is a marker of angiostenosis and aberrant expression of pankeratin AE1/AE3 has been described. Altered hepatic, renal, or thyroid functional tests have been observed; these function tests are useful tools in the staging of IVL; indeed, altered results are invariably associated with organ involvement by lymphoma cells [92, 93].

Table 4. Laboratory findings in IVL

	frequency (%)
Anemia (<12g/dl)	63
Leukocytopenia (<4000/μl)	24
Thrombocytopenia (<15000/μl)	29
Serum LDH high level	86
Serumβ2-microglobulin high level	82
ESR elevation	43
Hypoalubuminemia (<3.6 g/dl)	18
Serum monoclonal component	14

Table 5. Translocations in IVL reported in the literature

	chromosomal band	Translocation	Involved oncogene	Function
Molina A (96)	14q32, 18q21	t(14;18)(q32;q21)	BCL2	cell death
Ichikawa N (97)	12q11	t(X;12)(p21;q11)		
	3q10, 18q10	t(3;18)(q10;q10)		
Tsukadaira A (94)	14q32, 18q21	t(14;18)(q32;q21)	BCL2	cell death
Khoury H (95)	10p12, 22q	t(10;22)(p12;q?)		
	17p11, 22q	t(17;22)(p11;q?)		
	11p15, 14q32	t(11;14)(p15;q32)		
		t(11;14)		
	1q, 14q32	t(1;14)(q2?;q32)		
	11q15, 14q32	t(11;14)(q15;q32)		
Rashid R (98)	11q13, 14q32	t(11;14)(q13;q32)	CD44	
Kobayashi T (100)	14q32, 19q13	t(14;19)(q32;q13)	BCL3	
Cui J (102)	3q27, 14q32	t(3;14)(q27;q32)	BCL6/BCL5	transcriptional factor

Cytogenetic Analysis and Spectral Karyotyping [24, 94-102]

Previous reports of cytogenetic findings in IVL presented a unique case of IVL with complete premortem morphological, immunophenotypic, cytogenetic, as well as molecular cytogenetic evaluation. In particular, neoplastic lymphocytes were present in the peripheral blood, and the lymphomatous infiltrate in the kidney involved both the glomerular and peritubular capillaries simultaneously. The majority of cases were characterized by a complex karyotype with multiple numerical and structural changes. The numerical changes included monosomy of chromosomes 1, 4, 6, and 15 and trisomy 18. Structural changes included numerous deletions involving 1q22, 3q27, 6p15, 11q13, 14q32, 18q21, and 19q13 and duplications of 18q and 11q. Previous cytogenetic and/or molecular evidence of translocations involving a chromosomal band have been reported in IVL (Table 5).

Radiographic Findings

MRI (Figure 1) [71, 103-109]

In IVL, radiographic findings consistent with ischemic changes of the CNS have been reported. These changes are similar to changes consistent with CNS vasculitis. MRI appearances are nonspecific; the most suggestive findings are both asymmetrical, bilateral, contrast enhancing high-signal areas on T2 weighting and infarct-like lesions of the cortex and basal ganglia. In the most significant previous reports, MRI showed high signal lesions in the deep white matter, which appear to correlate pathologically with edema and gliosis. In infarct-like lesions correlated with recent or resolving infarcts usually reported pathologically, the diagnostic criteria were high-signal lesions in grey matter on T2-weighted images involving a vascular territory with little or no edema.

Patterns of abnormal MRI findings in IVL are: 1) infarct-like lesions, 2) nonspecific white matter lesions, 3) meningeal enhancement, 4) mass-like lesions, and 5) hyperintense lesions in the pons on T2WI.

The pathological features of the MRI in IVL are as follows:

1. The multiple pathological changes of MRI-diffusion reflect ischemic changes of small vessels, which are difficult to classify as a standard cerebral infarction.
2. The pathological changes of GD-MRI are adjacent areas of MRI-T2 or MRI-diffusion and spread over several weeks.

FDG/PET (Figure 2) [110-119]

FDG-PET/CT and random skin biopsy may be useful for the early diagnosis of IVL, because the tumor has a very high cellular density with an accelerated glucose metabolism and therefore shows a huge uptake of FDG into the tumor. FDG-PET can detect pathologically confirmed lesions as positive FDG-PET findings and the number of tumor cells in pathological specimens tended to be high when FDG-PET and biopsy findings matched. These findings suggested that the number of tumor cells per volume might be lower for IVL than for nodal lymphoma, with selective growth of tumor cells in the lumina of small vessels.

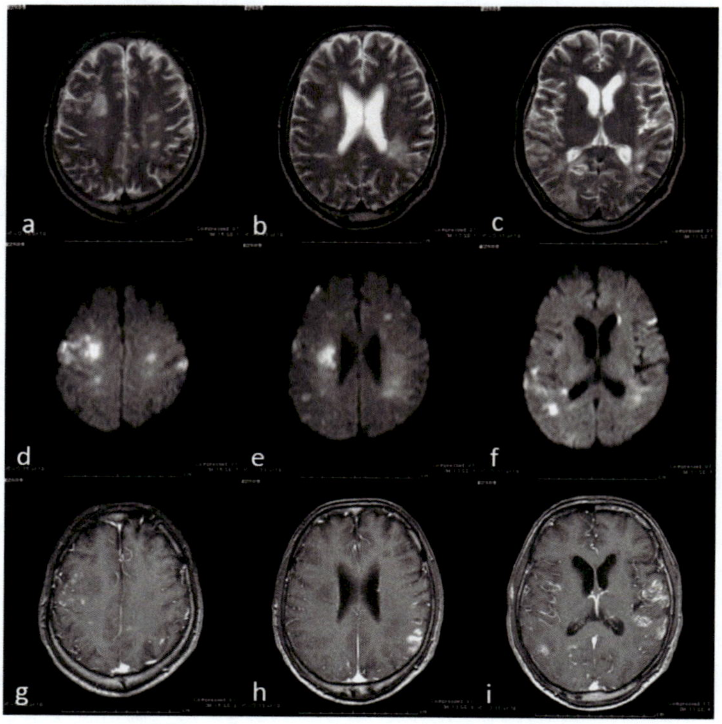

Figure 1. Brain MRI of IVL. Infarct-like lesions are observed in a IVL patients, appearing as multiple hyperintense spots on T2 image (a, b, c), Diffusion image (d, e, f) and T1 with gadolinium image (g, h, i) in white matter, including the periventricular areas.

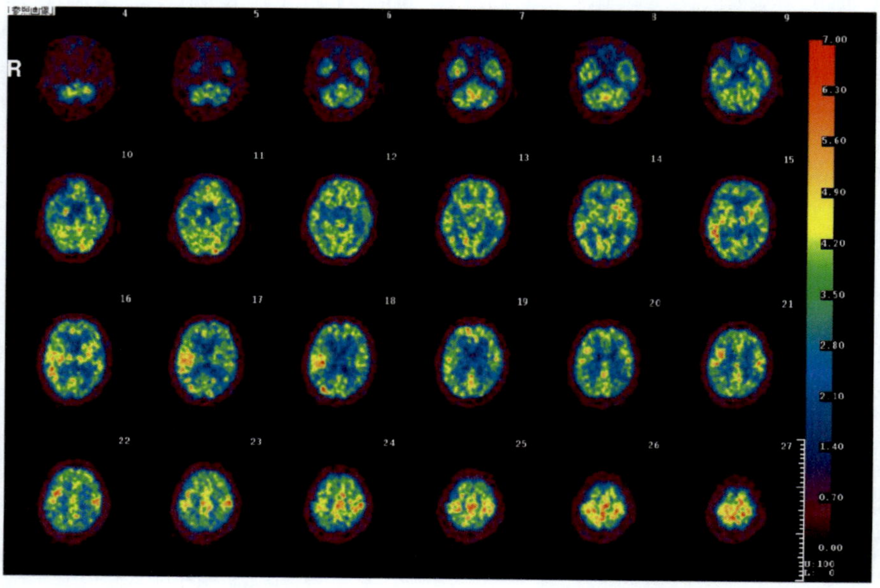

Figure 2. (Continued)

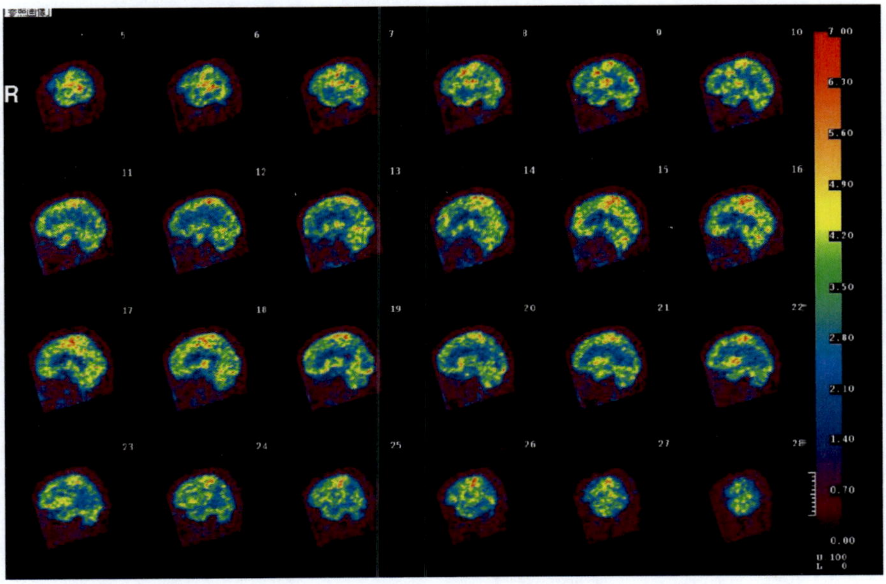

Figure 2 Brain FDG-PET of IVL. Positron emission tomography with ^{18}fluorodeoxyglucose (FDG-PET) images showing focally increase FDG uptake corresponding to the MRI lesions in white matter.

Pathological Findings [12, 16, 18, 24, 29, 94, 95, 120-123]

Tissue biopsy is mandatory for definitive diagnosis of IVL, and any affected organ has the potential to demonstrate microscopic evidence of the disease process. The tissues most commonly reported to be involved include bone marrow and peripheral blood, liver, spleen, skin, lung, and lymph node; however, other affected organs including heart, bowel, kidney, and CNS can potentially demonstrate microscopic evidence of the disease process (Table 6).

IVL is characterized by the proliferation of lymphoma cells within the lumina of small blood vessels, particularly capillaries and post-capillary venules. A tumor cell is circular, and the size of the cell is very similar to that of a lymphocyte. The nucleus of the tumor cell is enriched with chromatin with a clear nuclear membrane and nucleolus. The histological appearance of IVL involvement of brain, renal parenchyma, and thyroid has been shown, demonstrating the classic appearance of large malignant lymphocytes filling small vascular lumina. Lymphoma cells are included in the blood vessel with pathological changes such as thrombus formation, lymphocyte infiltration into the blood vessel wall, and fibrous thickening of the outer membrane of the small artery and the vein.

A summary of immunophenotypic features of IVL is as follows. Most of the tumor cells express B-cell antigens such as CD20 and are negative for CD3 epsilon (Figure 3). Occasionally, CD5 and CD10 can be expressed as well. Common antigens demonstrated to be frequently expressed by IVL cells include the following: CD79a, CD20, MUM1/IRF4, Bcl-2, CD19, immunoglobulin k light chain, CD5, Bcl-6, immunoglobulin l light chain (18%), CD10 (12%), and CD23 (4%).

Table 6. Tissue organ for definitive diagnosis of IVL

organ	Number of cases (N = 108)
bone marrow	88
liver	17
skin	16
lung	11
spleen	8
kidney	5
lymph node	3
adrenal gland	2
uterus	2
brain	1
testis	1
urinary duct	1
bladder	1

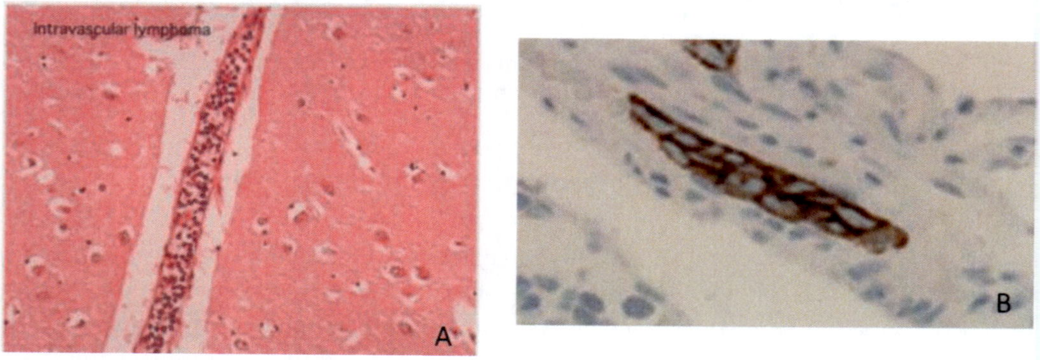

Figure 3 Microscopic findings of intravascular lymphocytes in central nervous system (frontal lobe). Large lymphoma cells fill the small vessels of the cerebral cortex. (A, ×100, H&E). Immunohistochemical staining of those cells shows positive cytoplasmic immunoreactivity to CD20. (B, × 200).

Treatment [10, 13, 25, 28, 122, 124-126]

Previously, the treatment of choice for all patients with IVL was combination chemotherapy. Cyclophosphamide, Adriamycin, Oncovin, and prednisone (CHOP) and CHOP-like chemotherapy have achieved positive objective responses; however, anthracycline-based chemotherapy has been associated with superior remission and overall survival rates. In previous reports, about half of the patients were diagnosed postmortem and the effect of steroid therapies was tentative.

Clinical outcomes of IVL were extremely dismal before the era of the anti-CD20 monoclonal antibody, rituximab. One important reason for such a dismal prognosis is the difficulty of timely and accurate diagnosis. Recently, in terms of the therapeutic aspects of IVL, diagnostic advances in detection of IVL using FDG-PET/CT or random skin biopsy have led to improvement in clinical outcomes by rituximab. The incidence of adverse reactions to rituximab can be markedly decreased if the tumor load is first reduced with an initial course of chemotherapy excluding rituximab. Future prospective studies of the timing of rituximab administration are warranted.

Several reports have shown efficacy for high-dose therapy with autologous stem-cell support (ASCT) in patients with IVL.

CONCLUSION

The most important factor for diagnosis of intravascular lymphoma is to suspect IVL. Although IVL usually involves fever, neurological symptoms, and skin symptoms but not lymphadenopathy, these symptoms are non-specific.

It is possible to identify the tumor cells from pathological specimens. For such identification the organs selected by the physician for biopsy are the key to accurate diagnosis.

Distinctive characteristics of IVL result in the tumor cells involving all types of organs, such as bone marrow, the CNS, skin, lung, adrenal gland, liver, kidney, spleen, thyroid, pituitary gland, and gastrointestinal tract, among others. Timely and accurate diagnosis is extremely important for patients with this disease, because appropriate treatment can improve clinical outcomes.

REFERENCES

[1] Tappeiner J, Pfleger L. [Angioendotheliomatosis proliferans systematisata. A clinically and pathohistologically new disease picture]. Der Hautarzt; Zeitschrift fur Dermatologie, Venerologie, und verwandte Gebiete. 1963 Feb;14:67-70.

[2] Jaffe ES. The 2008 WHO classification of lymphomas: implications for clinical practice and translational research. *Hematology/the Education Program of the American Society of Hematology Education Program.* 2009:523-31.

[3] Ponzoni M, Ferreri AJ, Campo E, Facchetti F, Mazzucchelli L, Yoshino T, et al. Definition, diagnosis, and management of intravascular large B-cell lymphoma: proposals and perspectives from an international consensus meeting. Journal of clinical oncology *: official journal of the American Society of Clinical Oncology*. 2007 Jul 20;25(21):3168-73.

[4] Domizio P, Hall PA, Cotter F, Amiel S, Tucker J, Besser GM, et al. Angiotropic large cell lymphoma (ALCL): morphological, immunohistochemical and genotypic studies with analysis of previous reports. *Hematological oncology*. 1989 May-Jun;7(3):195-206.

[5] Fredericks RK, Walker FO, Elster A, Challa V. Angiotropic intravascular large-cell lymphoma (malignant angioendotheliomatosis): report of a case and review of the literature. *Surgical neurology*. 1991 Mar;35(3):218-23.

[6] Ferreri AJ, Campo E, Seymour JF, Willemze R, Ilariucci F, Ambrosetti A, et al. Intravascular lymphoma: clinical presentation, natural history, management and prognostic factors in a series of 38 cases, with special emphasis on the 'cutaneous variant'. *British journal of haematology*. 2004 Oct;127(2):173-83.

[7] Ponzoni M, Ferreri AJ. Intravascular lymphoma: a neoplasm of 'homeless' lymphocytes? *Hematological oncology*. 2006 Sep;24(3):105-12.
[8] Zuckerman D, Seliem R, Hochberg E. Intravascular lymphoma: the oncologist's "great imitator." *The oncologist*. 2006 May;11(5):496-502.
[9] Shimada K, Kinoshita T, Naoe T, Nakamura S. Presentation and management of intravascular large B-cell lymphoma. *The lancet oncology*. 2009 Sep;10(9):895-902.
[10] Orwat DE, Batalis NI. Intravascular large B-cell lymphoma. *Archives of pathology and laboratory medicine*. 2012 Mar;136(3):333-8.
[11] Chihara T, Wada N, Ikeda J, Fujita S, Hori Y, Ogawa H, et al. Frequency of intravascular large B-cell lymphoma in Japan: study of the Osaka Lymphoma Study Group. *Journal of hematology and oncology*. 2011;4:14.
[12] Murase T, Yamaguchi M, Suzuki R, Okamoto M, Sato Y, Tamaru J, et al. Intravascular large B-cell lymphoma (IVLBCL): a clinicopathologic study of 96 cases with special reference to the immunophenotypic heterogeneity of CD5. *Blood*. 2007 Jan 15;109(2):478-85.
[13] Masaki Y, Dong L, Nakajima A, Iwao H, Miki M, Kurose N, et al. Intravascular large B cell lymphoma: proposed of the strategy for early diagnosis and treatment of patients with rapid deteriorating condition. *International journal of hematology*. 2009 Jun;89(5):600-10.
[14] Hong JY, Kim HJ, Ko YH, Choi JY, Jung CW, Kim SJ, et al. Clinical features and treatment outcomes of intravascular large B-cell lymphoma: a single-center experience in Korea. *Acta haematologica*. 2014;131(1):18-27.
[15] Kanda M, Suzumiya J, Ohshima K, Tamura K, Kikuchi M. Intravascular large cell lymphoma: clinicopathological, immuno-histochemical and molecular genetic studies. *Leukemia and lymphoma*. 1999 Aug;34(5-6):569-80.
[16] Ponzoni M, Arrigoni G, Gould VE, Del Curto B, Maggioni M, Scapinello A, et al. Lack of CD 29 (beta1 integrin) and CD 54 (ICAM-1) adhesion molecules in intravascular lymphomatosis. *Human pathology*. 2000 Feb;31(2):220-6.
[17] Kitagawa M, Matsubara O, Song SY, Kurashima C, Okeda R, Kasuga T. Neoplastic angioendotheliosis. Immunohistochemical and electron microscopic findings in three cases. *Cancer*. 1985 Sep 1;56(5):1134-43.
[18] Stroup RM, Sheibani K, Moncada A, Purdy LJ, Battifora H. Angiotropic (intravascular) large cell lymphoma. A clinicopathologic study of seven cases with unique clinical presentations. *Cancer*. 1990 Oct 15;66(8):1781-8.
[19] Glass J, Hochberg FH, Miller DC. Intravascular lymphomatosis. A systemic disease with neurologic manifestations. *Cancer*. 1993 May 15;71(10):3156-64.
[20] Bergmann M, Terzija-Wessel U, Blasius S, Kuchelmeister K, Kryne-Kubat B, Gerhard L, et al. Intravascular lymphomatosis of the CNS: clinicopathologic study and search for expression of oncoproteins and Epstein-Barr virus. *Clinical neurology and neurosurgery*. 1994 Aug;96(3):236-43.
[21] DiGiuseppe JA, Nelson WG, Seifter EJ, Boitnott JK, Mann RB. Intravascular lymphomatosis: a clinicopathologic study of 10 cases and assessment of response to chemotherapy. *Journal of clinical oncology: official journal of the American Society of Clinical Oncology*. 1994 Dec;12(12):2573-9.
[22] Demirer T, Dail DH, Aboulafia DM. Four varied cases of intravascular lymphomatosis and a literature review. *Cancer*. 1994 Mar 15;73(6):1738-45.

[23] Calamia KT, Miller A, Shuster EA, Perniciaro C, Menke DM. Intravascular lymphomatosis. A report of ten patients with central nervous system involvement and a review of the disease process. *Advances in experimental medicine and biology.* 1999;455:249-65.

[24] Murase T, Nakamura S, Kawauchi K, Matsuzaki H, Sakai C, Inaba T, et al. An Asian variant of intravascular large B-cell lymphoma: clinical, pathological and cytogenetic approaches to diffuse large B-cell lymphoma associated with haemophagocytic syndrome. *British journal of haematology.* 2000 Dec;111(3):826-34.

[25] Baehring JM, Longtine J, Hochberg FH. A new approach to the diagnosis and treatment of intravascular lymphoma. *Journal of neuro-oncology.* 2003 Feb;61(3):237-48.

[26] Sukpanichnant S, Visuthisakchai S. Intravascular lymphomatosis: a study of 20 cases in Thailand and a review of the literature. *Clinical lymphoma and myeloma.* 2006 Jan;6(4):319-28.

[27] Ferreri AJ, Dognini GP, Campo E, Willemze R, Seymour JF, Bairey O, et al. Variations in clinical presentation, frequency of hemophagocytosis and clinical behavior of intravascular lymphoma diagnosed in different geographical regions. *Haematologica.* 2007 Apr;92(4):486-92.

[28] Shimada K, Matsue K, Yamamoto K, Murase T, Ichikawa N, Okamoto M, et al. Retrospective analysis of intravascular large B-cell lymphoma treated with rituximab-containing chemotherapy as reported by the IVL study group in Japan. *Journal of clinical oncology* : official journal of the American Society of Clinical Oncology. 2008 Jul 1;26(19):3189-95.

[29] Matsue K, Asada N, Takeuchi M, Yamakura M, Kimura S, Odawara J, et al. A clinicopathological study of 13 cases of intravascular lymphoma: experience in a single institution over a 9-yr period. *European journal of haematology.* 2008 Mar;80(3):236-44.

[30] Kong YY, Dai B, Sheng WQ, Yang WT, Wang CF, Kong JC, et al. Intravascular large B-cell lymphoma with cutaneous manifestations: a clinicopathologic, immunophenotypic and molecular study of three cases. *Journal of cutaneous pathology.* 2009 Aug;36(8):865-70.

[31] Yin W, Li M, Gao Z, Huang F, Da J, Liu C. Intravascular large B-cell lymphoma with involvement of the abdominal subcutis: a case report and literature review. *International journal of hematology.* 2009 Apr;89(3):348-51.

[32] Park JH, Lee DY, Ko YH. Intravascular large B-cell lymphoma of the cutaneous variant in Korea. *The Journal of dermatology.* 2011 Feb;38(2):160-3.

[33] Wang L, Li C, Gao T. Cutaneous intravascular anaplastic large cell lymphoma. *Journal of cutaneous pathology.* 2011 Feb;38(2):221-6.

[34] Davey DD, Munn R, Smith LW, Cibull ML. Angiotrophic lymphoma. Presentation in uterine vessels with cytogenetic studies. *Archives of pathology and laboratory medicine.* 1990 Aug;114(8):879-82.

[35] Sill H, Hofler G, Kaufmann P, Horina J, Spuller E, Kleinert R, et al. Angiotropic large cell lymphoma presenting as thrombotic microangiopathy (thrombotic thrombocytopenic purpura). *Cancer.* 1995 Mar 1;75(5):1167-70.

[36] Murase T, Nakamura S, Tashiro K, Suchi T, Hiraga J, Hayasaki N et al. Malignant histiocytosis-like B-cell lymphoma, a distinct pathologic variant of intravascular

lymphomatosis: a report of five cases and review of the literature. *British journal of haematology*. 1997 Dec;99(3):656-64.

[37] Murase T, Nakamura S. An Asian variant of intravascular lymphomatosis: an updated review of malignant histiocytosis-like B-cell lymphoma. *Leukemia and lymphoma*. 1999 May;33(5-6):459-73.

[38] Geyer H, Karlin N, Palen B, Mesa R. Asian-variant intravascular lymphoma in the African race. Rare tumors. 2012 Jan 2;4(1):e10.

[39] Fung KM, Chakrabarty JH, Kern WF, Magharyous H, Gehrs BC, Li S. Intravascular large B-cell lymphoma with hemophagocytic syndrome (Asian variant) in a Caucasian patient. *International journal of clinical and experimental pathology*. 2012;5(5):448-54.

[40] Chapin JE, Davis LE, Kornfeld M, Mandler RN. Neurologic manifestations of intravascular lymphomatosis. *Acta neurologica Scandinavica*. 1995 Jun;91(6):494-9.

[41] Wahie S, Dayala S, Husain A, Summerfield G, Hervey V, Langtry JA. Cutaneous features of intravascular lymphoma. *Clinical and experimental dermatology*. 2011 Apr;36(3):288-91.

[42] Smadja D, Mas JL, Fallet-Bianco C, Meyniard O, Sicard D, de Recondo J, et al. Intravascular lymphomatosis (neoplastic angioendotheliosis) of the central nervous system: case report and literature review. *Journal of neuro-oncology*. 1991 Oct;11(2):171-80.

[43] Liszka U, Drlicek M, Hitzenberger P, Machacek E, Mayer H, Stockhammer G, et al. Intravascular lymphomatosis: a clinico-pathological study of three cases. *Journal of cancer research and clinical oncology*. 1994;120(3):164-8.

[44] Beristain X, Azzarelli B. The neurological masquerade of intravascular lymphomatosis. *Archives of neurology*. 2002 Mar;59(3):439-43.

[45] Hundsberger T, Cogliatti S, Kleger GR, Fretz C, Gahler A, Anliker M, et al. Intravascular lymphoma mimicking cerebral stroke: report of two cases. *Case reports in neurology*. 2011 Sep;3(3):278-83.

[46] Jitpratoom P, Yuckpan P, Sitthinamsuwan P, Chotinaiwattarakul W, Chinthammitr Y. Progressive multifocal cerebral infarction from intravascular large B cell lymphoma presenting in a man: a case report. *Journal of medical case reports*. 2011;5:24.

[47] Stahl RL, Chan W, Duncan A, Corley CC, Jr. Malignant angioendotheliomatosis presenting as disseminated intravascular coagulopathy. *Cancer*. 1991 Nov 15;68(10):2319-23.

[48] Lui PC, Wong GK, Poon WS, Tse GM. Intravascular lymphomatosis. *Journal of clinical pathology*. 2003 Jun;56(6):468-70.

[49] Ganguly S. Acute intracerebral hemorrhage in intravascular lymphoma: a serious infusion related adverse event of rituximab. *American journal of clinical oncology*. 2007 Apr;30(2):211-2.

[50] Passarin MG, Wen PY, Vattemi E, Buffone E, Ghimenton C, Bontempini L, et al. Intravascular lymphomatosis and intracerebral haemorrhage. Neurological sciences: official journal of the Italian Neurological *Society and of the Italian Society of Clinical Neurophysiology*. 2010 Dec;31(6):793-7.

[51] Marino D, Sicurelli F, Cerase A, Tripodi S, Cintorino M, Lazzi S, et al. Fulminant intravascular lymphomatosis mimicking acute haemorrhagic leukoencephalopathy. *Journal of the neurological sciences*. 2012 Sep 15;320(1-2):141-4.

[52] Haninger DM, Davis TA, Parker JR, Slone SP, Parker JC, Jr. Intravascular large B-cell lymphoma presenting as acute hemorrhagic cerebral infarct with delirium. *Annals of clinical and laboratory science*. 2013 Summer;43(3):305-10.

[53] Moussouttas M. Intravascular lymphomatosis presenting as posterior leukoencephalopathy. *Archives of neurology*. 2002 Apr;59(4):640-1.

[54] Gaul C, Hanisch F, Neureiter D, Behrmann C, Neundorfer B, Winterholler M. Intravascular lymphomatosis mimicking disseminated encephalomyelitis and encephalomyelopathy. *Clinical neurology and neurosurgery*. 2006 Jul;108(5):486-9.

[55] Ojeda VJ. Neoplastic angioendotheliosis of the spinal cord. Case report. *Acta neuropathologica*. 1983;62(1-2):164-6.

[56] Daniel SE, Rudge P, Scaravilli F. Malignant angioendotheliosis involving the nervous system: support for a lymphoid origin of the neoplastic cells. *Journal of neurology, neurosurgery, and psychiatry*. 1987 Sep;50(9):1173-7.

[57] Raroque HG, Jr., Mandler RN, Griffey MS, Orrison WW, Kornfeld M. Neoplastic angioendotheliomatosis. *Archives of neurology*. 1990 Aug;47(8):929-30.

[58] Dubas F, Saint-Andre JP, Pouplard-Barthelaix A, Delestre F, Emile J. Intravascular malignant lymphomatosis (so-called malignant angioendotheliomatosis): a case confined to the lumbosacral spinal cord and nerve roots. *Clinical neuropathology*. 1990 May-Jun;9(3):115-20.

[59] Harris CP, Sigman JD, Jaeckle KA. Intravascular malignant lymphomatosis: amelioration of neurological symptoms with plasmapheresis. *Annals of neurology*. 1994 Mar;35(3):357-9.

[60] Nakahara T, Saito T, Muroi A, Sugiura Y, Ogata M, Sugiyama Y, et al. Intravascular lymphomatosis presenting as an ascending cauda equina: conus medullaris syndrome: remission after biweekly CHOP therapy. *Journal of neurology, neurosurgery, and psychiatry*. 1999 Sep;67(3):403-6.

[61] Schwarz S, Zoubaa S, Knauth M, Sommer C, Storch-Hagenlocher B. Intravascular lymphomatosis presenting with a conus medullaris syndrome mimicking disseminated encephalomyelitis. *Neuro-oncology*. 2002 Jul;4(3):187-91.

[62] Davis TS. Intravascular lymphoma presenting with cauda equina syndrome: treated with CHOP and rituxan. *Leukemia and lymphoma*. 2003 May;44(5):887-8.

[63] Takizawa S, Shirasugi Y, Nakamura N, Nakagawa S, Tsuchiya T, Ando K, et al. An atypical form of Asian variant of intravascular large B-cell lymphoma presenting with myelopathy alone for 4 months prior to pancytopenia. *Internal medicine*. 2007;46(22):1879-80.

[64] Yang T, Tian L, Li Q, Liu Y, Zhang Q, Ma Z, et al. A case of intravascular B-cell lymphoma presenting as myelopathy and diagnosed post mortem. *Journal of the neurological sciences*. 2008 Sep 15;272(1-2):196-8.

[65] Savard M, Verreault S, Gould PV, Bernier V, Bouchard JP. Intravascular lymphoma with conus medullaris syndrome followed by encephalopathy. *The Canadian journal of neurological sciences Le journal canadien des sciences neurologiques*. 2008 Jul;35(3):366-71.

[66] Vital C, Heraud A, Vital A, Coquet M, Julien M, Maupetit J. Acute mononeuropathy with angiotropic lymphoma. *Acta neuropathologica*. 1989;78(1):105-7.

[67] Levin KH, Lutz G. Angiotropic large-cell lymphoma with peripheral nerve and skeletal muscle involvement: early diagnosis and treatment. *Neurology.* 1996 Oct;47(4):1009-11.

[68] Devlin T, Moll S, Hulette C, Morgenlander JC. Intravascular malignant lymphomatosis with neurologic presentation: factors facilitating antemortem diagnosis. *Southern medical journal.* 1998 Jul;91(7):672-6.

[69] Fallon KB, Oh SJ, Palmer CA. Intravascular malignant lymphomatosis diagnosed in both skeletal muscle and nerve biopsies. *Journal of clinical neuromuscular disease.* 2002 Dec;4(2):78-81.

[70] Oei ME, Kraft GH, Sarnat HB. Intravascular lymphomatosis. *Muscle and nerve.* 2002 May;25(5):742-6.

[71] De Bruecker Y, Demaerel P, Wilms G, Sciot R, Ballaux F, Robberecht W. A case of hemiparesis associated with cranial nerve lesions due to intravascular lymphomatosis(2003:4b). *European radiology.* 2003 Jul;13(7):1753-5.

[72] Koyama T, O'Uchi T, Matsue K. Neurolymphomatosis involving the trigeminal nerve and deep peroneal nerve in a patient with relapsed intravascular large B-cell lymphoma. *European journal of haematology.* 2010 Sep;85(3):275-6.

[73] Jiang QL, Pytel P, Rowin J. Disseminated intravascular large-cell lymphoma with initial presentation mimicking Guillain-Barre syndrome. *Muscle and nerve.* 2010 Jul;42(1):133-6.

[74] Roux S, Grossin M, De Bandt M, Palazzo E, Vachon F, Kahn MF. Angiotropic large cell lymphoma with mononeuritis multiplex mimicking systemic vasculitis. Journal of neurology, neurosurgery, and psychiatry. 1995 Mar;58(3):363-6.

[75] Yamada S, Tanimoto A, Nabeshima A, Tasaki T, Wang KY, Kitada S, et al. Diffuse large B-cell lymphoma presenting with neurolymphomatosis and intravascular lymphoma: a unique autopsy case with diverse neurological symptoms. *Diagnostic pathology.* 2012;7:94.

[76] Ramkumar B, Hutchison R, Khadim H, Gajra A. Intravascular large B-cell lymphoma--a diagnostic dilemma. *Clinical lymphoma, myeloma and leukemia.* 2013 Dec;13(6):e18-21.

[77] Konikkara JJ, Perurena OH, Warach S, Bauserman SC. A 62-year-old man with fluctuating neurological deficits and skin lesions. *JAMA neurology.* 2013 Jan;70(1):120-4.

[78] Kraus MD, Jones D, Bartlett NL. Intravascular lymphoma associated with endocrine dysfunction: a report of four cases and a review of the literature. *The American journal of medicine.* 1999 Aug;107(2):169-76.

[79] Kiyohara T, Kumakiri M, Kobayashi H, Shimizu T, Ohkawara A, Ohnuki M. A case of intravascular large B-cell lymphoma mimicking erythema nodosum: the importance of multiple skin biopsies. *Journal of cutaneous pathology. 2000* Sep;27(8):413-8.

[80] Gill S, Melosky B, Haley L, ChanYan C. Use of random skin biopsy to diagnose intravascular lymphoma presenting as fever of unknown origin. *The American journal of medicine.* 2003 Jan;114(1):56-8.

[81] Le K, Lim A, Bullpitt P, Wood G. Intravascular B-cell lymphoma diagnosed by skin biopsy. *The Australasian journal of dermatology.* 2005 Nov;46(4):261-5.

[82] Roglin J, Boer A. Skin manifestations of intravascular lymphoma mimic inflammatory diseases of the skin. *The British journal of dermatology.* 2007 Jul;157(1):16-25.

[83] Asada N, Odawara J, Kimura S, Aoki T, Yamakura M, Takeuchi M, et al. Use of random skin biopsy for diagnosis of intravascular large B-cell lymphoma. *Mayo Clinic proceedings*. 2007 Dec;82(12):1525-7.

[84] Le EN, Gerstenblith MR, Gelber AC, Manno RL, Ranasinghe PD, Sweren RJ, et al. The use of blind skin biopsy in the diagnosis of intravascular B-cell lymphoma. *Journal of the American Academy of Dermatology*. 2008 Jul;59(1):148-51.

[85] Kasuya A, Hashizume H, Takigawa M. Early diagnosis of recurrent diffuse large B-cell lymphoma showing intravascular lymphoma by random skin biopsy. *The Journal of dermatology*. 2011 Jun;38(6):571-4.

[86] Matsue K, Asada N, Odawara J, Aoki T, Kimura S, Iwama K, et al. Random skin biopsy and bone marrow biopsy for diagnosis of intravascular large B cell lymphoma. *Annals of hematology*. 2011 Apr;90(4):417-21.

[87] Ikoma N, Manabe Y, Yamaoka H, Akasaka E, Mabuchi T, Ozawa A, et al. Random skin biopsy of intravascular large B-cell lymphoma: a case report. *The Tokai journal of experimental and clinical medicine*. 2012 Sep;37(3):75-6.

[88] Higashi Y, Kawai K, Yonekura K, Takeda K, Kanzaki T, Utsunomiya A, et al. Indication for random skin biopsy for the diagnosis of intravascular large B cell lymphoma. *Dermatology*. 2012;224(1):46-50.

[89] Oomura M, Sakakibara N, Suzuki S, Wakita A, Mori Y, Kamimoto K. Intravascular lymphomatosis mimicking primary central nervous system lymphoma: a case report and literature review. *Case reports in neurology*. 2014 Jan;6(1):101-8.

[90] Kishi Y, Kami M, Kusumi E, Mineyama T, Kato D, Hamaki T, et al. Prostatic acid phosphatase: a possible diagnostic marker of intravascular large B-cell lymphoma. *Haematologica*. 2004 May;89(5):ECR13.

[91] Seki K, Miyakoshi S, Lee GH, Matsushita H, Mutoh Y, Nakase K, et al. Prostatic acid phosphatase is a possible tumor marker for intravascular large B-cell lymphoma. *The American journal of surgical pathology*. 2004 Oct;28(10):1384-8.

[92] Kawaguchi T, Ohwada C, Takeuchi M, Shimizu N, Sakaida E, Takeda Y, et al. Potential utility of serum soluble LR11 as a diagnostic biomarker for intravascular large B-cell lymphoma. *Leukemia and lymphoma*. 2014 Oct;55(10):2391-4.

[93] Coulibaly B, Mesturoux L, Petit B, Magy L, Labrousse F. Intravascular large B-cell lymphoma presenting as cauda equina syndrome and showing aberrant cytokeratin expression: a diagnostic challenge. *Pathology*. 2014 Apr;46(3):241-4.

[94] Tsukadaira A, Okubo Y, Ogasawara H, Urushibata K, Honda T, Miura I, et al. Chromosomal aberrations in intravascular lymphomatosis. *American journal of clinical oncology*. 2002 Apr;25(2):178-81.

[95] Khoury H, Lestou VS, Gascoyne RD, Bruyere H, Li CH, Nantel SH, et al. Multicolor karyotyping and clinicopathological analysis of three intravascular lymphoma cases. Modern pathology : an official journal of the United States and Canadian Academy of Pathology, Inc. 2003 Jul;16(7):716-24.

[96] Molina A, Lombard C, Donlon T, Bangs CD, Dorfman RF. Immunohistochemical and cytogenetic studies indicate that malignant angioendotheliomatosis is a primary intravascular (angiotropic) lymphoma. *Cancer*. 1990 Aug 1;66(3):474-9.

[97] Ichikawa N, Kobayashi H, Ito T, Saito H. Chromosomal aberrations detected after stimulation with lipopolysaccharide in a patient with Asian variant intravascular lymphomatosis. *Cancer genetics and cytogenetics*. 2000 Jul 1;120(1):83-4.

[98] Rashid R, Johnson RJ, Morris S, Dickinson H, Czyz J, O'Connor SJ, et al. Intravascular large B-cell lymphoma associated with a near-tetraploid karyotype, rearrangement of BCL6, and a t(11;14)(q13;q32). *Cancer genetics and cytogenetics.* 2006 Dec;171(2):101-4.

[99] Deisch J, Fuda FB, Chen W, Karandikar N, Arbini AA, Zhou XJ, et al. Segmental tandem triplication of the MLL gene in an intravascular large B-cell lymphoma with multisystem involvement: a comprehensive morphologic, immunophenotypic, cytogenetic, and molecular cytogenetic antemortem study. *Archives of pathology and laboratory medicine*. 2009 Sep;133(9):1477-82.

[100] Kobayashi T, Ohno H. Intravascular large B-cell lymphoma associated with t(14;19)(q32;q13) translocation. *Internal medicine*. 2011;50(18):2007-10.

[101] Yamamoto K, Yakushijin K, Okamura A, Hayashi Y, Matsuoka H, Minami H. Gain of 11q by an additional ring chromosome 11 and trisomy 18 in CD5-positive intravascular large B-cell lymphoma. Journal of clinical and experimental hematopathology : JCEH 2013;53(2):161-5.

[102] Cui J, Liu Q, Cheng Y, Chen S, Sun Q. An intravascular large B-cell lymphoma with a t(3;14)(q27;q32) translocation. *Journal of clinical pathology*. 2014 Mar;67(3):279-81.

[103] Williams RL, Meltzer CC, Smirniotopoulos JG, Fukui MB, Inman M. Cerebral MR imaging in intravascular lymphomatosis. AJNR American journal of neuroradiology. 1998 Mar;19(3):427-31. PubMed PMID: 9541293.

[104] Song DK, Boulis NM, McKeever PE, Quint DJ. Angiotropic large cell lymphoma with imaging characteristics of CNS vasculitis. *AJNR American journal of neuroradiology.* 2002 Feb;23(2):239-42.

[105] Martin-Duverneuil N, Mokhtari K, Behin A, Lafitte F, Hoang-Xuan K, Chiras J. Intravascular malignant lymphomatosis. *Neuroradiology*. 2002 Sep;44(9):749-54.

[106] Lozsadi DA, Wieshmann U, Enevoldson TP. Neurological presentation of intravascular lymphoma: report of two cases and discussion of diagnostic challenges. European journal of neurology : *the official journal of the European Federation of Neurological Societies*. 2005 Sep;12(9):710-4.

[107] Baehring JM, Henchcliffe C, Ledezma CJ, Fulbright R, Hochberg FH. Intravascular lymphoma: magnetic resonance imaging correlates of disease dynamics within the central nervous system. *Journal of neurology, neurosurgery, and psychiatry.* 2005 Apr;76(4):540-4.

[108] De Fino C, Arena V, Hohaus S, Di Iorio R, Bozzoli V, Mirabella M. Intravascular large B-cell lymphoma presenting as slowly progressive paraparesis with normal MRI features. *Journal of the neurological sciences.* 2012 Mar 15;314(1-2):171-4.

[109] Yamamoto A, Kikuchi Y, Homma K, O'Uchi T, Furui S. Characteristics of intravascular large B-cell lymphoma on cerebral MR imaging. *AJNR American journal of neuroradio*logy. 2012 Feb;33(2):292-6.

[110] Hoshino A, Kawada E, Ukita T, Itoh K, Sakamoto H, Fujita K, et al. Usefulness of FDG-PET to diagnose intravascular lymphomatosis presenting as fever of unknown origin. *American journal of hematology*. 2004 Jul;76(3):236-9.

[111] Odawara J, Asada N, Aoki T, Yamakura M, Takeuchi M, Ohuchi T, et al. 18F-Fluorodeoxyglucose positron emission tomography for evaluation of intravascular large B-cell lymphoma. *British journal of haematology.* 2007 Mar;136(5):684.

[112] Shimada K, Kosugi H, Shimada S, Narimatsu H, Koyama Y, Suzuki N, et al. Evaluation of organ involvement in intravascular large B-cell lymphoma by 18F-fluorodeoxyglucose positron emission tomography. *International journal of hematology.* 2008 Sep;88(2):149-53.

[113] Yamada S, Nishii R, Oka S, Higashi T, Yagi M, Satow T, et al. FDG-PET a pivotal imaging modality for diagnosis of stroke-onset intravascular lymphoma. *Archives of neurology.* 2010 Mar;67(3):366-7.

[114] Boslooper K, Dijkhuizen D, van der Velden AW, Dal M, Meilof JF, Hoogenberg K. Intravascular lymphoma as an unusual cause of multifocal cerebral infarctions discovered on FDG-PET/CT. *The Netherlands journal of medicine.* 2010 Jun;68(6):261-4.

[115] Matsue K, Hayama BY, Iwama K, Koyama T, Fujiwara H, Yamakura M, et al. High frequency of neurolymphomatosis as a relapse disease of intravascular large B-cell lymphoma. *Cancer.* 2011 Oct 1;117(19):4512-21.

[116] Hemmaway CJ, Danga A, Igbokwe U, Radunovic A. FDG-PET guided diagnosis of vaginal intravascular diffuse large B-cell lymphoma. *British journal of haematology.* 2012 Sep;158(6):678.

[117] Yamashita H, Suzuki A, Takahashi Y, Kubota K, Kano T, Mimori A. Intravascular large B-cell lymphoma with diffuse FDG uptake in the lung by 18FDG-PET/CT without chest CT findings. *Annals of nuclear medicine.* 2012 Jul;26(6):515-21.

[118] Kawai N, Okada M, Haba R, Yamamoto Y, Tamiya T. Insufficiency of positron emission tomography and magnetic resonance spectroscopy in the diagnosis of intravascular lymphoma of the central nervous system. *Case reports in oncology.* 2012 May;5(2):339-46.

[119] Wagner T, Brechemier D, Dugert E, Le Guellec S, Julian A, Hitzel A, et al. Diffuse pulmonary uptake on FDG-PET with normal CT diagnosed as intravascular large B-cell lymphoma: a case report and a discussion of the causes of diffuse FDG uptake in the lungs. Cancer imaging : *the official publication of the International Cancer Imaging Society.* 2012;12:7-12.

[120] Narimatsu H, Morishita Y, Saito S, Shimada K, Ozeki K, Kohno A, et al. Usefulness of bone marrow aspiration for definite diagnosis of Asian variant of intravascular lymphoma: four autopsied cases. *Leukemia and lymphoma.* 2004 Aug;45(8):1611-6.

[121] Imai H, Kajimoto K, Taniwaki M, Miura I, Hatta Y, Hashizume Y, et al. Intravascular large B-cell lymphoma presenting with mass lesions in the central nervous system: a report of five cases. *Pathology international.* 2004 Apr;54(4):231-6.

[122] Bouzani M, Karmiris T, Rontogianni D, Delimpassi S, Apostolidis J, Mpakiri M, et al. Disseminated intravascular B-cell lymphoma: clinicopathological features and outcome of three cases treated with anthracycline-based immunochemotherapy. *The oncologist.* 2006 Sep;11(8):923-8.

[123] Imai H, Shimada K, Shimada S, Abe M, Okamoto M, Kitamura K, et al. Comparative clinicopathological study of primary CNS diffuse large B-cell lymphoma and intravascular large B-cell lymphoma. *Pathology international.* 2009 Jul;59(7):431-7.

[124] Ferreri AJ, Dognini GP, Bairey O, Szomor A, Montalban C, Horvath B, et al. The addition of rituximab to anthracycline-based chemotherapy significantly improves outcome in 'Western' patients with intravascular large B-cell lymphoma. *British journal of haematology.* 2008 Oct;143(2):253-7.

[125] Kebir S, Kuchelmeister K, Niehusmann P, Nelles M, Kim Y, Thanendrarajan S, et al. Intravascular CNS lymphoma: Successful therapy using high-dose methotrexate-based polychemotherapy. *Experimental hematology and oncology*. 2012;1(1):37.
[126] Makino K, Nakata J, Kawachi S, Hayashi T, Nakajima A, Yokoyama M. Treatment strategy for reducing the risk of rituximab-induced cytokine release syndrome in patients with intravascular large B-cell lymphoma: a case report and review of the literature. *Journal of medical case reports*. 2013;7(1):280.

In: Primary Central Nervous System Lymphoma (PCNSL) ISBN: 978-1-63485-322-4
Editor: Ryuya Yamanaka

Chapter 19

PRIMARY CENTRAL NERVOUS SYSTEM POSTTRANSPLANT LYMPHOPROLIFERATIVE DISORDERS (PCNS-PTLD): INCIDENCE, MANAGEMENT AND OUTCOME

Masaya Honda**, *Michiaki Koga and Takashi Kanda
Department of Neurology and Clinical Neuroscience,
Yamaguchi University Graduate School of Medicine, Yamaguchi, Japan

ABSTRACT

Posttransplant lymphoproliferative disorder (PTLD) is a heterogeneous disease entity of lymphoid and plasmacytic proliferations which can occur after solid organ or bone marrow/stem cell transplantation. PTLD occasionally involves the central nervous system, however, primary occurrence in the central nervous system is quite rare. Epstein-Barr virus plays a causative role, and up to 90% of cases with PTLD are associated with this virus. The diagnosis of primary central nervous system (PCNS)-PTLD is made according to CT/MRI and physical findings. However, this is often challenging and a direct biopsy of the lesion is typically necessary for the definitive diagnosis. The optimal therapy for PCNS-PTLD remains unknown. A dose reduction or discontinuation of the immunosuppressive agents is effective for only a half of PTLD patients. CNS involvement is a poor prognostic factor, and an early diagnosis and initiation of chemotherapy or radiotherapy appears to be critical for maximizing a favorable outcome.

Keywords: posttransplant lymphoproliferative disorders, Epstein-Barr virus, central nervous system

* Corresponding Author address: Masaya Honda, Department of Neurology and Clinical Neuroscience, Yamaguchi University Graduate School of Medicine, Minamikogushi 1-1-1, Ube, Yamaguchi 7558505, Japan. Email: m.hon@yamaguchi-u.ac.jp.

INTRODUCTION

Posttransplant lymphoproliferative disorders (PTLD) are a heterogeneous disease entity of lymphoid and plasmacytic proliferations which can occur after solid organ or bone marrow/stem cell transplantation. The first case of PTLD was described in renal transplant in 1968 by Doak et al. [1]. According to the 2008 World Health Organization (WHO) classification, PTLD is divided into four major categories: early lesions, polymorphic PTLD, monomorphic PTLD and classical Hodgkin lymphoma-type PTLD according to morphologic, immunophenotypic, and molecular criteria. PTLD occasionally involves the central nervous system, however, primary occurrence in the central nervous system is quite rare. Schneck and Penn first reported two cases of primary central nervous system (PCNS)-PTLD after renal transplantation in 1970 [2].

INCIDENCE

The frequencies of PTLD occurrence are high (20-25%) among patients undergoing heart, lung, intestine, and multi-organ transplant, while those among renal and liver transplant recipients are lower (1-5%). Commonly affected organs include the lymph nodes, gastrointestinal tract, lung and liver, whereas CNS involvement is rare. A review of the Israel Penn International Transplant Tumor Registry showed that CNS involvement was observed in 15% of patients with PTLD, of whom a half show CNS involvement alone [3]. Pancreas and kidney transplant recipients showed the highest incidence of CNS involvement (27% and 18%, respectively).

The duration from transplantation to the diagnosis of PCNS-PTLD varied greatly among previous reports, ranging from 2 to 264 months [4-7]. In kidney transplant recipients, CNS involvement typically appears one year after transplantation.

DIAGNOSIS

PCNS-PTLD should be suspected if transplant recipients show mental status changes or new neurological abnormalities. The differential diagnosis in immunosuppressed patients is broad including infectious (e.g., abscess and toxoplasmosis) and neoplastic etiologies.

Diagnostic tests for PCNS-PTLD include gadolinium-enhanced brain MRI, a cerebral spinal fluid (CSF) analysis for EBV by PCR, cytology and flow cytometry. Brain CT/MRI typically show supratentorial multifocal lesions (hypodense on CT, hypointense on T1WI and hyperintense on T2WI on MRI) with a ring enhancement pattern, which mimics cerebral abscesses. However, approximately 60% of patients with PCNS-PTLD show abnormal but non-specific CSF findings, such as an elevated cell count or protein level. Cavaliere et al. reported that only one of 12 patients had definitive abnormal cytology findings, while another patient had abnormal flow cytometry findings [5].

Highly suggestive findings for the diagnosis of CNS-PTLD are the presence of gadolinium enhancing lesions on brain MRI, detection of EBV DNA in the CSF by PCR, and an increased EBV load in the peripheral blood. However, a brain biopsy is generally required for the diagnosis because supplementary assessments, including CSF and MRI evaluations, are generally nonspecific, and the definite diagnosis of PTLD is made according to the evaluation of pathological features.

TREATMENT

The optimal therapy for PCNS-PTLD has yet to be established. Regarding systemic PTLD, a reduction of immunosuppressive agents, antiviral therapies, monoclonal antibodies, chemotherapy, and radiation therapy has been used for PCNS-PTLD.

Initially, immunosuppressive agents which are used for the prevention of rejection should be reduced or discontinued, if possible, because immunosuppression is recognized to cause PTLD. In fact, a reduction of immunosuppressive agents leads to remission of polymorphic PTLD in approximately 50% of cases. However, PCNS-PTLD is often monomorphic, a more progressive state than polymorphic, thus more aggressive treatments such as chemotherapy and radiotherapy are needed.

Antiviral therapies, most commonly ganciclovir or acyclovir, have been used for EBV-driven malignancies. These drugs are capable of inhibiting lytic viral replication but have no effect on tumor cells due to the lack of thymidine kinase in latently infected B-cells. Two previous case reports have demonstrated the effect of antiviral therapies in CNS-PTLD.

Chemotherapy is the standard treatment in CNS lymphoma. Methotrexate (MTX) is highly effective in lymphomas and can pass through the blood-brain barrier [8]. Taj et al. reported that high-dose MTX was safe and effective in the treatment of PCNS-PTLD in pediatric liver transplant recipients [9].

Rituximab, a monoclonal antibody directed against CD20 expressed on B cells, is effective in PTLD without CNS involvement. However, the systemic administration of rituximab is not considered a promising treatment for PCNS-PTLD due to its large molecular size (145 kDa), which cannot pass through blood-brain barrier [10]. Alternatively, Bonney et al. reported successful treatment with intrathecal administration of rituximab in two children who developed isolated CNS-PTLD after hematopoietic stem cell transplantation [11].

Radiotherapy is also a potential option for PCNS-PTLD. Patients with PCNS-PTLD who received radiotherapy (alone or in combination with chemotherapy) showed a prolonged survival time (median 36 months) compared to those who did not (7 months) [6]. It was also reported that radiotherapy alone was efficacious in four (80%) out of five cases of CNS-PTLD.

PROGNOSIS

CNS involvement has been considered to be a poor prognostic factor for PTLD. A retrospective analysis by Cavaliere et al. demonstrated that the median survival of 33 patients with PCNS-PTLD was 47 months, and six patients died within one month after the diagnosis [5].

REFERENCES

[1] Doak PB, Montgomerie JZ, North JD, Smith F, (1968). Reticulum cell sarcoma after renal homotransplantation and azathioprine and prednisone therapy. *Br Med J.* 4, 74-748.

[2] Schneck SA, Penn I, (1970). Cerebral neoplasms associated with renal transplantation. *Arch Neurol.* 22, 226-233.

[3] Buell JF, Gross TG, Hanaway MJ, Trofe J, Roy-Chaudhury P, et al., (2005). Posttransplant lymphoproliferative disorder: significance of central nervous system involvement. *Transplant Proc.* 37, 954-955.

[4] Castellano-Sanchez AA, Li S, Qian J, Lagoo A, Weir E, et al., (2004). Primary central nervous system posttransplant lymphoproliferative disorders. *Am J Clin Pathol.* 121, 246-253.

[5] Cavaliere R, Petroni G, Lopes MB, Schiff D, (2010). Primary central nervous system post-transplant lymphoproliferative disorder: An International Primary Central Nervous System Lymphoma Collaborative Group report. *Cancer.* 116, 863-870.

[6] Snanoudj R, Durrbach A, Leblond V, Caillard S, Hurault De Ligny B, et al., (2003). Primary brain lymphomas after kidney transplantation: Presentation and outcome. *Transplantation.* 76, 930-937.

[7] Evens AM, Choquet S, Kroll-Desrosiers AR, Jagadeesh D, Smith SM, et al., (2013). Primary CNS Posttransplant Lymphoproliferative Disease (PTLD): An international report of 84 cases in the modern era. *Am J Transpl.* 13, 1512-1522.

[8] Nabors LB, Palmer CA, Julian BA, Przekwas AM, Kew CE, (2009). Isolated central nervous system posttransplant lymphoproliferative disorder treated with high-dose intravenous methotrexate. *Am J Transpl.* 9, 1243-1248.

[9] Taj MM, Messahel B, Mycroft J, Pitchard-Jones K, Baker A, et al., (2008). Efficacy and tolerability of high-dose methotrexate in central nervous system positive or relapsed lymphoproliferative disease following liver transplant in children. *Br J Haematol.* 140, 191-196.

[10] Evens AM, David KA, Helenowski I, Nelson B, Kaufman D, et al., (2010). Multicenter analysis of 80 solid organ transplantation recipients with posttransplantation lymphoproliferative disease: Outcomes and prognostic factors in the modern era. *J Clin Oncol.* 28, 1038-1046.

[11] Bonney DK, Htwe EE, Turner A, Kelsey A, Shabani A, et al., (2012). Sustained response to intrathecal rituximab in EBV associated post-transplant lymphoproliferative disease confined to the central nervous system following haematopoietic stem cell transplant. *Pediatr Blood Cancer.* 58, 459-461.

V. Outcomes and Quality of Life

In: Primary Central Nervous System Lymphoma (PCNSL) ISBN: 978-1-63485-322-4
Editor: Ryuya Yamanaka

Chapter 20

LONG-TERM QUALITY OF LIFE AND LEUCOENCEPHALOPATHY IN PRIMARY CNS LYMPHOMA

Junya Fukai**, *Koji Fujita, Yuji Uematsu and Naoyuki Nakao
Department of Neurological Surgery,
Wakayama Medical University School of Medicine,
Wakayama, Japan

ABSTRACT

Systemic high-dose methotrexate in combination with whole brain radiation therapy improved survival rates of the patients with primary CNS lymphoma. As patients with primary CNS lymphoma are living longer, survivors are at high risk of developing severe treatment-related complications, mainly disabling delayed neurotoxicity. After all, the long-term outcome, especially of elderly patients, is invariably dismal often accompanied by increased severe adverse effects such as cognitive dysfunction, leucoencephalopathy and impaired quality of life. Since high-dose methotrexate and whole brain radiation can each cause CNS damage, there is synergistic toxicity when these modalities are combined. It is important to recognize and avoid treatment-related complications in primary CNS lymphomas for a long-term period. In this chapter, we address delayed neuropsychological complications of methotrexate-based chemotherapy and whole brain radiation therapy and review the literature and our experience on long-term outcomes, such as cognitive function, MRI abnormality, and quality of life of primary CNS lymphoma survivors.

Keywords: long-term outcome, delayed neurotoxicity, quality of life, leucoencephalopathy

* Corresponding Author address: Department of Neurological Surgery, Wakayama Medical University School of Medicine, 811-1 Kimiidera, Wakayama, 641-0012, Japan, Email: junfukai@wakayama-med.ac.jp.

INTRODUCTION

Primary central nervous system (CNS) lymphoma is an aggressive cancer, seen more commonly in immunocompetent patients over 65 years of age (Nayak L., et al., 2015). Although prognosis remains poor, it has significantly improved over the past two decades as a result of better treatment strategies with a curative aim (Citterio G., et al., 2015). In many studies, younger age and better performance status are found to be predictive of improved overall and progression-free survival in patients with newly diagnosed primary CNS lymphoma (Ferreri A.J., et al., 2003) (Abrey L.E., et al., 2006) (Korfel A. and Schlegel U., 2013).

The treatment for newly diagnosed primary CNS lymphoma involves induction and consolidation phases (Nayak L., et al., 2015). High-dose methotrexate-based chemotherapy is typically used for induction. Consolidation involves additional treatment in the form of radiation, chemotherapy, or high-dose chemotherapy followed by autologous stem cell rescue to eliminate any residual disease. Historically, whole-brain radiation therapy was a treatment option. The addition of high-dose methotrexate (HD-MTX) to whole-brain radiation therapy (WBRT) has increased survival rates in primary CNS lymphoma. On the other hand, effective treatments often interfere with the patient's ability to function at prediagnosis levels. Now that patients can live longer, quality of life (QOL) has become the major concern in patients achieving long-term survival.

Neuropsychological deteriorations can be seen throughout the course of diagnosis and treatment in patients with primary CNS lymphoma. These can result from direct or indirect effects of primary CNS lymphoma or be treatment-related (Nayak L., et al., 2015). The latter, namely, neurological complications can be seen as a consequence of chemotherapy and radiation therapy in patients with primary CNS lymphoma. Although neurological complications can occur at any time in the course of the disease, some toxicities of chemo-radiotherapy may develop for years or even decades after completion of treatment. Therefore, these toxicities are likely to be seen with increasing frequency as patients with primary CNS lymphoma are living longer and receiving multiple courses of antineoplastic regimens, some of which are life-long (Nolan C.P. and DeAngelis, L.M., 2015).

Neurotoxicity from treatment, such as cognitive dysfunction, occur months to years after diagnosis. In patients older than 60 years treated with WBRT, virtually all long-term survivors develop this complication, although, in patients younger than 60 years, neurotoxicity rates ranging from 26% to 63% have been reported (Harder H., et al., 2004) (Gavrilovic I.T., et al., 2006) (Doolittle N.D., et al., 2013). These complications can diminish the patient's quality of life and eventually shorten survival (Nolan C.P. and DeAngelis, L.M., 2015). Delayed treatment-related neurotoxicity emerged as a significant disabling complication of the combined treatment (Batchelor T. and Loeffler J.S., 2006) (Gavrilovic I.T., et al., 2006) (Morris P.G., and Abrey L.E., 2009) (Abrey L.E., Yahalom J., et al., 2000) (Ferreri A.J., et al., 2003) (Harder H., et al., 2004) (Correa D.D., et al., 2007) (Correa D.D., et al., 2012) (Lai R., et al., 2004) (Doolittle N.D., et al., 2013). Neuropsychological and neuroimaging outcomes have been identified as indicators of neurotoxicity (Harder H., et al., 2004) (Correa D.D., et al., 2007) (Correa D.D., et al., 2012) (Fliessbach K., et al., 2003) (Fliessbach K., et al., 2005) (Juergens A., et al., 2010) (Correa D.D., et al., 2004) (Neuwelt E.A., et al., 2005) (Weller M., 2011) (Doolittle N.D., et al., 2013).

Patients with treatment-related neurotoxicity often demonstrate MRI abnormalities, which appear to correlate with cognitive dysfunction after combined therapy (Harder H., et al., 2004) (Correa D.D., et al., 2012) (Correa D.D., et al., 2004) (Doolittle N.D., et al., 2013). In this chapter, we address delayed neuropsychological complications of methotrexate-based chemotherapy and whole brain radiation therapy and review the literature and our experience on long-term outcomes, such as cognitive function, MRI abnormality, and quality of life (QOL) of primary CNS lymphoma survivors.

DELAYED NEUROTOXICITY

Methotrexate-Based Chemotherapy

Since MTX has poor blood-brain barrier penetration, the drug's potential for CNS toxicity depends upon its method of administration, either intravenous (IV) at high doses greater than 1 g/m^2 or directly into the cerebro-spinal fluid through a lumber puncture or Ommaya reservoir (Nayak L., et al., 2015). CNS toxicity may occur within hours (acute), days to weeks (subacute), or months to years (chronic) after administration. MTX toxicity may range from an acute aseptic meningitis or encephalopathy to a delayed and often debilitating leucoencephalopathy with dementia. The combination of WBRT with either high-dose IV MTX or intrathecal (IT) MTX increases the risk of delayed leucoencephaolpathy. MTX and WBRT can each cause CNS damage, but there is synergistic toxicity when these modalities are combined (Correa D.D., et al., 2012). Indeed, in a randaomized phase 3 study to investigate whether first-line chemotherapy based on HD-MTX was non-inferior to the same chemotherapy regimen followed by WBRT for overall survival, treatment-related neurotoxicity in patients with sustained complete response was more common in patients receiving WBRT (22/45, 49%) than in those who did not (9/34, 26%) (Thiel E., et al., 2010).

A delayed multifocal leucoencephalopathy can be the most debilitating form of MTX neurotoxicity (Correa D.D., et al., 2012). This chronic syndrome is usually seen after repeated high doses of IV MTX or IT MTX and occurs 6 months to years after cessation of treatment.

Symptoms typically include personality and behavioral changes (Nayak L., et al., 2015). In the most extreme form, a severe dementia may develop. MRI typically shows bilateral periventricular white matter changes often occurring prior to symptom onset. This pattern of leucoencephalopathy more commonly occurs with the concomitant use of HD IV MTX or IT MTX with radiation therapy, particularly when the radiation is given prior to the MTX. The radiation therapy may disrupt the blood-brain barrier and result in increased permeability of the white matter to the MTX.

By the way, some patients with cancer who have received chemotherapy other than MTX develop neurocognitive dysfunction that is more subtle than the severe impairment seen in delayed MTX leucoencephalopathy (Ahles T.A., 2012). They describe issues primarily with short-term memory and concentration and an inability to resume high-level tasks they were performing before their diagnosis and treatment (Nolan C.P. and DeAngelis, L.M., 2015). This entity has been called chemo brain. Many studies that describe chemo brain report a significant decline in short-term memory and execute function that is not proportionate to mood disorders such as anxiety and depression. On the other hand, some studies also show that patients with untreated cancer are more cognitively impaired than a comparable control group, raising an interesting issues regarding the cancer itself and other comorbidities of cognitive function (Mandelblatt J.S., et al., 2014) (Ahles T.A., et al, 2010).

Probable risk factors for chemo brain are high-dose as opposed to standard-dose chemotherapy, pretreatment lower IQ and level of education, older age, and female gender (Nolan C.P. and DeAngelis, L.M., 2015). Although most of the symptoms of chemo brain are self-limited, affecting patients predominantly during treatment or shortly thereafter, in some patients, symptoms may persist for decades after cessation of treatment. The exact pathophysiology of chemo brain is unknown, but it may be related to reduction of progenitor cells in the hippocampus and frontal subcortical white matter.

Whole-Brain Radiation Therapy

Patients who survive longer than 6 months may become vulnerable to long-term radiation injury (Nolan C.P. and DeAngelis, L.M., 2015). The curative dose of radiation therapy on any neoplasm is limited by potential damage to normal tissue unavoidable contained within portal.

Risk factors include those specific to radiation, such as total dose, dose per fraction, treatment duration, and volume of tissue treated, as well as patient-specific factors including age, gender, comorbid conditions, and previous or concurrent chemotherapy. Radiation injury may occur at any time: acute (during or immediately after treatment), subacute (within 6 months of treatment), or delayed (6 months to years after treatment). Early and subacute injury is often reversible, whereas delayed injury is not.

Delayed radiation toxicity occurring months to years after treatment can be irreversible and disabling. It manifests primarily as either radiation necrosis in patients with primary or metastatic brain tumors treated with external beam radiation therapy and radiosurgery or as a diffuse leucoencephalopathy with cortical atrophy in some patients in whom a large volume of brain tissue is treated with radiation, most commonly WBRT (Greene-Schloesser D., et al., 2012) (Nolan C.P. and DeAngelis, L.M., 2015).

Cognitive impairment can occur in up to 90% of patients who survive more than 6 months after WBRT (Nolan C.P. and DeAngelis, L.M., 2015). Approximately 2% to 5% of these patients will develop dementia. The degree of cognitive impairment ranges from mild deficits in short-term memory and attention to dementia. These clinical findings are not associated with radiographic evidence of necrosis. Brain MRI displays sulcal atrophy, ventricular dilatation, and white matter hyperintensity (leucoencephalopathy). Leucoencephalopathy occurs in patients with primary CNS lymphoma treated with WBRT, particularly elderly patients and those treated with concomitant cytotoxic therapy such as MTX or cytarabine. Although the exact pathogenesis of delayed cognitive dysfunction after radiation therapy remains unknown, evidence exists for both direct injury to brain parenchyma and vasculature as well as an indirect neuroinflammatory process involving cytokines and reactive oxygen species (Greene-Schloesser D., et al., 2013). Since MTX and WBRT can each cause CNS damage through vascular injury, neuronal loss, inflammation, demyelination, and necrosis and can disrupt hippocampal neurogenesis, there is synergistic toxicity when these modalities are combined (DeAngelis L. and Posner J.B., 2009).

LONG-TERM OUTCOME

In the literature, there are several studies focusing on long-term outcome of patients with primary CNS lymphoma, such as cognitive function, neuroimaging and quality of life (McAllister L.D., et al., 2000) (Fliessbach K., et al., 2003) (Lai R., 2004) (Harder H., et al., 2004) (Correa D.D., 2004) (Fliessbach K., 2005) (Correa D.D., 2007) (Correa D.D., et al., 2009) (Juergens A., et al., 2010) (Correa D.D., et al., 2012) (Doolittle N.D., et al., 2013). The results of these studies are similar in that patients treated with HD-MTX and WBRT did poorly on cognitive assessment as well as on quality-of-life measures and additionally had MRI evidence of extensive white matter abnormalities (Taphoorn M.J., 2004) (Correa D.D., et al., 2012) (Abrey L.E., 2012) (Nayak L., et al., 2015).

Cognitive Function

Because formal psychometric evaluations are not routinely performed, the true risk of this complication has likely been underestimated (Doolittle N.D., et al., 2013). Cognitive dysfunction after combined therapy has been discussed in correlation with MRI abnormalities often demonstrated in patients with treatment-related neurotoxicity (Harder H., et al., 2004) (Correa D.D., 2004) (Correa D.D., et al., 2012). Although neuropsychological and neuroimaging outcomes have been identified as indicators of neurotoxicity, these indicators have been evaluated in a standardized fashion in only a few relatively small studies (Fliessbach K., et al., 2003) (Correa D.D., 2004) (Harder H., et al., 2004) (Fliessbach K., 2005) (Correa D.D., 2007) (Juergens A., et al., 2010) (Weller M., 2011) (Correa D.D., et al., 2012). Therefore, a test battery evaluating cognition and QOL was developed by the International PCNSL Collaborative Group investigators and recommended for prospective trials (Correa D.D., 2007).

Using this standardized neurocognitive battery designed to evaluate neurotoxicity in multinational primary CNS trials, Doolittle and his colleagues prospectively performed the neuropsychological assessment for a large number of primary CNS lymphoma survivors in complete remission (n = 80) with a long median follow-up of 5.5 years (2-26 years) (Correa D.D., 2007) (Doolittle N.D., et al., 2013). This tests measure attention and executive function (Wechsler Adult Intelligence Scale—III Digit Span subtest (Digits Forward, Digits Backward), Trail Making Test Parts A and B, and Brief Test of Attention), verbal memory (Hopkins Verbal Learning Test–Revised), and motor skills (Grooved Pegboard Test, Dominant and Nondominant). As a result, 19% of the long-term survivors showed impairment in multiple cognitive domains, including 47% of those treated with WBRT. This group had poorer attention/executive function, motor skills, and composite scores (the number of SDs above or below the mean for a population of similar age) than patients not treated with WBRT. Of interest, verbal memory and composite scores improved as the length of the interval from diagnosis to long-term evaluation increased, suggesting that verbal memory may improve as disease free survival increases. Notably, 8 (12%) of 65 survivors treated with chemotherapy without WBRT showed cognitive impairment in multiple domains even after complete disease remission. This study might provide the longest reported follow-up data in primary CNS lymphoma, although survivors were evaluated at different time points since completing therapy. This primary CNS lymphoma test battery allowed standardized collection of cognitive data and the findings are valuable as a comparison series of long-term survivorship for future PCNSL studies.

The results of previous studies are similar in that patients treated with the combined modality therapy had impairments across several neuropsychological domains (Taphoorn M.J. and Klein M., 2004) (Correa D.D., et al., 2012) (Abrey L.E., 2012). Still, previous studies have a limitation including lack of pre- and post-treatment baseline and long-term follow-up neurocognitive evaluations with the identical test battery on most of the survivors. The investigators could not evaluate changes over time in long-term primary CNS lymphoma survivors. Further longitudinal studies on late cognitive adverse effects are warranted to prove "changes over time" by serial follow-up from diagnosis to progression.

More frequently, single-drug and multidrug HD-MTX-based regimens without WBRT have been used in an effort to increase survival while avoiding the risk of delayed neurotoxicity (Doolittle N.D., et al., 2013). Considering the risk of chemo brain, it might be relevant to assess the possible cognitive adverse effects of these therapies, particularly in the elderly, although prospective studies involving patients treated with HD-MTX alone reported either preserved or improved cognitive functions in most patients (Correa D.D., et al., 2007) (Juergens A., et al., 2010).

Neuroimaging

MRI abnormalities are often demonstrated in patients with treatment-related neurotoxicity. In the literature, it is reported that MRI abnormalities appear to correlate with cognitive dysfunction after WBRT + HD-MTX therapy but may not correlate with cognitive decline after MTX-based therapy alone (Fliessbach K., et al., 2003) (Harder H., et al., 2004) (Correa D.D., 2004) (Fliessbach K., 2005) (Neuwelt E.A., et al., 2005).

Correa et al. measured white matter (WM) disease and cortical global atrophy (GA) on brain MRI scans in primary CNS lymphoma survivors treated with HD-MTX plus WBRT or HD-MTX alone (Correa D.D., 2012). WM abnormalities were rated on a fluid-attenuated inversion recovery sequence and included: no WM change (grade 0), minimal patchy WM foci (grade 1), start of confluence of WM disease (grade 2), large confluent areas (grade 3), confluence with cortical and subcortical involvement (grade 4), leucoencephalopathy (grade 5), and possible radiation necrosis (grade 6). GA was rated on T1-weighted MRI scans and included: no atrophy (grade 0), mild atrophy (grade 1), moderate atrophy (grade 2), and severe atrophy (grade 3). In this study, 50 primary CNS lymphoma patients in disease remission underwent a post-treatment baseline evaluation, and 33 patients completed a follow-up evaluation with mean time interval of 16.2 months for patients treated with the combined modality regimen and 14.1 months for patients treated with chemotherapy alone. On the baseline evaluation, more extensive WM abnormalities (grades 2–6) were evident in 67% of patients who received WBRT + HD-MTX and in 54% of patients treated with chemotherapy alone. Moderate to severe GA (grades 2–3) was evident in 44% of patients who received WBRT + HD-MTX and in 54% of patients treated with chemotherapy alone. There were no significant differences between the 2 treatment groups on extent of WM disease or GA. Next, a comparison of WM ratings between the posttreatment baseline and follow-up showed that there was an increase in WM disease among patients who received

WBRT + HD-MTX. Notably, there were no significant changes in WM ratings among patients treated with HD-MTX alone or in GA ratings for either treatment modality group. As the result of neuropsychological assessment in this cohort, patients treated with WBRT + HD-MTX had impairment across most cognitive tests, including selective attention, motor speed, set-shifting, verbal learning, delayed recall, and recognition memory, while patients treated with chemotherapy alone did not meet criteria for cognitive impairment. Moreover, there were no significant changes between the initial and follow-up evaluations on any of the cognitive tests, except for an improvement in attention among patients treated with HD-MTX alone.

These results support previous studies reporting that MRI abnormalities correlate with cognitive dysfunction after combined therapy. The authors also stated that treatment with HD-MTX alone is not associated with MRI abnormalities and cognitive decrements in primary CNS lymphoma patients, even among the elderly. As the next step, it would be necessary to investigate delayed neurotoxicity in a larger cohort of survivors treated with enhanced chemotherapy alone within the longer follow-up period.

Quality of Life

Regarding QOL of primary CNS lymphoma survivors, there is not a standardized fashion to assess but a few reports in the literature (Harder H., et al., 2004) (Correa D.D., 2012) (Doolittle N.D., et al., 2013).

In the Doolittle's study, QOL of patients was assessed by using the European Organization for Research and Treatment of Cancer (EORTC) QOL Questionnaire–30 (QLQ-C30) and Brain Cancer Module–20 (Aaronson N.K., et al., 1993) (Doolittle N.D., et al., 2013). The EORTC QLQ-C30 measures 5 functional scales (physical, role, emotional, cognitive, and social) and global health status / QOL. The EORTC QOL Questionnaire Brain Cancer Module–20 assesses items such as visual disorders, communication deficit, and future uncertainty. This study showed scores at a time point after completing therapy as a long-term QOL outcome according to treatment group (HD-MTX-based regimens with or without WBRT). As a result, the long-term survivors showed poorer global QOL, and poorer physical, role, emotional, and social function. Each QLQ-C30 functional scale of the WBRT group was significantly lower than that of the non-WBRT groups. Because this study does not include pre- and post-treatment baseline evaluations, QOL changes, especially decline, over time cannot be demonstrated.

In the Correa's study, QOL and mood were assessed using the Functional Assessment of Cancer Therapy-Brain (FACT-BR, version 4) and the Beck Depression Inventory (BDI) (Correa D.D., 2012). A comparison of mean scores on a self-report measure of QOL (FACT-BR) between treatment groups showed that patients who received HD-MTX alone had significantly lower mean scores compared with patients treated with WBRT + HD-MTX (low scores indicate fewer complaints). Patients treated with HD-MTX alone had lower scores, indicating more intact QOL than that of patients treated with WBRT. The 2 groups did not differ significantly on a measure of depression (BDI), and mean scores did not indicate depressed mood. There were no significant changes between baseline and follow-up in the FACT-BR or BDI scores for either treatment group.

Considering the correlation between QOL and neuropsychological and neuroimaging outcomes, lower QOL was positively associated with cognitive decline and inversely corresponded with MR abnormalities. These findings support several reports that treatment-related cognitive deficits can be of sufficient severity to interfere with QOL in primary CNS survivors.

Wakayama Medical University Hospital Series

Background

As combined chemotherapy and radiation improve survival rates and patients live longer, concerns mount about the long-term outcome and delayed nerurotoxicity in treatment of primary CNS lymphoma. Development of delayed white matter abnormalities indicative of leucoencephalopathy have been correlated with cognitive dysfunction, poor performance status and low quality of life.

Objective

We retrospectively reviewed data on the outcome of primary CNS lymphoma patients treated at Wakayama medical university hospital (WMUH). Especially, we focused on the serial change of neuroimaging and quality of life, and analyzed the correlation between leucoencephalopathy and performance status.

Methods

Fifty-two primary CNS lymphoma patients treated at WMUH between 1993 and 2014 were included in this analysis. In these patients, 32 patients who received HD-MTX and WBRT underwent annual evaluation of brain magnetic resonance imaging (MRI) and Karnofsky performance status (KPS).

According to the Monaco's grading scale, we evaluated the development of delayed white matter changes using fluid attenuated image recovery (FLAIR) magnetic resonance images: grade 1, 1/4 little or no white matter hyperintensity; grade 2, 1/4 limited periventricular hyperintensity; and grade 3, 1/4 diffuse white matter hyperintensity (Monaco E.A. 3rd, et al., 2013). Local white matter changes from specific tumors were not incorporated. Figure 1 shows representative MRIs.

The general function of patients was measured with the Karnofsky Performance Status scale (KPS) (Karnofsky D.A., 1949) (Mor V, et al., 1984).

Additionally, data regarding age, gender, number of the lesion, chemotherapy, radiation, response, survival and cause of death were able to be collected.

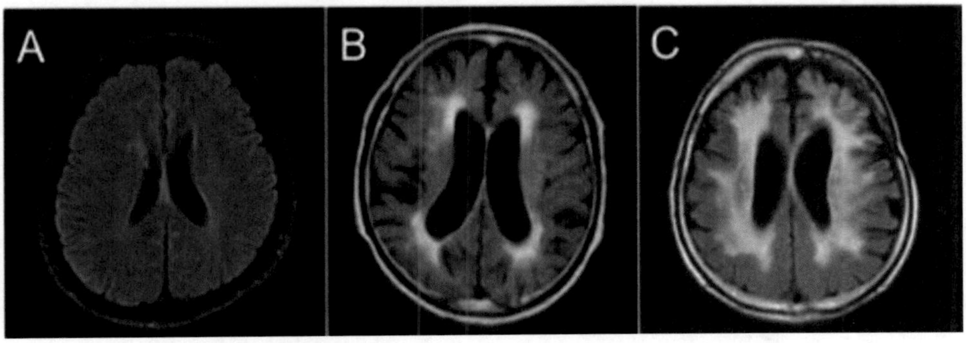

Figure 1. Representative fluid-attenuated inversion recovery magnetic resonance images are shown for (A) grade 1, (B) grade 2, and (C) grade 3 leucoencephalopathy.

Overall survival (OS) and progression-free survival (PFS) were analyzed in univariate and multivariate analysis. Univariate analysis was calculated with the logrank test. Multivariate analysis was done by Cox proportional hazard survival model under specification of hazard ratio (HR). The association between leucoencephalopathy grade and KPS scale was assessed by using the Pearson correlation coefficient. The correlation between leucoencephalopathy grade and outcome (survival, tumor-related death and tumor-unrelated death) was assessed by using the Yates Chi square test. A $p < 0.05$ was considered to be significant. Statistical calculations were performed with the Excel®Statistical Program File ystat2013.

Results

Patient demographics and characteristics are summarized overall (n = 52) in Table 1 (33 males and 19 females). The overall median age was 65.1 years (29-87). Thirty-two patients were treated with HD-MTX + WBRT (+ local irradiation), 4 with local irradiation only and 16 with others. The median follow-up period was 36 months (minimum, 13 months; maximum, 136 months).

As shown in Table 2, mean overall survival and progression-free survival periods are 34.1 and 23.6 months, respectively. In univariate analysis, HD-MTX and WBRT (with local irradiation) were significantly associated with better OS and PFS (Table 3) In multivariate analysis for OS and PFS, leucoencephalopathy was revealed as an unfavorable prognositc factor (Table 4).

In thirty-seven patients whose data were able to be collected, distribution of leucoencephalopathy grading at initial diagnosis, after induction treatment and at the latest assessment was shown in Figure 2. At the initial diagnosis, there were no patients with grade 3 leucoencephalopathy. On the latest imaging, thirteen patients (35%) showed grade 3, which indicates development of delayed white matter change.

KPS scale scores of 52 patients at the time of the latest MR assessment were shown in Table 5 and the association between leucoencephalopathy grade and Karnofsky performance status scale was analyzed in Figure 3. As a result, the inverse correlation between white matter change and performance status was demonstrated.

Table 1. Demographics and characteristics of the study cohort

	n = 52
Gender, n (%)	
male	33 (64)
female	19 (36)
Age at diagnosis, year	
median	65
range	29 – 87
Lesion, n	
single	32
multiple	20
Induction treatment, n	
HD-MTX + WBRT (+ local)	32
WBRT	4
others	16
Chemotherapeutic agent, n	
MTX	33
steroid	6
other	7
none	6
Radiation modality, n	
whole brain	30
whole brain + local	7
local	5
stereotactic radiosurgery	3
none	7
Follow-up period, months	
median	36
range	13 - 136

Abbreviations: HD-MTX, high-dose methotrexate; WBRT, +.

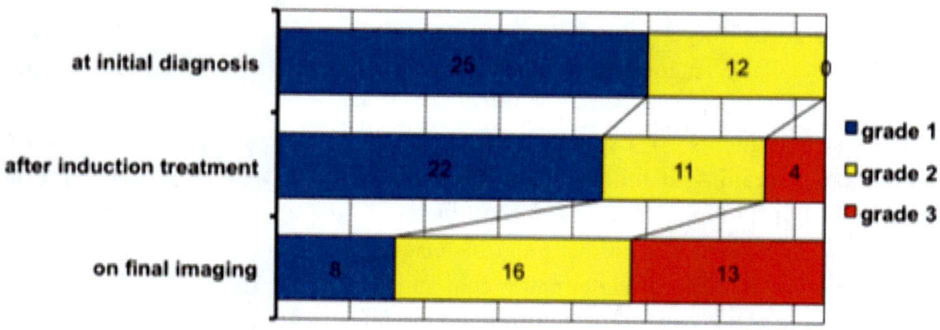

Figure 2. Distribution of leucoencephalopathy grade at initial diagnosis, after induction treatment and on final imaging in 37 patients. At the initial diagnosis, there were no patients with grade 3 leucoencephalopathy. On final imaging, thirteen patients (35%) showed grade 3, which indicates development of delayed white matter change.

Table 2. Clinical results of the study cohort

	n = 52
Initial response, n	
CR	36
PR	14
SD	1
PD	1
Recurrence, n	
+	27
-	25
Progression-free survival, months	
median	16.0
mean	23.6
Overall survival, months	
median	26.0
mean	34.1
Outcome	
alive	14
dead	38
Cause of death	
tumor-related	31
tumor-unrelated	7

Table 3. Univariate analysis of prognostic factors for overall survival and progression-free survvival

	Overall survival	Progression-free survival
Gender	0.036	0.060
Number of lesion	0.807	0.925
HD-MTX + WBRT	0.002	0.001
Chemotherapy	0.024	0.018
Radiation (WBRT)	< 0.001	< 0.001
Initial treatment response	< 0.001	0.002
Recurrence	0.343	-

Abbreviations: HD-MTX, high-dose methotrexate; WBRT, whole-brain radiotherapy.

Table 4. Multivariate analysis of prognostic factors for overall survival and progression-free survival

	Overall survival (hazard ratio)	Progression-free survival (hazard ratio)
Gender	0.725 (0.753)	0.043 (0.140)
Age at initial diagnosis	0.066 (1.076)	0.097 (1.080)
Karnofsky performance status at initial diagnosis	0.818 (1.005)	0.134 (0.960)
Chemotherapy (no methotrexate)	0.937 (1.089)	0.753 (2.676)
Radiation (whole brain radiation therapy)	0.400 (0.239)	0.582 (0.167)
Initial treatment response (no complete response)	0.038 (7.837)	0.084 (8.410)
Leucoencephalopathy	0.049 (0.104)	0.039 (0.006)

Table 5. Karnofsky performanse status scale score on final imaging in 52 patients

Karnofsky performance status scale	n = 52
90, 100	23
70, 80	10
50, 60	14
30, 40	3
10, 20	2

During the observation period, 21 of 37 patients followed have died. In these patients, fifteen patients died due to tumor progression and six due to tumor-unrelated causes (5, pneumonia; 1, renal insufficiency) (Figure 4). Distribution of leucoencephalopathy grading of these patients was also shown in Figure 4. A significantly larger proportion of patients with grades 3 leucoencephalopathy were apparent in patients with tumor-unrelated causes of death. The correlation between grade 3 leucoencephalopathy and tumor-unrelated death proved to be statistically significant.

Figure 5 depicts annual changes of white matter abnormality of 21 patients whose MRI were obtained annually. In the patients with grade 3 leucoencepahlopathy at the time of analysis, white matter change had progressed to grade 2 leucoencephalopathy for three years after initial diagnosis and all patients with grade 3 died within 4 years (Figure 5).

Discussion and Conclusion

HD-MTX plus WBRT significantly improved OS and PFS of primary CNS lymphoma patients in our study cohort. However, leucoencephalopathy could developed despite good tumor control, resulting in worse performance status and tumor-unrelated death.

A prospective study would be necessary to correlate these findings with neurocognition and quality of life. It should be considered how to increase survival while avoiding the risk of delayed neurotoxicity in the development of novel treatment strategy.

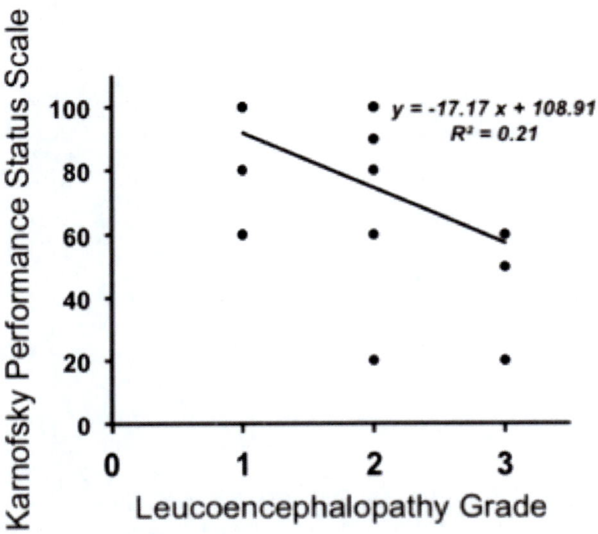

Figure 3. Correlation analysis between leucoencephalopathy grade and Karnofsky performance status scale on final imaging in 52 patients. The inverse correlation between white matter change and performance status was demonstrated.

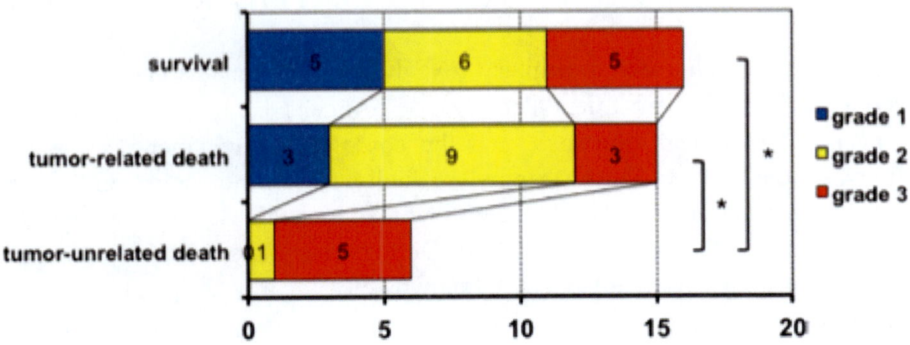

*Statistically significant in chi-square analysis.

Figure 4. Distribution of leucoencephalopathy grade on final imaging in the patients' outcome at the time of analysis. During the observation period, 21 of 37 patients followd have died. In to tumor-unrelated causes (5, Pneumonia; 1, renal insufficiency), A significantly larger proportion of patients with grade 3 leucoencephalopathy were apparent in patients with tumor-unrelated causes of death. The correlation between grade 3 leucoencephalopathy and tumor-unrelated death proved to be statistically significant.

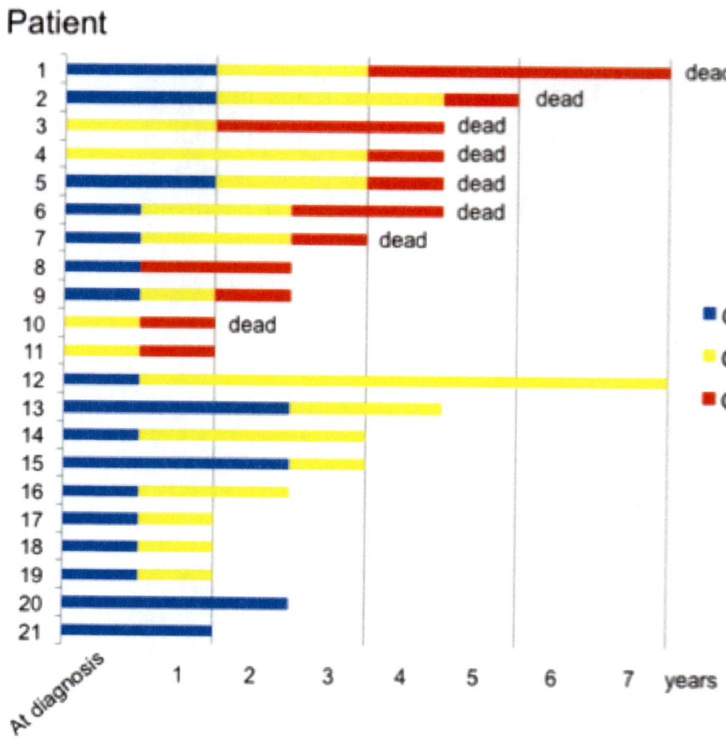

Figure 5. Graph depicts annual change of leucoencephalopathy grade in 21 patients. In the patients with grade 3 leucoencephalopathy at the time of analysis, white matter change had progressed to grade 2 leucoencephalopathy for three years after initial diagnosis and all patients with grade 3 died within 4 years.

NOVEL TREATMENT STRATEGY AND DELAYED NEUROTOXICITY

The best therapeutic approach to primary CNS lymphoma remains uncertain, with few randomized trials to guide treatment decisions (DeAngelis L.M., 2015). The choice of cytostatic agents; the role of rituximab; and the consolidative treatment in the form of chemotherapy, whole-brain radiation therapy, or high-dose chemotherapy and autologous stem cell transplantation are feasible, but questions that several ongoing randomized trials will attempt to answer (Nayak L., et al., 2015). On the other hand, survivor patients are at high risk of developing severe treatment-related toxicity, mainly disabling neurotoxicity, raising the question of whether to intensify therapy to improve the cure rate or to downgrade treatment to reduce side effects (Citterio G., 2015).

Recently updated results from a phase III trial (G-PCNSL-SG-1) do not support the use of radiotherapy in primary CNS lymphoma, although the analyses had several limitations (Korfel A., 2015) (DeAngelis L.M., 2015). Consolidative whole-brain radiation therapy may benefit disease-free survival, but, owing to the concern of neurotoxicity, impaired quality of life in survivors, and lack of conclusive evidence that it improves overall survival, the focus has been on treating patients with chemotherapy alone, particularly with the use of consolidative high-dose chemotherapy and autologous stem cell transplantation (Nayak L., et al., 2015). Actual front-line therapy consists of HD-MTX-based chemotherapy, mostly in combination with high-dose cytarabine and/or alkylating agents. The use of high-dose chemotherapy supported by autologous stem-cell transplantation is increased (Citterio G., 2015). However, as shown in the randomised phase 3 trial, treatment-related neurotoxicity in patients with sustained complete response was not uncommon in patients who received high-dose chemotherapy without radiation (9/34, 26%) but common in those receiving WBRT (22/45, 49%) (Thiel E., 2010). As a next step, it should be investigated whether intensified chemotherapy to improve the cure rate might increase chemo brain and delayed neurotoxicity.

By the way, there is a literature describing that chemotherapy and radiation therapy have very different toxicity profiles in patients receiving these modalities for primary CNS lymphoma (Nolan C.P. and DeAngelis L.M., 2015). The vulnerability can be often dependent on individual predisposition as well as comorbid conditions. Recognition of these interrelated factors can identify patients at highest risk for neurologic complications of therapy, and intensified management of premorbid conditions may reduce an individual's risk. Enhanced efforts to identify genetic predispositions to neurotoxicity must help militate against these complications in the future. More vigorous preventive and therapeutic strategies are necessary to maintain neurocognitive function and preserve QOL of survivors.

Conclusion

HD-MTX in combination with WBRT improved survival rates of the patients with primary CNS lymphoma, although single-drug and multidrug HD-MTX-based regimens without WBRT have been used in an effort to increase survival. Since patients with primary CNS lymphoma are living longer, survivor patients are at high risk of developing severe treatment-related toxicity, mainly disabling neurotoxicity. After all, the long-term outcome, especially of elderly patients, is invariably dismal often accompanied by increased severe adverse effects such as cognitive dysfunction, leucoencephalopathy and impaired quality of life. It is important to recognize and avoid treatment-related complications. Further modification and improvement of therapeutic regimens is critical to diminish long-term consequences of nervous system injury and improve a patient's QOL.

References

Aaronson N.K., Ahmedzai S., Bergman B., Bullinger M., Cull A., Duez N. J., Filiberti A., Flechtner H., Fleishman S. B., de Haes J.C. J. M., Kaasa S., Klee M., Osoba D., Razavi D., Rofe P.B., Schraub S., Sneeuw K., Sullivan M., Takeda F. for the European Organization for Research and Treatment of Cancer Study Group on Quality of Life, (1993). The European Organization for Research and Treatment of Cancer QLQC30 QLQC30: a quality-of-life instrument for use in international clinical trials in oncology. *J Natl Cancer Inst.* 85, 365–376.

Abrey L.E., DeAngelis L.M., Yahalom J., (1998). Long-term survival in primary CNS lymphoma. *J Clin Oncol.* 16, 859-63.

Abrey L.E., Yahalom J., DeAngelis L.M., (2000). Treatment for primary CNS lymphoma: the next step. *J Clin Oncol.* 3144–3150.

Abrey L.E., Ben-Porat L., Panageas K.S., Yahalom J., Berkey B., Curran W., Schultz C., Leibel S., Nelson D., Mehta M., DeAngelis L.M., (2006). Primary central nervous system lymphoma: the Memorial Sloan-Kettering Cancer Center prognostic model. *J Clin Oncol.* 24, 5711-5.

Abrey L.E., (2012). The impact of chemotherapy on cognitive outcomes in adults with primary brain tumors. *J Neurooncol.* 108, 285–290.

Ahles T.A., Saykin A.J., McDonald B.C., Li Y., Furstenberg C.T., Hanscom B.S., Mulrooney T.J., Schwartz G.N., Kaufman P.A., (2010). Longitudinal assessment of cognitive changes associated with adjuvant treatment for breast cancer: impact of age and cognitive reserve. *J Clin Oncol.* 28, 4434-40. doi: 10.1200/JCO.2009.27.0827.

Ahles T.A., (2012). Brain vulnerability to chemotherapy toxicities. *Psychooncology.* 21, 1141-8. doi: 10.1002/pon.3196.

Batchelor T., Loeffler J.S., (2006). Primary CNS lymphoma. *J Clin Oncol.* 24, 1281–1288.

Citterio G., Reni M., Ferreri A.J., (2015). Present and future treatment options for primary CNS lymphoma. *Expert Opin Pharmacother.* Sep 15:1-11.

Correa D.D., DeAngelis L.M., Shi W., Thaler H., Glass A., Abrey L.E., (2004). Cognitive functions in survivors of primary central nervous system lymphoma. *Neurology.* 62, 548-55.

Correa D.D., Maron L., Harder H., Klein M., Armstrong C.L., Calabrese P., Bromberg J.E., Abrey L.E., Batchelor T.T., Schiff D., (2007). Cognitive functions in primary central nervous system lymphoma: literature review and assessment guidelines. *Ann Oncol.*18, 1145–51.

Correa D.D., Rocco-Donovan M., DeAngelis L.M., Dolgoff-Kaspar R., Iwamoto F., Yahalom J., Abrey L.E., (2009). Prospective cognitive follow-up in primary CNS lymphoma patients treated with chemotherapy and reduced-dose radiotherapy. *J Neurooncol.* 91; 315-21. doi: 10.1007/s11060-008-9716-0. Epub 2008 Nov 1.

Correa D.D., Shi W., Abrey L.E., Deangelis L.M., Omuro A.M., Deutsch M.B., Thaler H.T., (2012). Cognitive functions in primary CNS lymphoma after single or combined modality regimens. *Neuro Oncol.* 14, 101-8.

DeAngelis L., Posner J.B., (2009). Side effects of radiation therapy. In: DeAngelis, L., Posner, J.B., eds. Neurologic Complications of Cancer. 2nd ed. New York: Oxford University Press, 551–555.

DeAngelis L.M., (2015). Neuro-oncology: Primary CNS lymphoma treatment--the devil is in the details. *Nat Rev Neurol.* 11, 314-5. doi: 10.1038/nrneurol.2015.64.

Doolittle N.D., Korfel A., Lubow M.A., Schorb E., Schlegel U., Rogowski S., Fu R., Dósa E., Illerhaus G., Kraemer D.F., Muldoon L.L., Calabrese P., Hedrick N., Tyson R.M., Jahnke K., Maron L.M., Butler R.W., Neuwelt E.A., (2013). Long-term cognitive function, neuroimaging, and quality of life in primary CNS lymphoma. *Neurology.* 81, 84-92.

Ferreri A.J., Blay J.Y., Reni M., Pasini F., Spina M., Ambrosetti A., Calderoni A., Rossi A., Vavassori V., Conconi A., Devizzi L., Berger F., Ponzoni M., Borisch B., Tinguely M., Cerati M., Milani M., Orvieto E., Sanchez J., Chevreau C., Dell'Oro S., Zucca E., Cavalli F., (2003). Prognostic scoring system for primary CNS lymphomas: the International Extranodal Lymphoma Study Group experience. *J Clin Oncol.* 21, 266-72.

Ferreri A.J., Abrey L.E., Blay J.Y., Borisch B., Hochman J., Neuwelt E.A., Yahalom J., Zucca E., Cavalli F., Armitage J., Batchelor T., (2003). Summary statement on primary central nervous system lymphomas from the Eighth International Conference on Malignant Lymphoma, Lugano, Switzerland, June 12 to 15, 2002. *J Clin Oncol.* 21, 2407–2414.

Fliessbach K., Urbach H., Helmstaedter C., Pels H., Glasmacher A., Kraus J A., Klockgether T., Schmidt-Wolf I., Schlegel U., (2003). Cognitive performance and magnetic resonance imaging findings after high-dose systemic and intraventricular chemotherapy for primary central nervous system lymphoma. *Arch Neurol.* 60, 563–568.

Fliessbach K., Helmstaedter C., Urbach H., Althaus A., Pels H., Linnebank M., Juergens A., Glasmacher A., Schmidt-Wolf I.G., Klockgether T., Schlegel U., (2005). Neuropsychological outcome after chemotherapy for primary CNS lymphoma: a prospective study. *Neurology.* 64, 1184-8.

Gavrilovic I.T., Hormigo A., Yahalom J., DeAngelis L.M., Abrey L.E., (2006). Long-term follow-up of high-dose methotrexate-based therapy with and without whole brain irradiation for newly diagnosed primary CNS lymphoma. *J Clin Oncol.* 24, 4570–4574.

Greene-Schloesser D., Robbins M.E., Peiffer A.M., Shaw E.G., Wheeler K.T., Chan M.D., (2012). Radiation-induced brain injury: A review. *Front Oncol.* 2, 73. doi: 10.3389/fonc.2012.00073. eCollection 2012.

Greene-Schloesser D, Moore E., Robbins M.E., (2013). Molecular pathways: radiation-induced cognitive impairment. *Clin Cancer Res.*19, 2294-300. doi: 10.1158/1078-0432.CCR-11-2903.

Harder H., Holtel H., Bromberg J.E., Poortmans P., Haaxma-Reiche H., Kluin-Nelemans H.C., Menten J., van den Bent M.J., (2004). Cognitive status and quality of life after treatment for primary CNS lymphoma. *Neurology.* 62, 544-7.

Hoang-Xuan K., Bessell E., Bromberg J., Hottinger A.F., Preusser M., Rudà R., Schlegel U., Siegal T., Soussain C., Abacioglu U., Cassoux N.., Deckert M., Dirven C.M., Ferreri A.J., Graus F., Henriksson R., Herrlinger U., Taphoorn M., Soffietti R., Weller M.; European Association for Neuro-Oncology Task Force on Primary CNS Lymphoma., (2015). Diagnosis and treatment of primary CNS lymphoma in immunocompetent patients: guidelines from the European Association for Neuro-Oncology. *Lancet Oncol.* 16, e322-32. doi: 10.1016/S1470-2045(15)00076-5.

Janelsins M.C., Kesler S.R., Ahles T.A., Morrow G.R., (2014). Prevalence, mechanisms, and management of cancer-related cognitive impairment. *Int Rev Psychiatry* 26, 102-13. doi: 10.3109/09540261.2013.864260.

Juergens A., Pels H., Rogowski S., Fliessbach K., Glasmacher A., Engert A., Reiser M., Diehl V., Vogt-Schaden M., Egerer G., Schackert G., Reichmann H., Kroschinsky F., Bode U., Herrlinger U., Linnebank M., Deckert M., Fimmers R., Schmidt-Wolf I.G., Schlegel U., (2010). Long-term survival with favorable cognitive outcome after chemotherapy in primary central nervous system lymphoma. Ann Neurol;67:182–189.

Karnofsky D.A., (1949). Evaluation of chemotherapy agents. Colombia University Press, NY.

Korfel A., Schlegel U., (2013). Diagnosis and treatment of primary CNS lymphoma. *Nat Rev Neurol.* 9, 317-27. doi: 10.1038/nrneurol.2013.83.

Korfel A., Thiel E., Martus P., Möhle R., Griesinger F., Rauch M., Röth A., Hertenstein B., Fischer T., Hundsberger T., Mergenthaler H.G., Junghanß C., Birnbaum T., Fischer L., Jahnke K., Herrlinger U., Roth P., Bamberg M., Pietsch T., Weller M., (2015).

Randomized phase III study of whole-brain radiotherapy for primary CNS lymphoma. *Neurology.* 84, 1242-8. doi: 10.1212/WNL.0000000000001395.

Korfel A., (2015). A focus on pharmacotherapy for primary central nervous system lymphoma. *Expert Rev Hematol.* 8, 559-62. doi: 10.1586/17474086.2015.1066672. Epub 2015 Jul 9.

Lai R., Abrey L.E., Rosenblum M.K., DeAngelis L.M., (2004). Treatment-induced leukoencephalopathy in primary CNS lymphoma: a clinical and autopsy study. *Neurology.* 62, 451–456.

Lee Y.W., Cho H.J., Lee W.H., Sonntag W.E., (2012). Whole brain radiation-induced cognitive impairment: pathophysiological mechanisms and therapeutic targets. *Biomol Ther (Seoul).* 20, 357-70. doi: 10.4062/biomolther.2012.20.4.357. Review.

Mandelblatt J.S., Jacobsen P.B., Ahles T., (2014). Cognitive effects of cancer systemic therapy: implications for the care of older patients and survivors. *J Clin Oncol.* 32, 617-26. doi: 10.1200/JCO.2014.55.1259. Epub 2014 Jul 28.

McAllister L.D., Doolittle N.D., Guastadisegni P.E., Kraemer D.F., Lacy C.A., Crossen J.R., Neuwelt E.A., (2000). Cognitive outcomes and long-term follow-up results after enhanced chemotherapy delivery for primary central nervous system lymphoma. *Neurosurgery.* 46:51–60; discussion 60–61.

Morris P.G., Abrey L.E., (2009). Therapeutic challenges in primary CNS lymphoma. *Lancet Neurol.* 581–592.

Monaco E.A. 3rd, Faraji A.H., Berkowitz O., Parry P.V., Hadelsberg U., Kano H., Niranjan A., Kondziolka D., Lunsford L.D., (2013). Leukoencephalopathy after whole-brain radiation therapy plus radiosurgery versus radiosurgery alone for metastatic lung cancer. *Cancer.*119, 226-32. doi: 10.1002/cncr.27504.

Mor V, Laliberte L, Morris JN, Wiemann M (1984) The Karnofsky performance status scale: an examination of its reliability and validity in a research setting. *Cancer.* 53; 2002–2007.

Nayak L., Pentsova E., Batchelor T.T., (2015). Primary CNS lymphoma and neurologic complications of hematologic malignancies. *Continuum (Minneap Minn).* 21, 355-72.

Neuwelt E.A., Guastadisegni P.E., Varallyay P., Doolittle N.D., (2005). Imaging changes and cognitive outcome in primary CNS lymphoma after enhanced chemotherapy delivery. *AJNR Am J Neuroradiol.* 26, 258–265.

Neuwelt E.A., Schiff D., (2015). Primary CNS lymphoma: a landmark trial and the next steps. *Neurology.* 84; 1194-5. doi: 10.1212/WNL.0000000000001407.

Nolan C.P., DeAngelis, L.M., (2015). Neurologic Complications of Chemotherapy and Radiation Therapy. *Continuum (Minneap Minn).* 21, 429-51.

Omuro A.M., Ben-Porat L.S., Panageas K.S., Kim A.K., Correa D.D., Yahalom J., Deangelis L.M., Abrey L.E., (2005). Delayed neurotoxicity in primary central nervous system lymphoma. *Arch Neurol.* 62, 1595-600.

Omuro A., Taillandier L., Chinot O., Sierra Del Rio M., Carnin C., Barrie M., Soussain C., Tanguy M.L., Choquet S., Leblond V., Hoang-Xuan K.; ANOCEF Group (French Neuro-Oncology Association), (2011). Primary CNS lymphoma in patients younger than 60: can whole-brain radiotherapy be deferred? *J Neurooncol.* 104, 323-30. doi: 10.1007/s11060-010-0497-x.

Taphoorn M.J., Klein M., (2004). Cognitive deficits in adult patients with brain tumours. *Lancet Neurol.* 3, 159–68.

Thiel E., Korfel A., Martus P., Kanz L., Griesinger F., Rauch M., Röth A., Hertenstein B., von Toll T., Hundsberger T., Mergenthaler H.G., Leithäuser M., Birnbaum T., Fischer L., Jahnke K, Herrlinger U., Plasswilm L., Nägele T., Pietsch T., Bamberg M., Weller M., (2010). High-dose methotrexate with or without whole brain radiotherapy for primary CNS lymphoma (G-PCNSL-SG-1): a phase 3, randomised, non-inferiority trial. *Lancet Oncol.* 11, 1036-47. doi: 10.1016/S1470-2045(10)70229-1. Epub 2010 Oct 20.

Weller M., (2011). Neurocognitive function: an emerging surrogate endpoint for neuro-oncology trials. *Neuro Oncol.* 13, 565.

In: Primary Central Nervous System Lymphoma (PCNSL)
Editor: Ryuya Yamanaka
ISBN: 978-1-63485-322-4

Chapter 21

LONG-TERM OUTCOME AND SUPPORTIVE CARE IN PATIENTS WITH PRIMARY CENTRAL NERVOUS SYSTEM LYMPHOMA

Ryuya Yamanaka[1,*], Saori Yoshioka[2], Sawako Fujimoto[3] and Yoko Iwawaki[2]

[1]Laboratory of Molecular Target Therapy for Cancer, Graduate School for Medical Science, Kyoto Prefectural University of Medicine, Kyoto, Japan
[2]Department of Cancer Nursing, Graduate School of Nursing for Health Care Science, Kyoto, Japan
[3]Palliative care unit, Kyoto Prefectural University of Medicine, Kyoto, Japan

ABSTRACT

Data on the long-term follow-up for patients with primary central nervous system lymphoma (PCNSL) are limited. We experienced late relapse and development of neurotoxicity among long-term follow-up patients. Novel treatment strategies should be developed to prevent delayed neurotoxicity. Patient follow-up should also be prolonged in PCNSL patients, because central nervous system (CNS) and systemic relapse can occur as late as 10 years after the initial onset of disease. A multidisciplinary team with well-trained neuro-oncologists is necessary to provide palliative care to patients with PCNSL early in the course of the disease. It is also important for families and caregivers to develop coping strategies and provide psychosocial support. It is also imperative to sufficiently train all types of healthcare professionals for the palliative care of PCNSL patients.

Keywords: end of life issue, long-term follow-up, neurotoxicity, primary central nervous system lymphoma, relapse, supportive care

* Corresponding author: Ryuya Yamanaka. Laboratory of Molecular Target Therapy for Cancer, Graduate School for Medical Science, Kyoto Prefectural University of Medicine, 465 Kajii-cho, Kamigyoku, Kyoto 602-8566, Japan. Email:ryaman@koto.kpu-m.ac.jp.

Introduction

Primary central nervous system lymphoma (PCNSL) is an extranodal non-Hodgkin's lymphoma (NHL) that primarily manifests in the brain, the eye, and the spinal cord, or in the leptomeninges [1]. Most PCNSLs are high-grade B-cell-type NHLs with less favorable prognoses compared to systemic NHLs [1]. The incidence of PCNSL has reportedly been increasing; however, this could partly be due to a better understanding of the disease [2]. Several therapeutic regimens targeting PCNSL were published in the last decade. The overall survival for PCNSL patients has been improved from 10 to 79 months after the introduction of high-dose methotrexate (HD-MTX) containing chemotherapy with or without irradiation [3-16]. It is widely accepted that MTX is the most effective agent against PCNSL; however, more effective chemotherapy protocols should be developed and a role for whole brain irradiation (WBIR) should be established. In this chapter, we describe issues concerning the long-term outcome and supportive care in PCNSL patients.

Does PCNSL Really Originate from CNS?

The CNS has been a controversial site of origin for PCNSL as it is thought to lack a regular lymphatic system. Only a few studies so far reported a connection between the CNS and the lymphatic system. The nasal route through the olfactory nerves to the nasal lymphatics, or the arachnoid villi associated with superior and inferior sagittal sinuses were believed to be a direct connection between cerebrospinal fluid (CSF) and cervical lymphatics [17, 18]. Recently, functional lymphatic vessels lining the dural sinuses, connected to deep cervical lymph nodes of the CNS and able to carry both fluid and immune cells, were also discovered [19, 20]. These findings may indicate CNS as the origin of neoplastic lymphoma cells. However, in our series [21], a few systemic lymphomas were verified at autopsy just a few months after PCNSL onset. A few years or longer after complete remission of CNS lymphoma, some cases developed systemic lymphomas [21]. Bernstein et al. reported CNS relapse occurred in patients with systemic NHL shortly after initial treatment, suggesting that such patients had subclinical CNS involvement at diagnosis [22]. The early and delayed recurrence may be explained by undetectable systemic lymphoma at initial diagnosis; some CNS lymphomas may be derived from systemic lymphomas. O'Neill et al. [23] reported that systemic lymphoma was suspected in 4% of PCNSL patients at diagnosis, which might have differentiated from secondary CNS lymphomas metastasized from nodal lymphomas. It is recommended to include physical examination, bone marrow biopsy, testicular sonography, and CT scan of the chest, abdomen, and pelvis in the systemic staging [24]. The 18-FDG PET-CT imaging is not yet routinely practiced in ruling out systemic lymphomas; however, should be evaluated further.

The Importance of Long-Term Follow-Up in Patients

There are only a few reports of PCNSL patient follow-up for more than 10 years [25, 26]. Most of the data published on PCNSL are from an average observation period of 5 years or less. The information on late relapse and neurotoxicity of long-term survivors is limited and overall survival data are likely to be overestimated. Thiel et al. [14] suggested that whole brain radiation therapy (WBRT) could be referred from first-line treatment of PCNSL. Delayed neurotoxicity was more common in patients who received WBRT than in those who did not. It is accepted that HD-MTX combined with WBRT had been a major risk factor for delayed neurotoxicity in long-term PCNSL survivors. The neuropathological process of delayed neurotoxicity is based on microangiopathy leading to diffuse white matter injury with clinical manifestation of cognitive impairment. Since formal psychometric evaluations are not routinely performed, cognitive complications have been underestimated. As treatment has increased survival rates, it is necessary to evaluate the improvement in patients' quality of life and cognitive function. A test battery evaluating cognition and quality of life was developed by the investigators of the International PCNSL Collaborative Group, and was proposed for prospective clinical trials [27]. Continued development of better treatment strategies is necessary for the prevention of delayed neurotoxicity.

In our experience [21], most relapses occurred within the first few years of disease; however, approximately 15% of CNS and systemic late relapse occurred after achieving complete remission. Late relapses that occurred more than 5 years after the initial onset of disease have only been discussed in a few studies [28-30]. Nayak et al. [30] reported 10 late relapses among 230 patients. This is likely because of the activation of clinically inactive tumors, or the possible development of therapy-induced secondary lymphoma in these patients. Nevertheless, molecular analyses showed that one case of relapsing tumor was clonally related to the original tumor [30]. Since our experience is that CNS and systemic recurrence could occur as late as 10 years after the initial onset of PCNSL, we would like to propose the importance of long-term follow-up in patients with PCNSL.

SUPPORTIVE CARE AND END-OF LIFE ISSUES

There have been proposals for improving the quality of care at the end-of-life in cancer patients; however, many cancer patients could not receive appropriate supportive care in the last stage of their disease [31]. Patients with advanced cancer have significant symptoms and limited quality of life. Early initiation of supportive care improves the quality of life and prolongs survival in cancer patients. Supportive care also plays an important role in the management of patients with brain tumor. A subset of end-of life problems is specific to patients with brain tumors. Although the management of PCNSL is advancing, only a small percentage of patients are able to overcome the disease. PCNSL progression or therapy related uncontrolled symptoms and spiritual issues arise when patients face the end stages of their illness. Supportive care is usually administered late in the course of the disease, when intervention proves less effective in improving the patient's quality of life. Supportive care is offered by a care team consisting of doctors, nurses, pharmacologists, rehabilitation therapists, social workers, nutritional experts, and other healthcare professionals for patients and families. Clinical symptoms such as pain, fatigue, cognitive deterioration, sleep disorder, and other general complaints are controlled by adequate supportive management of patients. The most frequent symptoms encountered in brain tumor patients in their last month were drowsiness (85%), dysphagia (85%), headache (36%), epilepsy (30%), delirium (15%), and death rattle (12%) [32]. Most patients usually have a peaceful death with loss of consciousness; however, in some instances, the multidrug approach to pain control is required for patients with meningeal spread of PCNSL. The presence of delirium or cognitive disorder may alter "peaceful death" [32]. A multidisciplinary team with well-trained neuro-oncologists is necessary to perform palliative care for patients with brain tumor early in the course of the disease [32]. Patients can catch up with their daily lives through appropriate management of their symptoms and the resulting improvement in the quality of life. Hospice care at home, as well as hospice facilities are specific forms of palliative care for patients with life-limiting illnesses. Common symptoms in PCNSL patients are motor and sensory impairment, cognitive and personality changes, communication disorders, seizures, and delirium. These symptoms depend on the location and size of the tumor and brain edema. Family members may feel that the patient is no longer the same person. It is difficult for families and caregivers to take care of terminal patients; they suffer from physical as well as psychological distress. The importance of specific issues such as nutrition and hydration is emphasized in brain tumor patients, and families are encouraged to avoid prolonging a useless situation [32]. We have to address and respect the patients' wishes at the end of life. It is also important for families and caregivers to develop coping strategies and provide psychosocial support. Education of all types of healthcare professionals for the palliative care of brain tumor patients including PCNSL is imperative.

REFERENCES

[1] Panageas KS, Elkin EB, DeAngelis LM, Ben-Porat L, Abrey LE. Trends in survival from primary central nervous system lymphoma, 1975-1999: a population-based analysis. *Cancer*. 2005;104(11):2466-2472.

[2] Olson JE, Janney CA, Rao RD, Cerhan JR, Kurtin PJ, Schiff D, Kaplan RS, O'Neill BP. The continuing increase in the incidence of primary central nervous system non-Hodgkin lymphoma: a surveillance, epidemiology, and end results analysis. *Cancer*. 2002;95(7): 1504-1510.

[3] Abrey LE, Yahalom J, DeAngelis LM. Treatment for primary CNS lymphoma: The next step. *J Clin Oncol*. 2000; 18:3144-3150.

[4] Bessell EM, López-Guillermo A, Villá S, Verger E, Nomdedeu B, Petit J, Byrne P, Montserrat E, Graus F. Importance of radiotherapy in the outcome of patients with primary CNS lymphoma: An analysis of the CHOD/BVAM regimen followed by two different radiotherapy treatments. *J Clin Oncol*. 2002; 20:231-236.

[5] DeAngelis LM, Seiferheld W, Schold SC, Fisher B, Schultz CJ; Radiation Therapy Oncology Group Study 93-10. Combination chemotherapy and radiotherapy for primary central nervous system lymphoma: Radiation Therapy Oncology Group Study 93-10. *J Clin Oncol*. 2002; 20:4643-4648.

[6] Herrlinger U, Schabet M, Brugger W, Kortmann RD, Küker W, Deckert M, Engel C, Schmeck-Lindenau HJ, Mergenthaler HG, Krauseneck P, Benöhr C, Meisner C, Wiestler OD, Dichgans J, Kanz L, Bamberg M, Weller M. German Cancer Society Neuro-Oncology Working Group NOA-03 multicenter trial of single-agent high-dose

methotrexate for primary central nervous system lymphoma. *Ann Neurol.* 2002; 51: 247-252.

[7] Batchelor T, Carson K, O'Neill A, Grossman SA, Alavi J, New P, Hochberg F, Priet R. Treatment of primary CNS lymphoma with methotrexate and deferred radiotherapy: A report of NABTT 96-07. *J Clin Oncol.* 2003; 21:1044-1049.

[8] Poortmans PM, Kluin-Nelemans HC, Haaxma-Reiche H, Van't Veer M, Hansen M, Soubeyran P, Taphoorn M, Thomas J, Van den Bent M, Fickers M, Van Imhoff G, Rozewicz C, Teodorovic I, van Glabbeke M; European Organization for Research and Treatment of Cancer Lymphoma Group. High-dose methotrexate-based chemotherapy followed by consolidating radiotherapy in non-AIDS-related primary central nervous system lymphoma: European Organization for Research and Treatment of Cancer Lymphoma Group Phase II Trial 20962. *J Clin Oncol.* 2003; 21:4483-4488.

[9] Korfel A, Martus P, Nowrousian MR, Hossfeld DK, Kirchen H, Brücher J, Stelljes M, Birkmann J, Peschel C, Pasold R, Fischer L, Jahnke K, Thiel E; German primary central nervous system lymphoma Study Group (G-PCNSL-SG). German primary central nervous system lymphoma Study Group (G-PCNSL-SG). Response to chemotherapy and treating institution predict survival in primary central nervous system lymphoma. *Br J Haematol.* 2005; 128:177-183.

[10] Omuro AM, DeAngelis LM, Yahalom J, Abrey LE. Chemoradiotherapy for primary CNS lymphoma: An intent-to-treat analysis with complete follow-up. *Neurology.* 2005; 64:69-74.

[11] Ferreri AJ, Dell'Oro S, Foppoli M, Bernardi M, Brandes AA, Tosoni A, Montanari M, Balzarotti M, Spina M, Ilariucci F, Zaja F, Stelitano C, Bobbio F, Corazzelli G, Baldini L, Ponzoni M, Picozzi P, Caligaris Cappio F, Reni M. MATILDE regimen followed by radiotherapy is an active strategy against primary CNS lymphomas. *Neurology.* 2006; 66(9):1435-1438.

[12] Ferreri AJ, Reni M, Foppoli M, Martelli M, Pangalis GA, Frezzato M, Cabras MG, Fabbri A, Corazzelli G, Ilariucci F, Rossi G, Soffietti R, Stelitano C, Vallisa D, Zaja F, Zoppegno L, Aondio GM, Avvisati G, Balzarotti M, Brandes AA, Fajardo J, Gomez H, Guarini A, Pinotti G, Rigacci L, Uhlmann C, Picozzi P, Vezzulli P, Ponzoni M, Zucca E, Caligaris-Cappio F, Cavalli F; International Extranodal Lymphoma Study Group (IELSG). High-dose cytarabine plus high-dose methotrexate versus high-dose methotrexate alone in patients with primary CNS lymphoma: A randomised phase 2 trial. *Lancet.* 2009; 374:1512-1520.

[13] Pels H, Juergens A, Glasmacher A, Schulz H, Engert A, Linnebank M, Schackert G, Reichmann H, Kroschinsky F, Vogt-Schaden M, Egerer G, Bode U, Schaller C, Lamprecht M, Hau P, Deckert M, Fimmers R, Bangard C, Schmidt-Wolf IG, Schlegel U. Early relapses in primary CNS lymphoma after response to polychemotherapy without intraventricular treatment: Results of a phase II study. *J Neurooncol.* 2009;91: 299-305.

[14] Thiel E, Korfel A, Martus P, Kanz L, Griesinger F, Rauch M, Röth A, Hertenstein B, von Toll T, Hundsberger T, Mergenthaler HG, Leithäuser M, Birnbaum T, Fischer L, Jahnke K, Herrlinger U, Plasswilm L, Nägele T, Pietsch T, Bamberg M, Weller M. High-dose methotrexate with or without whole brain radiotherapy for primary CNS lymphoma (G-PCNSL-SG-1): a phase 3, randomised, non-inferiority trial. *Lancet Oncol.* 2010;11(11):1036-1047.

[15] Wieduwilt MJ, Valles F, Issa S, Behler CM, Hwang J, McDermott M, Treseler P, O'Brien J, Shuman MA, Cha S, Damon LE, Rubenstein JL. Immuno-chemotherapy with intensive consolidation for primary CNS lymphoma: A pilot study and prognostic assessment by diffusion-weighted MRI. *Clin Cancer Res.* 2012; 18:1146-1155.

[16] Morris PG, Correa DD, Yahalom J, Raizer JJ, Schiff D, Grant B, Grimm S, Lai RK, Reiner AS, Panageas K, Karimi S, Curry R, Shah G, Abrey LE, DeAngelis LM, Omuro A. Rituximab, methotrexate, procarbazine, and vincristine followed by consolidation reduced-dose whole-brain radiotherapy and cytarabine in newly diagnosed primary CNS lymphoma: final results and long-term outcome. *J Clin Oncol.* 2013;31(31):3971-3979.

[17] Kida S, Pantazis A, Weller RO. CSF drains directly from the subarachnoid space into nasal lymphatics in the rat. Anatomy, histology and immunological significance. *Neuropathol Appl Neurobiol.* 1993;19(6):480-488.

[18] Walter BA, Valera VA, Takahashi S, Ushiki T. The olfactory route for cerebrospinal fluid drainage into the peripheral lymphatic system. *Neuropathol Appl Neurobiol.* 2006; 32(4):388-396.

[19] Louveau A, Smirnov I, Keyes TJ, Eccles JD, Rouhani SJ, Peske JD, Derecki NC, Castle D, Mandell JW, Lee KS, Harris TH, Kipnis J. Structural and functional features of central nervous system lymphatic vessels. *Nature.*2015; 523, 337-341.

[20] Aspelund A, Antila S, Proulx ST, Karlsen TV, Karaman S, Detmar M, Wiig H, Alitalo K. A dural lymphatic vascular system that drains brain interstitial fluid and macromolecules. *J Exp Med.* 2015;212(7):991-999.

[21] Yamanaka R, Morii K, Shinbo Y, Homma J, Sano M, Tsuchiya N, Yajima N, Tamura T, Hondoh H, Takahashi H, Kakuma T, Tanaka R. Results of treatment of 112 cases of primary CNS lymphoma. *Jpn J Clin Oncol.* 2008;38(5):373-380.

[22] Bernstein SH, Unger JM, Leblanc M, Friedberg J, Miller TP, Fisher RI. Natural history of CNS relapse in patients with aggressive non-Hodgkin's lymphoma: a 20-year follow-up analysis of SWOG 8516 -- the Southwest Oncology Group. *J Clin Oncol.* 2009;27 (1):114-119.

[23] O'Neill BP, Dinapoli RP, Kurtin PJ, Habermann TM. Occult systemic non-Hodgkin's lymphoma (NHL) in patients initially diagnosed as primary central nervous system lymphoma (PCNSL): how much staging is enough? *J Neurooncol.* 1995;25(1):67-71.

[24] Hoang-Xuan K, Bessell E, Bromberg J, Hottinger AF, Preusser M, Rudà R, Schlegel U, Siegal T, Soussain C, Abacioglu U, Cassoux N, Deckert M, Dirven CM, Ferreri AJ, Graus F, Henriksson R, Herrlinger U, Taphoorn M, Soffietti R, Weller M; European Association for Neuro-Oncology Task Force on Primary CNS Lymphoma. Diagnosis and treatment of primary CNS lymphoma in immunocompetent patients: guidelines from the European Association for Neuro-Oncology. *Lancet Oncol.* 2015;16(7):e322-332.

[25] Gavrilovic IT, Hormigo A, YahalomJ, DeAngelis LM, Abrey LE. Long-term follow-up of high-dose methotrexate-based therapy with and without whole brain irradiation for newly diagnosed primary CNS lymphoma. *J Clin Oncol.* 2006;24(28):4570-4574.

[26] Ferreri AJ, Ciceri F, Brandes AA, Montanari M, Balzarotti M, Spina M, Ilariucci F, Zaja F, Stelitano C, Bobbio F, Corazzelli G, Baldini L, Reni M. MATILDE chemotherapy regimen for primary CNS lymphoma: results at a median follow-up of 12 years. *Neurology.* 2014;82(15):1370-1373.

[27] Correa DD, Maron L, Harder H, Klein M, Armstrong CL, Calabrese P, Bromberg JE, Abrey LE, Batchelor TT, Schiff D. Cognitive functions in primary central nervous system lymphoma: literature review and assessment guidelines. *Ann Oncol*. 2007;18(7): 1145-1151.

[28] Yamasaki T, Shima N, Yamabe H, Nagaoka S, Moritake K, Kikuchi H. Primary malignant lymphoma of the central nervous system--report of four long-term survivors. *Neurol Med Chir* (Tokyo). 1995;35(9):655-662.

[29] Herrlinger U, Hebart H, Kanz L, Dichgans J, Weller M. Relapse of primary CNS lymphoma after more than 10 years in complete remission. *J Neurol*. 2005;252(11): 1409-1410.

[30] Nayak L, Hedvat C, Rosenblum MK, Abrey LE, DeAngelis LM. Late relapse in primary central nervous system lymphoma: clonal persistence. *Neuro Oncol*. 2011;13 (5):525-529.

[31] Taillibert S, Laigle-Donadey F, Sanson M. Palliative care in patients with primary brain tumors. *Curr Opin Oncol*. 2004;16(6):587-592.

[32] Pace A, Di Lorenzo C, Guariglia L, Jandolo B, Carapella CM, Pompili A. End of life issues in brain tumor patients. *J Neurooncol*. 2009;91(1):39-43.

INDEX

#

A

B

C

D

E

F

P

Q

R